Quantitative Evaluation of HIV Prevention Programs

The Institution for Social and Policy Studies at Yale University

The Yale ISPS Series

Quantitative Evaluation of HIV Prevention Programs

**Edited by Edward H. Kaplan
and Ron Brookmeyer**

Yale University Press

New Haven and London

Contributors

Massimo Arcà, M.Sc., Department of Epidemiology, Azienda Sanitaria Locale Roma E (ASL RME), Rome, Italy.

Sally Blower, Ph.D., Department of Biomathematics, University of California, Los Angeles.

Margaret L. Brandeau, Ph.D., Department of Management Science and Engineering, Stanford University, Stanford, California.

Ron Brookmeyer, Ph.D., Department of Biostatistics, Johns Hopkins University, Bloomberg School of Public Health, Baltimore, Maryland.

Michael P. Busch, M.D., Ph.D., Blood Centers of the Pacific, San Francisco, California.

Giulia Cesaroni, M.Sc., Department of Epidemiology, ASL RME, Rome, Italy.

Marina Davoli, M.D., M.Sc., Department of Epidemiology, ASL RME, Rome, Italy.

Julia M. Dayton, Ph.D., Department of Epidemiology and Public Health, School of Medicine, Yale University, New Haven, Connecticut.

Donna M. Edwards, Ph.D., Sandia National Laboratories, Livermore, California.

M. Elizabeth Halloran, M.D., D.Sc., Department of Biostatistics, Rollins School of Public Health, Emory University, Atlanta, Georgia.

David R. Holtgrave, Ph.D., Division of HIV/AIDS Prevention, Centers for Disease Control and Prevention, Atlanta, Georgia.

Michael G. Hudgens, Ph.D., Fred Hutchinson Cancer Research Center, Seattle, Washington.

Robert S. Janssen, M.D., Director, Division of HIV/AIDS Prevention, Centers for Disease Control and Prevention, Atlanta, Georgia.

James G. Kahn, M.D., M.P.H., Institute for Health Policy Studies, Department of Epidemiology and Biostatistics, Center for AIDS Prevention Studies, and AIDS Research Institute, University of California, San Francisco.

Edward H. Kaplan, Ph.D., William N. and Marie A. Beach Professor, School of Management, and Department of Epidemiology and Public Health, School of Medicine, Yale University, New Haven, Connecticut.

Katia Koelle, B.S., Department of Biomathematics, University of California, Los Angeles.

Ira M. Longini, Jr., Ph.D., Department of Biostatistics, Rollins School of Public Health, Emory University, Atlanta, Georgia.

Elliot Marseille, Dr. P.H., Health Strategies International, Institute for Health Policy Studies, and AIDS Research Institute, University of California, San Francisco.

Michael H. Merson, M.D., Dean and Anna M. R. Lauder Professor, Department of Epidemiology and Public Health, School of Medicine, Yale University, New Haven, Connecticut.

John Mills, M.D., Australian National Centre in HIV Virology Research, and the Macfarlane Burnet Center for Medical Research, Victoria, Australia.

Douglas K. Owens, M.D., M.S., Center for Quality Management in HIV Care, Veterans' Affairs Palo Alto Health Care System, and Center for Primary Care and Outcomes Research, Stanford University, Stanford, California.

Nancy S. Padian, Ph.D., Department of Obstetrics and Gynecology, University of California, San Francisco.

Carlo A. Perucci, M.D., Department of Epidemiology, ASL RME, Rome, Italy.

Tomas Philipson, Ph.D., Irving B. Harris Graduate School of Public Policy Studies, University of Chicago.

Steven D. Pinkerton, Ph.D., Center for AIDS Intervention Research, Medical College of Wisconsin, Milwaukee, Wisconsin.

Harold Pollack, Ph.D., School of Public Health, University of Michigan, Ann Arbor, Michigan.

Joseph Saba, M.D., Axios International, Dublin, Ireland; formerly with UNAIDS, Geneva, Switzerland.

Glen A. Satten, Ph.D., Division of HIV/AIDS Prevention, Centers for Disease Control and Prevention, Atlanta, Georgia.

Ross D. Shachter, Ph.D., Department of Management Science and Engineering, Stanford University, Stanford, California.

Stephen C. Shiboski, Ph.D., Department of Epidemiology and Biostatistics, University of California, San Francisco.

Teresa Spadea, M.Sc., M. Phil., Department of Epidemiology, Azienda Sanitaria Locale 5, Grugliasco (To), Italy.

Susan Stramer, Ph.D., National Reference Laboratory for Infectious Diseases, American Red Cross, Atlanta, Georgia.

Annette D. Verster, M.A., ITACA, Rome, Italy.

Published with assistance from the Louis Stern Memorial Fund.

Set in Adobe Garamond and Stone Sans types by The Composing Room of Michigan, Inc. Printed in the United States of America.

Library of Congress Cataloging-in-Publication Data
Kaplan, Edward Harris.
    Quantitative evaluation of HIV prevention programs / edited by Edward H. Kaplan and Ron Brookmeyer.
      p. cm.
    Includes bibliographical references and index.
    ISBN 0-300-08751-9 (cloth : alk. paper)
    1. AIDS (Disease)—Prevention—Congresses.   2. AIDS (Disease)—Prevention—Government policy—Evaluation—Congresses.   I. Brookmeyer, Ron.
    RA643.8 .K37   2001
    362.1'969792—dc21   2001039022

A catalogue record for this book is available from the British Library.

10 9 8 7 6 5 4 3 2 1

Contents

Foreword

Donald L. Thomsen, Jr.

In 1974, the Societal Institute of the Mathematical Sciences (SIMS) held what turned out to be the first in a series of Research Application Conferences (RACs) for the purpose of exploring in depth selected societal fields in light of their receptivity to mathematical/statistical analysis. The RACs were well received and have been held every two to three years ever since, going on now for over twenty-five years and coinciding with the twenty-fifth anniversary of SIMS. Societal fields which have benefited from this kind of attention include energy, human exposure, and health topics such as AIDS; human exposure covers a wide range of environmental issues and is a field to which SIMS has given considerable effort.

Altogether, fourteen SIMS RACs have been held. Proceedings have followed each of the first thirteen as rapidly as possible so that researchers could have access to recent results as soon as possible. A bibliography of the first thirteen conferences appears below.

The fourteenth conference, held in July 1998 at the Domaine de Divonne Hotel (Divonne-les-Bains, France) was on "The Quantitative Evaluation of HIV Prevention Programs." This AIDS conference was supported in part by the National Institute on Drug Abuse.

SIMS wishes to acknowledge the untiring efforts of the two editors of this volume, who also served as cochairs of the meeting: Professor Edward H. Kaplan (Yale University, School of Management and Department of Epidemiology and Public Health, School of Medicine) and Professor Ron Brookmeyer (Department of Biostatistics, Johns Hopkins University. Bloomberg School of Public Health). SIMS would also like to acknowledge the enthusiastic support and continuing encouragement on the part of NIDA's project officer, Dr. Peter I. Hartsock.

RESEARCH APPLICATION CONFERENCES

1. Levin SA (editor). *Ecosystems Analysis and Prediction.* Philadelphia: SIAM, 1975.
2. Ludwig D, Cooke KL (editors). *Epidemiology.* Philadelphia: SIAM, 1975.
3. Roberts FS (editor). *Energy: Mathematics and Models.* Philadelphia: SIAM, 1976.
4. Whittemore AS (editor). *Environmental Health: Quantitative Methods.* Philadelphia: SIAM, 1977.
5. Shugart Jun HH (editor). *Time Series and Ecological Processes.* Philadelphia: SIAM, 1978.
6. Breslow NE, Whittemore AS (editors). *Energy and Health.* Philadelphia: SIAM, 1979.
7. Buckmaster JD (editor). *Fluid Mechanics in Energy Conversion.* Philadelphia: SIAM, 1980.
8. Prentice RL, Whittemore AS (editors). *Environmental Epidemiology: Risk Assessment.* Philadelphia: SIAM, 1984.
9. Prentice RL, Thompson DJ (editors). *Atomic Bomb Survivor Data: Utilization and Analysis.* Philadelphia: SIAM, 1984.
10. Moolgavkar SH, Prentice RL (editors). *Modern Statistical Methods in Chronic Disease Epidemiology.* New York: Wiley, 1986.
11. Moolgavkar SH (editor). *Scientific Issues in Quantitative Cancer Risk Assessment.* Boston: Birkhäuser, 1990.
12. Jewell NP, Dietz K, Farewell VT (editors). *AIDS Epidemiology: Methodological Issues.* Boston: Birkhäuser, 1992.
13. Dietz K, Bacchetti P, Pagano M (editors). *Quantitative Methods for Studying AIDS, Statistics in Medicine* 13 (19–20), 1994.

Introduction

Edward H. Kaplan and Ron Brookmeyer

The epidemic of human immunodeficiency virus (HIV), the cause of
the acquired immune deficiency syndromes (AIDS), has led to the infection of an estimated 58 million people worldwide, 22 million of
whom have already died (Merson and Dayton, Chapter 1, this volume). HIV and AIDS have reduced life expectancies by more than 10
years in hard hit countries such as Burkina Faso and Côte d'Ivoire, and
by 22 years in Zimbabwe.[1] The impact of this epidemic reaches beyond those directly infected with HIV. Children with HIV-infected
parents become orphans, while networks of friends and families suffer
as loved ones become infected and ill. Economies are stripped of pro-
ductive participants, and scarce societal resources must be redirected
from other public pursuits toward HIV/AIDS-specific activities such as
medical care for HIV- and AIDS-afflicted persons.

The severe consequences of HIV infection and AIDS indicated above
have led public health practitioners to focus on the *prevention* of new
HIV infections. Given all that has been learned regarding HIV transmission routes, it seems plausible that specific interventions could be
designed to block the spread of new infections. Indeed, since HIV can

be transmitted only via direct contact with infectious blood, blood products (e.g., plasma), or bodily fluids (e.g., semen, breast milk, saliva), a menu of prevention options has evolved. Implemented interventions have focused on changing individual HIV risk behaviors via counseling and education (e.g., safer sex, needle hygiene), the use of biological/medical advances (e.g., HIV screening of blood and plasma donors, zidovodine treatment for infected pregnant women), and "prevention technologies" (e.g., condoms, spermicides/microbicides, and sterile syringes). In addition, laboratory researchers continue their quest to produce an HIV vaccine.

Are HIV prevention programs succeeding in their goal of reducing the rate of new HIV infections? Is the public health return on HIV prevention programs sufficiently large to warrant continued investment? Despite the large literature discussing HIV prevention in theory and practice,[2,3] it is difficult to provide even order of magnitude estimates of the impact of most HIV prevention programs, let alone a summary cost-effectiveness statement. Which HIV prevention programs are more cost-effective? How much money should be spent on different programs in different locations? Which new programs are worth trying out, further planning, or abandoning altogether? Very little has been written regarding these topics (though the World Bank report *Confronting AIDS* is a notable exception.)[1]

As the term *HIV prevention* implies, the overriding goal is to prevent the occurrence of new HIV infections, by either blocking transmission from those already infected or protecting susceptible people from becoming infected. It therefore seems reasonable to assume that evaluations of HIV prevention programs should focus on whether such programs are indeed preventing the spread of new infections.

Unfortunately, a major problem in evaluating HIV prevention programs results from the difficulties inherent in directly measuring the rate of new HIV infections (the HIV *incidence rate*). Indeed, a U.S. National Research Council panel studying the evaluation of HIV prevention programs has stated that "HIV incidence data would not be a sensitive indicator for populations in which HIV infection was rare. . . . Furthermore, HIV incidence data are not only difficult to obtain, but they are also difficult to interpret. HIV incidence rates require extremely large samples and protracted testing to determine a program's effectiveness. Moreover, the rates can reflect other conditions unrelated to the effects of the program, such as the absence or saturation of the infection in a given locale."[4]

For many prevention programs, evaluation has been based on the study of changes in self-reported risky behaviors in response to an intervention. For example, programs where drug injectors report reductions in needle sharing (a very risky behavior with respect to the transmission of HIV and other viruses) or participants report increases in the use of condoms are considered successful. Other studies have sought to estimate the preventive impact of a program by looking at changes in HIV *prevalence* (that is, the fraction of the population that is infected with HIV). Under certain circumstances, such studies might well uncover programs that do successfully reduce the rate of new HIV infections. Under other circumstances, however, misleading (and potentially *very* misleading) results could be obtained.

This book addresses the quantitative evaluation of HIV prevention programs. The focus on evaluating HIV prevention distinguishes it from other books that have explored quantitative aspects of the HIV/AIDS epidemic. For example, Brookmeyer and Gail[5] describe quantitative approaches to AIDS epidemiology with an emphasis on statistical methods, while Kaplan and Brandeau[6] present articles discussing AIDS policy modeling, forecasting, infectivity and disease progression, and risky behavior. Holtgrave[7] contains several applications of cost-effectiveness analysis to HIV prevention, while Philipson and Posner[8] pursue a microeconomic model of risky behavior and its implications for public HIV intervention programs. This is the first book that brings together several quantitative methods for the purpose of evaluating HIV prevention.

Recent advances in the economic, statistical, and mathematical aspects of epidemic modeling combined with increasing scrutiny of HIV prevention decisions led the volume editors to organize a unique conference tightly focused around the quantitative evaluation of HIV prevention programs. Sponsored by the Societal Institute for the Mathematical Sciences (SIMS) with financial support from the United States National Institute on Drug Abuse (NIDA), a group of experts assembled in Divonne-les-Bains, France, on July 6–8, 1998 (immediately following the 12th World AIDS Conference in nearby Geneva). The participants included behavioral scientists, biologists, economists, epidemiologists, health service researchers, operations researchers, policy makers, and statisticians. All, however, were (and remain) concerned about the conduct and consequences of HIV prevention evaluations. The chapters in this book derive directly from the proceedings of this conference. They fall naturally into four categories: setting the context and developing concepts for HIV prevention (Part I), cost-effectiveness and resource allocation (Part II), HIV prevention case studies (Part III), and the development of new methods for the quantitative study of new problems in HIV prevention (Part IV).

Part I begins with Chapter 1, by Michael H. Merson and Julia M. Dayton, which provides an overview of HIV prevention programs in developing countries. Merson and Dayton report recent estimates of the extent of HIV infection and AIDS worldwide, and summarize the results of existing HIV program evaluations. The chapter addresses structural interventions, those that "change laws, policies, and standard operating procedures in a society," and links these to national-level responses to HIV and AIDS.

Chapter 2, by David R. Holtgrave and Steven D. Pinkerton, directly addresses the "big picture" questions in HIV prevention decision making: Are HIV prevention programs worth the investment? What do HIV prevention programs really cost? How can we estimate the impact of a national "rollout" of a prevention program before actual implementation? Is the national HIV prevention effort making a difference in the epidemic? Viewed within the U.S. context from the perspective of the Centers for Disease Control and Prevention, the authors provide several "minicases" to illustrate their approach to these policy questions.

Returning to the evaluation of HIV prevention programs, in Chapter 3 Ron Brookmeyer provides a tour of the key statistical issues that surface in empirical HIV prevention studies. The chapter portrays the strengths and weaknesses of alternative study designs, including randomized controlled trials (at the individual or community level), natural experiments, and observational studies. The uses of surveillance data and associated epidemic modeling are also noted. The chapter highlights the special care required to choose and interpret summary measures for evaluating HIV prevention programs.

In a companion chapter (the closing chapter of Part I), Chapter 4, Nancy S. Padian and Stephen C. Shiboski survey epidemiological issues in evaluating HIV prevention programs. The chapter focuses on causal criteria: only interventions that can be causally linked to reductions in the rate of new HIV infections merit policy implementation. These criteria have led to the primacy of the randomized trial in influencing policy makers. These points are illustrated by examining the case histories of different HIV prevention studies.

Part II is devoted to studies that combine economic analysis with epidemic modeling to address questions of cost-effectiveness and resource allocation. Margaret L. Brandeau leads off in Chapter 5 with a model that frames these issues and offers a methodology for resolving them. She formally considers two problems. The first is the optimal investment problem: What is the right amount of money, free from budget constraints, to invest in a given program? (Note that the answer could be "nothing.") The second is the resource allocation problem: How should a fixed prevention budget be divided among available prevention activities? Both problems are approached within the assumptions of a standard epidemic model. The chapter discusses both exact and approximate solutions to these problems, and develops practical guidelines for decision makers based on the models.

In Chapter 6, Harold Pollack examines the cost-effectiveness of methadone treatment for injection drug users as an HIV prevention program. The analysis begins with a descriptive model of HIV transmission among drug users but then embeds the operations of a methadone program into the model. Combining empirical observations regarding the cost and operational properties of methadone programs (e.g., time spent in programs, recidivism to drug use) with the epidemic model enables estimates of the cost per HIV infection averted on account of methadone treatment. Across a wide array of model parameter values, the analysis suggests that methadone treatment can prevent new infections at a cost of $100,000 to $300,000 per infection averted.

In Chapter 7, the final chapter of this section, Douglas K. Owens, Donna M. Edwards, and Ross D. Shachter examine the cost-effectiveness of potential HIV vaccines. In a manner similar to Pollack's chapter, the authors first develop an HIV epidemic model for a cohort of homosexual men, and then incorporate the presumed workings of vaccines with different levels of effectiveness. The model considers both preventive vaccines (those that protect susceptibles from infection) and vaccines designed to lessen the likelihood of transmission from the already infected. The models suggest that vaccines of even modest efficacy provide substantial health benefits, and can also reduce health expenditures. If both types of vaccines become available, the model suggests how such vaccines should be deployed, depending upon the characteristics of the epidemic in the population vaccinated.

Part III reports three HIV prevention case studies. Each of these chapters evaluates a real program (or collection of programs) that has been implemented. These chapters study how such programs affect HIV transmission by combining observed data with HIV transmission models. The credibility of such evaluations rests largely with the credibility of the underlying models.

Chapter 8, by Massimo Arcà and coauthors, presents a model-based evaluation of the harm reduction program in Rome, Italy. This large-scale program involved street outreach, needle exchange, condom distribution, and several other activities. Over a two-year period, this program contacted more than 5,000 drug users. Building on earlier work, the authors constructed an HIV epidemic model in the absence of the program, and then included program operations in an expanded model to estimate the impact of the program. The model suggests that over a two-year period, the program prevented between 120 and 200 new HIV infections at a cost of approximately $30,000 to $40,000 per infection prevented.

In Chapter 9, Edward H. Kaplan reports his analysis of Israel's ban on Ethiopian blood donors. Fearing the possibility that Ethiopian Israelis, who were believed to have a 50-fold higher chance of HIV infection relative to non-Ethiopian Israelis, might inadvertently contaminate Israel's blood supply with HIV infection, Israel's blood bank discarded all donations from Ethiopian Israelis without informing the donors. Using recently developed snapshot incidence estimators (similar to that reported in Chapter 14 by Glen A. Satten and colleagues), Kaplan was able to estimate the incidence of new infections among Ethiopian Israelis. Combining this with data regarding the number of Ethiopian versus non-Ethiopian Israeli donors, the chapter shows that the ban prevented at most one infectious donation every 10 years. An economic analysis suggests that the ban could not be judged cost-beneficial if the social costs of banning Ethiopian Israeli donors exceed $234,000 annually, or $3.90 per Ethiopian Israeli per year.

In Chapter 10, the final chapter of Part III, James G. Kahn, Elliot Marseille, and Joseph Saba evaluate several combinations of formula and breastfeeding with the overall goal of maximizing life expectancy. This case study presents an interesting trade-off: though preventing maternal-infant HIV transmission is obviously of great importance, withholding breast milk can actually increase non-HIV sources of mortality (due to the loss of maternal antibodies transmitted via breastfeeding). The analysis requires constructing infant mortality curves corresponding to both breastfeeding from HIV-infected mothers and formula feeding. Possible strategies include always breastfeeding, never breastfeeding, or breastfeeding for some specified period and then switching to formula feeding. In seven of eight geographic settings, the optimal strategy appears to be formula feeding. The authors estimate that adopting the model-based recommendations would prevent between 2 and 19 fatal events per 100 children.

Part IV is concerned with new quantitative methodologies for evaluating HIV prevention programs. In Chapter 11, Tomas Philipson addresses an interesting and overlooked issue in community-level HIV prevention trials. In the usual randomized controlled trial, one compares control and experimental groups to determine whether the prevention mechanism in question has had an effect. Philipson considers the case where individual outcomes (e.g., becoming infected with HIV or not) depend not only upon whether one is in the control or experimental arm of the study, but also upon the overall number of persons in each arm. For example, in a vaccine trial, the likelihood that an unvaccinated person would become infected could well depend upon the fraction of all persons in the population who are vaccinated. It is important to determine the difference between so-called private effects (in the vaccine example, protection offered by the vaccine itself) and external effects (which would be induced by the number of persons vaccinated in the population). This is particularly important when estimating the populationwide impact of an intervention that has been evaluated in smaller studies. Philipson proposes two-stage randomization schemes for sorting out these effects, and illustrates in the context of HIV prevention community trials in Africa.

In Chapter 12, Ira M. Longini, Jr., Michael G. Hudgens, and M. Elizabeth Halloran propose a research design for estimating both the protective and infectivity-reducing effects of vaccines. Results from such a trial could provide better data for the economic vaccine model presented earlier by Owens and colleagues. The novel feature of the research design is the incorporation of steady sexual partners of participants already enrolled in an otherwise standard trial. Following the structure of the Bangkok Metropolitan Administration cohort of injecting drug users, the authors simulate HIV transmission within this trial structure to investigate whether their design is sufficiently powerful to estimate both vaccine effects. The results suggest that the proposed design can in fact detect such effects, while standard analysis absent their design modification would lead to biased results.

Sally Blower, Katia Koelle, and John Mills provide a different vaccine analysis in Chapter 13. They develop an epidemic model for HIV, and then show how various vaccines under discussion would interrupt HIV transmission. Importantly, however, these authors also consider the impact of behavioral changes that might accompany mass vaccination programs on the resulting levels of HIV in the population. For example, if the mere existence of an effective vaccine leads those vaccinated to increase risk taking in sexual behavior, which in turn could lead to increased exposure to HIV, then the resulting reductions in HIV transmission would be less, and perhaps much less, than otherwise anticipated. This chapter also discusses current obstacles to HIV vaccine development and reviews current HIV vaccine strategies.

Glen A. Satten and colleagues report in Chapter 14 a major breakthrough in our ability to estimate HIV incidence and identify recent HIV infections. These authors explain how scientists at the Centers for Disease Control have "detuned" standard HIV antibody tests in a manner that stretches the "window period" between HIV infection and the development of detectable antibodies by 129 days over the usual test. Using the standard and detuned tests together leads to a procedure for identifying early HIV infections: those testing positive on the standard test but negative on the detuned test must have become infected recently. A simple formula for estimating HIV incidence from a single sample follows, and the authors validate their method using data from a cohort study of gay men in San Francisco and repeat blood donors (both populations where HIV incidence can be directly observed). Their model produces an impressive match with the data. The authors also suggest how this tool can be used to evaluate prevention programs within the context of a controlled trial.

In Chapter 15, the final chapter of Part IV (and the book), Stephen C. Shiboski and Nancy S. Padian consider the importance of evidence for time-varying HIV infectivity for HIV prevention programs. Recent attention has focused on the implications of possibly increased HIV transmission from recently infected persons. If the recently infected are in fact more likely to transmit, then prevention programs that seek to prevent transmission via targeting the already infected are less likely to be effective, because those *recently* infected would be both more likely to transmit and more difficult to find. However, it is by no means certain that the ability to transmit HIV is much higher for those in the early stages of HIV infection. This chapter presents a framework for evaluating the epidemiological evidence regarding the importance of primary infection, provides a set of tools with which such evidence can be quantified and summarized, and presents the results of applying these tools to available data.

The evaluation of HIV prevention programs presents many challenges. Also, though evaluations remain imperfect, strategic HIV prevention decisions will continue to be made. The chapters in this book share the goal of making sense out of HIV prevention studies with an eye toward better decision making in this realm. Our belief is that research of this nature will become only more important in the years ahead.

REFERENCES

1. World Bank. *Confronting AIDS: Public Priorities in a Global Epidemic.* Rev. ed. New York: Oxford University Press, 1999.
2. Normand J, Vlahov D, Moses LE (editors). *Preventing HIV Transmission: The Role of Sterile Needles and Bleach.* Washington DC: National Academy Press, 1995.
3. Auerbach JD, Wypijewska C, Brodie HKH (editors). *AIDS and Behavior: An Integrated Approach.* Washington DC: National Academy Press, 1994.

4. Coyle SL, Boruch RF, Turner CF (editors). *Evaluating AIDS Prevention Programs*. Washington DC: National Academy Press, 1991, p. 6.

5. Brookmeyer R, Gail MH. *AIDS Epidemiology: A Quantitative Approach*. Oxford: Oxford University Press, 1994.

6. Kaplan EH, Brandeau ML (editors). *Modeling the AIDS Epidemic: Planning, Policy and Prediction*. New York: Raven Press, 1994.

7. Holtgrave DR (editor). *Handbook of Economic Evaluation of HIV Prevention Programs*. New York: Plenum Press, 1998.

8. Philipson TJ, Posner A. *Private Choices and Public Health: The AIDS Epidemic in an Economic Perspective*. Cambridge: Harvard University Press, 1993.

Part One Evaluating HIV Prevention Programs: Context and Concepts

Chapter 1 Overview of HIV Prevention Programs in Developing Countries

Michael H. Merson and Julia M. Dayton

In this chapter we review the global epidemiology of HIV infection, particularly in developing countries. We summarize what has been learned about the efficacy of behavioral and medical interventions to prevent HIV infection in these countries, and offer a few ideas about how modeling could assist in planning public health prevention programs.

EPIDEMIOLOGY OF HIV IN DEVELOPING COUNTRIES

General Epidemiology

The United Nations Combined AIDS Program (UNAIDS) estimates that as of the end of 2000 a total of 57.9 million adults and children worldwide have been infected by HIV. About 36.1 million of these individuals have already died from AIDS, and 21.8 million are still living with HIV. Over 90 percent of those living with HIV are in developing countries (Table 1.1). 4.7 million adults and 600,000 children are be-

Table 1.1. Estimated Number of People Living with AIDS Worldwide, December 2000

People with HIV or AIDS	Regional Total
Developing World	
Sub-Saharan Africa	25.3 million
South and Southeast Asia	5.8 million
Latin America	1.4 million
East Asia and Pacific	640,000
Caribbean	390,000
Eastern Europe and Central Asia	700,000
North Africa and Middle East	400,000
Industrialized World	
North America	920,000
Western Europe	540,000
Australia and New Zealand	15,000

Source: UNAIDS, AIDS Epidemic Update: December 2000. Geneva: World Health Organization, 2000.

lieved to have acquired HIV during 2000, and almost all of these were living in developing countries.[1]

HIV is a sexually transmitted disease (STD) that affects mostly adults in the prime of life (15 to 49 years). It is transmitted mainly by sex or other direct contact with bodily fluids of an infected person. Most adult transmission in the developing world is by heterosexual sex, though transmission by sex between men occurs often more commonly than realized and in all countries. The second most important mode of transmission is the sharing of unsterilized needles and syringes among injection drug users (IDUs), a practice which is common in many countries in Asia, Eastern Europe, and South America, particularly in Brazil and Argentina. Parenteral transmission also occurs by blood transfusion or medical injection, but these account for a relatively small percentage of infections. Mother-to-child transmission is a third mode of transmission, and is most common in sub-Saharan Africa, the region with the greatest number of HIV-infected women.[2]

How the Epidemic Spreads

The extent to which an infectious disease spreads in a population depends on its *reproductive rate*, that is, the average number of susceptible people infected by an infected person over his or her lifetime.[3] In order for an epidemic to be maintained, its reproductive rate must be greater than one. The greater the reproductive rate, the more rapidly it will spread. The amount of time a person remains infectious, his or her risk of transmission per sexual contact, and the rate of acquisition of new partners all affect the reproductive rate of any STD, including HIV. Biological, behavioral, and economic factors influence these three variables.

BIOLOGICAL FACTORS

Recent evidence suggests that the average probability of transmission from an infected person to a noninfected person (called *infectivity*) is greatest during primary infection, the time between exposure to HIV and the appearance of HIV antibodies, and when an infected person is in the advanced stages of the disease and has developed AIDS (as indicated by a low CD4 T-lymphocyte count).[4] Untreated STDs also increase the risk of HIV transmission, particularly genital ulcer disease.[5,6] Simulations of the initial ten years of the HIV epidemic in Uganda indicate that over 90 percent of HIV infections can be attributed to STDs.[7] Male circumcision has been shown to have a protective effect against HIV transmission.[4,8]

BEHAVIORAL FACTORS

The rate of partner change, the number of concurrent partners, and mixing patterns influence the reproductive rate. Both the average rate of partner change in a population and the variation across individuals are important.[9] The greater the number of partners, the faster the spread of HIV. In almost all societies, most individuals have few sexual partners during their lifetime, but a small number have many partners. However, this latter group may be sufficient to sustain an epidemic and gradually extend its spread to the rest of the population. The number of concurrent partners appears to be more important than the total number of sexual partners.[10] The more mixing between high-risk individuals (those with many partners) and low-risk individuals (those with few sexual partners), the faster the epidemic will spread in the general population.[11] This is likely to occur, for example, in countries with an active commercial sex industry.

ECONOMIC FACTORS

Poverty may also increase transmission. Impoverished women are more vulnerable and less effective in negotiating safe sex with partners and more likely to engage in sex work. Poverty may motivate men to migrate for work, putting them at risk for having more sexual partners while away from the family. Empirical analysis by the World Bank of national-level aggregate data supports these hypotheses.[9]

Factors that accompany economic growth, particularly improved infrastructure and increased travel, can facilitate spread of the epidemic. One reason is that an open economy facilitates the movement of individuals. Economic growth may also contribute to a shift from more conservative to more liberal social attitudes, which may lead to greater individual freedom and more risky sexual activity.

WOMEN ARE AT GREATER RISK THAN MEN

Although globally more men than women have been infected with HIV (with the exception of sub-Saharan Africa), new infections are increasing faster among women. Women are also becoming infected at a younger age than men.[12] Biological, behavioral, and social factors explain these gender differences. Like other STDs, HIV is more easily transmitted from men to women than from women to men. Young women and girls are particularly vulnerable, as they have more cervicovaginal fragility. Recent studies in several African populations found that women aged 15 to 19 are five or six times more likely to be HIV-positive than men of the same age.[66] Females are also more likely than males to have nonsymptomatic STDs, and, since these STDs are likely to go untreated, females have an elevated risk for HIV infection. Social factors, such as a lack of control over the conditions under which they have sex, can also contribute to increased risk for HIV infection. This applies to a spectrum of sexually active females—from sex workers to monogamous, married women.[12]

Impact on Mortality Rates, Life Expectancy, and Population Growth

AIDS causes a large share of mortality in developing countries: at the end of 2000, a total of 17.5 million adults and 4.3 million children under the age of 15 had died since the beginning of the epidemic.[1] By 1990, AIDS was the third leading cause of adult death in the developing world (following tuberculosis and other infectious diseases), but its share of mortality is growing much faster than any other disease.[13] In African countries with the most severe epidemics, over half of adult mortality is attributed to AIDS.[14] It has been estimated that HIV will be the second largest contributor to prime-age adult death in developing countries by the year 2020, accounting for over one-third of adult deaths from infectious disease.[14] Infant mortality rates are higher owing to AIDS, with countries that had significantly reduced infant mortality and with high HIV prevalence rates being relatively more affected. For example, by the year 2010, infant mortality rates in Zimbabwe are estimated to be twice as high as they would have been without AIDS.[15]

The HIV epidemic is also decreasing life expectancy rates in developing countries, reversing important gains made in recent decades. Life expectancies have been reduced by 4 to 26 years in those countries most severely affected by the epidemic.[15] AIDS is also expected to reduce population growth rates in many countries, but rates will remain positive in the year 2010 (although some will be near zero). AIDS has also caused absolute declines in population size, and it is estimated that there are 16 million fewer people today in the 21 most affected countries in sub-Saharan Africa.[15]

Stages of the Epidemic

There is wide variation in patterns of the epidemic across countries and regions of the developing world. A useful way to compare the severity of the epidemic in different countries is to use data on the prevalence of HIV infection among populations who do or do not engage in high-risk behavior. Based on these criteria, the World Bank delineated a typology of "stages" of the epidemic (Figure 1.1):[9]

- *Nascent:* HIV prevalence is less than 5 percent in all known subpopulations presumed to practice high-risk behavior.
- *Concentrated:* HIV prevalence has surpassed 5 percent in one or more subpopulations presumed to practice high-risk behavior, but prevalence among women attending urban antenatal clinics is less than 5 percent.
- *Generalized:* HIV prevalence has surpassed 5 percent in one or more subpopulations at high risk and among women attending urban antenatal clinics.

Sub-Saharan Africa has been most severely affected, with an estimated 25.3 million people living with HIV at the end of 2000. There were 3.8 million new infections in 2000, the most for any region. Heterosexual transmission accounts for over 90 percent of all HIV infections in the region. As discussed earlier, the average age of those contracting HIV has been decreasing, and rates of newly acquired HIV are highest among young women (and to a lesser extent, young men) aged 15 to 24.[66]

At least 20 countries in this region have generalized epidemics. This includes most countries in southern Africa, where HIV is currently spreading most rap-

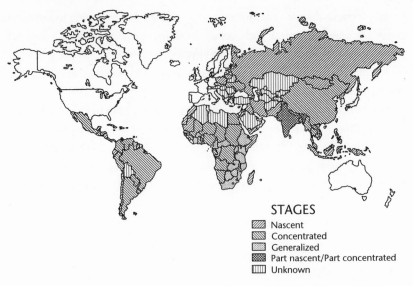

STAGES
- ▨ Nascent
- ▧ Concentrated
- ░ Generalized
- ▓ Part nascent/Part concentrated
- ▥ Unknown

Figure 1.1. Stages of the AIDS epidemic in the developing world, 1997. *Source:* World Bank, 1999.

idly, probably owing to the recent increase in ease of transportation and economic growth. In South Africa, the epidemic exploded in the 1990s, as indicated by an increase in the prevalence from 4.2 percent among urban antenatal clinic attendees in 1991 to 16 percent among antenatal clinic attendees nationwide in 1997. In Botswana, Namibia, Swaziland, and Zimbabwe, 20 to 26 percent of people aged 15 to 49 are living with HIV today. The West African countries of Côte d'Ivoire and Burkina Faso also have generalized epidemics, but HIV rates appear to be stabilizing in this region.

The AIDS epidemic is also generalized in most countries in East Africa, which was one of the first areas to suffer from AIDS. There is evidence that prevalence is declining in at least one East African country, Uganda, particularly among young people living in urban areas (see below). A few sub-Saharan African countries—Cape Verde, Madagascar, Mauritania, Mauritius, and Somalia—are still at the nascent stage of the epidemic.

In South and Southeast Asia, 5.8 million persons were estimated to be living with HIV at the end of 2000 and infection rates are increasing rapidly in this region. Most countries in the region, including China, India, and Malaysia, have concentrated epidemics. However, levels of infection and modes of transmission vary greatly across the region. Thailand has been most severely affected. In

Bangkok the prevalence among IDUs rose from 1 percent in late 1987 to over 30 percent eight months later.[16] In parallel to the epidemic among IDUs, HIV was transmitted among sex workers and their clients, and then to the general population. By mid-1993, the prevalence was 35 percent among IDUs, 29 percent among brothel-based sex workers, and 1 percent among pregnant women.[17] Rates were much higher in the northern part of the country. Since 1993, the overall epidemic has declined, as reflected by a decrease in prevalence among young army conscripts and childbearing women, as discussed later in this chapter.

There are two major epidemics in China, where about half a million people were infected at the end of 1999, up from 200,000 at the end of 1996.[66,18] One epidemic is occurring among IDUs, who are mostly in the southwest region of the country. As of 1999, prevalence rates in IDU populations reached as high as 70 to 80 percent in some areas, and were on average 30 to 50 percent in this region.[19] The other, newer epidemic is among heterosexuals, mainly along the economically prosperous eastern seaboard, where STDs are also increasing.

In India, prevalence rates in some populations are over ten times those in neighboring China. Although surveillance is limited, it is estimated that about 4 million people were living with HIV at the end of 1999, making India the country with the second highest number of HIV-infected persons (South Africa is higher).[66] In at least 5 states, more than 1 percent of pregnant women are now infected. In Mumbai (formerly Bombay) the percentage of patients at STD clinics who were HIV-infected rose from 23 percent in 1994 to 56 percent in 1999. In Tamil Nadu, prevalence of HIV was as high as 6.5 percent in antenatal clinics in one city. In the northeast, transmission is mainly by needle sharing among IDUs. Manipur State reported 6 percent of the AIDS cases in 1997, all among IDUs, 73 percent of whom were infected by 1996.[20]

In Cambodia, HIV infection has spread to the general population, with 3.76 percent of married women of reproductive age infected with HIV in 1998.[66] In Myanmar, infection among sex workers increased from 4 percent in 1992 to over 20 percent in 1996, and two-thirds of IDUs and about 2 percent of pregnant women were found to be infected in 1996.[21] In Vietnam, over 18 percent of high-risk groups and 0.1 percent of women attending urban antenatal clinics were HIV-infected in 1997.[9]

The epidemic is nascent in other countries of the region. It is not clear why the epidemic has not spread more widely in the Philippines, Indonesia, and Singapore, where the virus has been for several years and sex work is common. One possible explanation regards differences in the commercial sex industry.

Evidence suggests that the intensity of epidemics associated with sex workers is determined primarily by the number of sex partners (clients) per sex worker, the frequency of use of commercial sex by men, and the rate of regular condom use in commercial sex. In Indonesia and the Philippines, it is thought that there are fewer customers per sex worker and a smaller percentage of men engaging in commercial sex.[20] Countries like the Philippines, Bangladesh, and Indonesia also have much less intravenous drug use. Another potential explanation for the low rates in Indonesia is the widespread availability of STD treatment.

In Latin America, about 1.4 million people were estimated to be living with HIV as of December 2000.[1] More than half of the countries in Latin America have concentrated epidemics, including Brazil and Mexico. In several countries of the region, including Brazil, Mexico, and the countries of the Southern Cone (Argentina, Chile, Paraguay, and Uruguay), HIV infections were initially concentrated among men who have sex with men and among IDUs.[22] Although data are scarce for both these population groups, as many as 30 percent of Mexican men who have sex with men may be infected.[23] Rates among IDUs vary from 5 to 11 percent in Mexico to close to 50 percent in Argentina and Brazil.[23] More recently, heterosexual transmission has become predominant and now accounts for the majority of all HIV transmission in adults.

In the Caribbean, most transmission early in the epidemic was also by sex between men, but heterosexual transmission is now the primary mode of transmission. HIV rates are generally higher here than in other parts of Latin America and are on the rise. In Haiti, HIV prevalence increased from 2 percent in 1989 to 5 percent of the adult rural population in 1994,[24] and by 1996 (the most recent surveillance data available) almost 6 percent of pregnant women were HIV-infected.[66] In the Dominican Republic, the most recent data from one surveillance site indicated an HIV prevalence of 8 percent among pregnant women.[23]

Reliable data about the extent of the epidemic are scarce from Eastern Europe and the former Soviet Union, but what is available suggests that most countries have nascent epidemics. The exception is Ukraine, where the epidemic is concentrated because of a high prevalence among IDUs. There are signs, however, that the epidemic is spreading most quickly in independent states of the former Soviet Union, where the population living with HIV doubled between the end of 1997 and the end of 1999.[66] The spread of the epidemic is most extensive in Russia and Belarus, and to a lesser extent in Moldova, the Baltic States, the Caucasus, and Kazakhstan.[25] Increasing incidence rates among IDUs in some of the major cities, like those in Ukraine, suggest that the epidemic may be spreading rapidly among this group in other countries as well. The potential for spread by sexual transmission also exists, as STD rates are also increasing dramatically in many countries. For example, between 1988 and 1996, there was a 62-fold increase in the incidence of syphilis reported in Russia.[26] In Central Europe, the increase is much lower and (with the exception of Poland) homosexual transmission is most common, whereas in the Balkan countries HIV cases resulting from heterosexual contact were reported more frequently.[25]

Although data are scarce for North Africa and the Middle East, existing information suggests that the epidemic is in the nascent stage in these regions. There is, however, evidence of rapid transmission among drug users in Bahrain and Egypt,[9] and in Tunisia and Pakistan.[66]

According to the World Bank, at the end of 1999, about 80 percent of the population of developing countries lived in areas where the epidemic was either nascent or concentrated, and not yet generalized.[9] Thus, there is still hope of preventing a generalized epidemic in many places, but it is imperative to act quickly to prevent this from occurring.

EVALUATION OF HIV/AIDS PREVENTION INTERVENTIONS IN DEVELOPING COUNTRIES

The goal of HIV prevention is to minimize the number of new HIV infections. This suggests the need to focus prevention interventions on individuals who are likely to transmit HIV infection to many others—that is, those with many sexual or needle-sharing partners. Behavioral research in developing countries has identified several groups who are at particularly high risk: sex workers and their clients, IDUs, truck drivers, fishermen, military personnel, men who have sex with men, and people with STDs. Collecting information about incidence and prevalence among high-risk populations and about their characteristics and behaviors is a critical first step in HIV prevention.

Three broad approaches to prevention of HIV transmitted sexually or through injection drug use can be applied: influencing individuals to engage in less risky behavior; STD treatment; and altering the larger social and policy environment in which people live. The first two approaches have been the most widely implemented, but the third approach, which involves structural and environmental changes, could potentially effect change on a much larger scale.

Table 1.2. Interventions for HIV Prevention in Developing Countries

	Number of Studies
Behavioral change	
Targeted condom promotion	6
Communitywide risk reduction	3
School-based education	2
Harm reduction among IDUS	2
Voluntary counseling and testing	10
STD treatment with or without condom promotion	6
Structural and environmental interventions	5

Source: M. Merson, J. Dayton, and K. O'Reilly, Effectiveness of HIV prevention interventions in developing countries, *AIDS*, 2000; 14 (Suppl. 2): S68–84.

Behavioral Change at the Individual Level

We recently reviewed published evaluations of 34 behavioral prevention interventions undertaken in 18 developing countries (Table 1.2).[27] Sixteen of these interventions aimed to change individual behavior through targeted condom promotion or voluntary counseling and testing (VCT). Condom promotion interventions significantly increased condom use when targeted to high-risk groups, such as sex workers and their clients, truckers, and factory workers. In most of the studies we reviewed, rates of condom use increased at least twofold when evaluated six months after program implementation. A study in Indonesia also showed that easy accessibility to condoms (by either free distribution or sale) was important for increasing condom use.

We found that the effectiveness of VCT programs in preventing HIV transmission was mixed. It was most effective in increasing and sustaining condom use and maintaining low seroconversion rates in uninfected partners, when directed at discordant couples. In other situations, such as when only one sexual partner received VCT or among childbearing women, the effectiveness of VCT was unclear and more evaluation is needed. Some of the studies found more evidence of behavior change as a result of VCT among HIV-infected individuals than in uninfected persons, but more analysis is needed in this area.

We found very few studies that evaluated behavior change interventions directed at other risk groups in developing countries, such as men who have sex with men, youth, IDUS, and HIV-infected individuals. Such studies are urgently needed, as are evaluations of other types of behavior change interventions, like the popular opinion leader model, which has been effective in industrialized countries.[28,29]

STD Treatment: Alone and Combined with Targeted Condom Promotion

We further examined the effectiveness of STD treatment and interventions that combined STD treatment with condom promotion. The most convincing evidence of the effectiveness of STD treatment has come from a randomized, controlled trial in Mwanza, Tanzania. The intervention provided community-based STD care (including training of primary health care workers in STD syndromic case management, making available effective antibiotics and promoting health care seeking behavior by those infected) and reduced HIV incidence by 42 percent after 2 years.[30] This decrease was the result of a reduction in the duration and hence the prevalence of symptomatic STDs in a population where HIV prevalence was not high.[31,32] These results were corroborated by a controlled clinical study in Malawi in which men with HIV infection and urethritis were shown to have eightfold higher HIV concentrations in semen as compared with men without urethritis. Two weeks after antibiotic therapy, the HIV level decreased significantly in both gonococcal and nongonococcal urethritis patients, although the decline was less dramatic for the latter.[33] Additional evidence from a clinical study among female sex workers in Abidjan also showed that cervicovaginal shedding of HIV-1 was associated with ulcerative and nonulcerative STDs and decreased significantly following treatment.[34] Published results of a study of the effectiveness of mass STD treatment in Rakai, Uganda, found no effect of STD treatment on HIV incidences after 20 months, suggesting little short-term impact of such treatment in a mature epidemic.[31,35]

Available evidence from studies in Congo (formerly Zaire), Bolivia, South Africa, and Kenya suggests that combining STD treatment with targeted condom promotion has been highly effective in reducing the spread of STDs and HIV in those settings.[36-39] At issue now is the treatment protocol for syndromic case management of STDs among women in resource-poor settings, given the overtreatment that occurs with the use of available protocols.[40,41]

Structural and Environmental Interventions

Structural interventions change laws, policies, and standard operating procedures in a society, and environmental interventions alter living conditions, resources, and opportunities.[42] These approaches to promoting healthier behavior have been used successfully in the United States, for example, to reduce motorcycle injuries and automobile accidents by, respectively, mandating helmet use and decreasing speed limits and increasing seat belt use. Although not many structural and environmental interventions in developing countries have been implemented or evaluated, they hold the promise of being effective in reducing HIV transmission.

The most prominent example of a structural intervention in HIV prevention in a developing country is the 100 percent condom use policy in Thailand, which mandates and enforces condom use at all commercial sex establishments (see below). Other countries have implemented smaller-scale structural interventions. For example, in Brazil, the removal of high taxes on imported condoms helped to lower the price of condoms and to increase consumption.[43] In the Dominican Republic, a pilot program increased condom use by making condoms available in hotel rooms.[44] Other structural interventions that have the potential to reduce HIV transmission include syringe exchange, taxes on the consumption of commodities associated with risky behavior (e.g., alcoholic beverages sold at bars), and subsidies for condoms.

Environmental interventions that can prevent HIV infections include programs and policies that allow spouses and families to move with migrant laborers, empower women (e.g., by expanding their educational opportunities), and make STD treatment and condoms more widely available.[42,43] The most widely implemented programs of the latter type have been condom social marketing programs. They not only promote the sale and use of condoms, but also strive to make them available in more convenient locations and their use more socially acceptable. In over 40 developing countries that have received social marketing assistance from a number of international organizations since 1984, condom sales have increased exponentially, with a cumulative total of almost 4.8 billion condoms sold as of 1998.[45] In many countries these programs have paved the way for more aggressive advertising and promotion of all brands of condoms and encouraged market diversity and expansion of the condom sector in general.[46]

Despite these achievements, the studies in this review that assessed the effects of social marketing on behavior provided mixed results, with evidence of reduction in some risky sexual behaviors but not others.[47–49] Where behavior did change, it was not known which components of the multifaceted social marketing programs were most influential or whether individuals who purchased and used condoms were those most at risk for HIV infection. More rigorous evaluations are needed and some are already under way, including assessments of social marketing interventions targeted to youth in Guinea, and condom consumer profile surveys in Côte d'Ivoire, Rwanda, and Kenya.[50]

Other potentially important environmental interventions include promoting policies that encourage spouses and families to move with migrant laborers and expanding education for women and girls. Policies that make STD treatment more widely available and more accessible would also help to reduce the spread of HIV by, for example, expanding the over-the-counter availability of STD treatment and improving the training of pharmacists in treating STDs.

National-Level Response:
Combining Interventions

As discussed earlier in this chapter, the epidemic in Thailand spread exponentially during the 1980s. Although the government response did not start until 1989, it was massive and led by the prime minister. It began with a nationwide condom advertising campaign and was soon followed by the 100 percent condom use policy. In addition, STD services and over-the-counter antibiotics were widely available. The enormous increase in condom use and the paralleled STD and HIV declines strongly suggest that this multifaceted government response helped prevent many HIV infections in Thailand.[51] Between 1989 and 1995, the number of male STD cases presented at government clinics decreased 85 percent. There was a corresponding increase in condom use in brothels, from 14 percent in 1989 to 85 percent in 1991 to 91 percent in 1993.[52] At the same time, studies in large cohorts of 21-year-old enlisted men from northern Thailand at the time of conscription showed that HIV prevalence had decreased from 10.4 and 12.5 percent in the 1991 and 1993 cohorts, respectively, to 6.7 percent in the 1995 cohort.[53] Data have demonstrated significant declines in STD and HIV incidence among the 1991 and 1993 cohorts during their two-year period of military service.[54] A study of women giving birth at a hospital in Northern Thailand also confirms this trend; a rapid rise in HIV prevalence was observed from 1990 to 1994 and was followed by a sharp decline from 1994 to 1997.[55]

There are strong indications that HIV incidence has also declined in Uganda. In Nsambya (Kampala) and Jinja, HIV prevalence among pregnant women decreased 53 percent and 79 percent, respectively, in 15- to 19-year-olds between 1991 and 1996. At the same time, nationwide sexual abstinence has increased among males and females aged 15 to 19 and men and women in urban areas report increased use of condoms during the last sexual intercourse of risk.[56] Evidence from antenatal clinic-based sentinel surveillance in West Uganda between 1991 and 1997 indicates that HIV prevalence also declined markedly in younger age groups in this part of the country.[57] These positive behavioral changes have been linked to various individual and community-based interventions implemented during the past 10 years in the country, which include: interventions promoting monogamy and abstinence; a social marketing campaign; improved STD treatment; and the large number of people who have been counseled and tested for HIV. The importance of a multifaceted AIDS prevention program has been confirmed by a recent study that has identified the marked heterogeneity in risk factors for HIV, suggesting that a variety of approaches are needed to promote prevention in diverse circumstances.[58] Declines in HIV prevalence in Tanzania and Zambia suggest that a similar phenomenon may be occurring in these countries.[59,60]

In Senegal, HIV prevalence remained low and stable between 1989 and 1996.[61,62] Behavioral surveys indicate high condom use, with 60 percent of men and 40 percent of women ages 15 to 24 reporting that they used a condom with their most recent casual partner. These findings have been attributed to the existing norms in Senegalese society, which encourage conservative sexual behavior, combined with a strong political response that started early in the epidemic and included widely available STD treatment, sex education in primary and secondary schools, condom promotion, and social marketing. The positive interaction between the existing sexual norms in Senegal and HIV prevention interventions suggests that identifying and promoting "protective" social norms could also be effective in other countries.

POTENTIAL USES OF MODELING
IN HIV PREVENTION

Four factors are particularly helpful in determining the appropriate mix of prevention interventions in a particular setting: information on the epidemiology of HIV and the stage of the epidemic; knowledge of what types of interventions are effective; information about the cost-effectiveness of specific interventions; and the level of resources available for HIV prevention. The mix of interventions will necessarily vary from country to country; no single combination of interventions is appropriate in all settings.

The epidemiology of HIV suggests two clear messages for prevention.[9] First, it is imperative to *act early* in the epidemic, when HIV spreads exponentially. As noted earlier, viral load is also highest during the first few months of infection, so that early in the epidemic a large proportion of those infected may be highly infectious. And, from a budgetary perspective, it is far less costly to prevent HIV than to treat people with AIDS. Second, it is crucial to target interventions initially to those with the highest-risk behavior. This will have the greatest impact in terms of the number of new HIV infections prevented, as individuals with large numbers of sexual and needle-sharing partners who do not use condoms or clean injecting equipment are those most likely to become infected and then spread HIV. Changing the behavior of these individuals, even if only a relatively few members of society, is essential to curbing the epidemic.

Policy makers and program planners may use modeling in their HIV prevention programs in other ways.

- *Forecasting:*   They can use modeling to forecast the course of an epidemic if no interventions are undertaken. Such predictions can include information on morbidity, impact on child and adult mortality, average life span, and direct and indirect costs to the nation.

- *Estimating the importance of risk factors:*   Modeling may be helpful in estimating the importance of a risk factor in HIV prevention. As noted above, aggressive STD treatment reduced HIV incidence in Mwanza, where the HIV epidemic was not mature. However, mass antibiotic treatment for STDs did not have an impact on HIV incidence in Uganda, where the epidemic is more mature.[35] Earlier modeling efforts predicted this latter outcome.[7]

- *Predicting the impact of a prevention intervention:*   Modeling can predict the impact of specific prevention interventions on the course of the HIV epidemic. These include STD treatment and promoting condom use among high-risk persons with different patterns of sexual behavior.[9]

- *Predicting the impact of a biomedical intervention:*   Modeling can be used to estimate the impact of biomedical interventions. For example, from information now available, one can predict the impact of antiretroviral agents on perinatal transmission and on mortality from HIV infection. Once the effect of these drugs on HIV shedding in sperm and cervico-vaginal fluid is better known, modeling could be useful in predicting the impact that use of these drugs will have on HIV transmission and incidence. Also, modeling has been used to predict the impact of AIDS vaccines on the rate of new infections.[63]

- *Predicting the impact of a mixture of interventions:*   Modeling has been used to predict the impact of a mixture of interventions on the course of the epidemic.[57,64,65] Such efforts have allowed policy makers to compare the cost of HIV prevention to prevention of other diseases, for example, through comparative calculations of the cost of averting an infection. Analyses of this type have shown HIV prevention to be relatively cost-effective,[64] giving further support to the need for public health officials and politicians to overcome the various social and cultural barriers and constraints to HIV prevention.

The chapters in Parts II through IV of this book provide excellent examples of the modeling applications mentioned above.

REFERENCES

1. UNAIDS. AIDS Epidemic Update: December 2000. Geneva: World Health Organization, 2000.
2. Quinn T, Ruff A, Halsey N. Special considerations for developing countries. In: Pizzo P, Wilfert C, eds. *Pediatric AIDS: The Challenge of HIV Infection in Infants, Children and Adolescents.* Baltimore: Williams and Wilkins, 1994.
3. May M, Anderson R. Transmission dynamics of HIV infection. *Nature* 1987; 326:137–142.
4. Royce R, Sena A, Cates W Jr, Cohen M. Sexual transmission of HIV. *N Engl J Med* 1997; 336:1072–1078.
5. Hayes R, Mosha F, Nicoll A, et al. A community trial of the impact of improved sexually transmitted disease treatment on the HIV epidemic in rural Tanzania: Design. *AIDS* 1995; 9:919–926.
6. Laga M, Manoka A, Kivuvu M. Non-ulcerative sexually transmitted diseases as risk factors for HIV-1 transmission in women: Results from a cohort study. *AIDS* 1993; 7:95–102.
7. Robinson N, Mulder D, Auvert B, Hayes R. Proportion of HIV infections attributable to other sexually transmitted diseases in a rural Ugandan population: Simulation model estimates. *International Journal of Epidemiology* 1997; 26:180–189.
8. Kelly R, Kiwanuka N, Wawer M, et al. Age of male circumcision and risk of prevalent HIV infection in rural Uganda. *AIDS* 1999; 13:399–405.
9. World Bank. *Confronting AIDS: Public Priorities in a Global Epidemic.* Rev. ed. New York: Oxford University Press, 1999.
10. Morris M, Podhisita C, Wawer M, Handcock M. Bridge populations in the spread of HIV/AIDS in Thailand. *AIDS* 1996; 10:1265–1271.
11. Anderson R. The spread of HIV and sexual mixing patterns. In: Mann J, Tarantola D, eds. *AIDS in the World II: Global Dimensions, Social Roots, and Responses.* New York: Oxford University Press, 1996.
12. Vuylsteke B, Sunkutu R, Laga M. Epidemiology of HIV and sexually transmitted infections in women. In: Mann J, Tarantola D, eds. *AIDS in the World II: Global Dimensions, Social Roots, and Responses.* New York: Oxford University Press, 1996.
13. Murray C, Lopez A. The global burden of disease. In: Murray C, Lopez A, eds. *The Global Burden of Disease: A Comprehensive Assessment of Mortality and Disability from Diseases, Injuries, and Risk Factors in 1990 and Projected to 2020.* Vol. 1. Cambridge, MA: Harvard University Press, 1996.
14. Mulder D, Nunn A, Kamali A, Nakiyingi J, Wagner H, Kengeya-Kayondo J. Two-year

HIV-1 associated mortality in a Ugandan rural population. *Lancet* 1994; 343:1021–1023.

15. Stanecki K, Way P. A special chapter focusing on HIV/AIDS in the developing world. In: McDevitt T, ed. *World Population Profile: 1998*. Bureau of the Census, US Department of Commerce, 1999.

16. Weniger B, Limpakarnjanarat K, Ungchusak K, et al. The epidemiology of HIV infection and AIDS in Thailand. *AIDS* 1991; 5:S71–85.

17. Brown T, Sittitrai W, Vanichseni S, Thisyakorn U. The recent epidemiology of HIV and AIDS in Thailand. *AIDS* 1994; 8:S131–141.

18. UNAIDS. *Report on the Global HIV/AIDS Epidemic*. Geneva: World Health Organization, 1998.

19. Wu Z. Epidemiology of HIV/AIDS in China. In: Wu Z, Qi G, Zhang J, eds. *Epidemiology and Interventions of AIDS in China*. Beijing: Science Press, 1999:39–56.

20. Monitoring the AIDS Epidemic (MAP). The status and trends of the HIV/AIDS/STDs epidemics in Asia and the Pacific. Report for the Fourth International Conference on AIDS in Asia and the Pacific. Manila, Philippines, 1997.

21. UNAIDS. *Report on the Global HIV/AIDS Epidemic*. Geneva: World Health Organization, 1997.

22. Mertens T, Low-Beer D. HIV and AIDS: Where is the epidemic going? *Bulletin of the World Health Organization* 1996; 74;121–129.

23. UNAIDS. *AIDS Epidemic Update: December 1998*. Geneva: World Health Organization, 1998.

24. UNAIDS. *The Status and Trends of the Global HIV/AIDS Pandemic: Final Report*. Geneva: World Health Organization, 1996.

25. Dehne KL, Khodakevich L, Hamers FF, Schwartlander B. The HIV/AIDS epidemic in eastern Europe: Recent patterns and trends and their implications for policy-making. *AIDS* 1999; 13:741–749.

26. Tichonova L, Borisenko K, Ward H, Meheus A, Gromyko A, Renton A. Epidemics of syphilis in the Russian Federation: Trends, origins, and priorities for control. *Lancet* 1997; 350:210–213.

27. Merson M, Dayton J, O'Reilly K. Effectiveness of HIV prevention interventions in developing countries. *AIDS* 2000; 14(Suppl. 2):568–584.

28. Kelly J. Community-level interventions are needed to prevent new HIV infections. *American Journal of Public Health* 1999; 89;299–301.

29. Sikkema K, Kelly J, Winett R, et al. Outcomes of a randomized community-level HIV prevention intervention for women living in 18 low-income housing developments. *American Journal of Public Health* 2000; 90:57–63.

30. Grosskurth H, Mosha F, Todd J, et al. Impact of improved treatment of STDs on HIV infection in rural Tanzania: Randomized controlled trial. *Lancet* 1995; 346:530–536.

31. Hitchcock P, Fransen L. Preventing HIV infection: Lessons from Mwanza and Rakai. *Lancet* 1999; 353:513–515.

32. Mayaud P, Mosha F, Todd J, et al. Improved treatment services significantly reduce the prevalence of sexually transmitted diseases in rural Tanzania: Results of a randomized controlled trial. *AIDS* 1997; 11:1873–1880.

33. Cohen M, Hoffman I, Royce R, et al. Reduction of concentration of HIV-1 in semen after treatment of urethritis: Implications for prevention of sexual transmission of HIV-1. *Lancet* 1997; 349:1868–1873.

34. Ghys P, Fransen K, Diallo M, et al. The associations between cervicovaginal HIV shedding, sexually transmitted diseases and immunosuppression in female sex workers in Abidjan, Cote d'Ivoire. *AIDS* 1997; 11:F85–93.

35. Wawer M, Sewankambo N, Serwadda D, et al. Control of sexually transmitted diseases for AIDS prevention in Uganda: A randomized community trial. *Lancet* 1999; 353;525–535.

36. Laga M, Alary M, Nzila N, et al. Condom promotion, sexually transmitted diseases treatment, and declining incidence of HIV-1 infection in female Zairian sex workers. *Lancet* 1994; 344;246–248.

37. Levine W, Revollo R, Kaune V, et al. Decline in sexually transmitted disease prevalence in female Bolivian sex workers: Impact of an HIV prevention project. *AIDS* 1998; 12: 1899–1906.

38. Steen R, Vuylsteke B, DeCoito T, et al. Evidence of declining STD prevalence in a South African mining community following a core-group intervention. *Sexually Transmitted Diseases* 2000; 27:1–8.

39. Jackson D, Rakwar J, Richardson B, et al. Decreased incidence of sexually transmitted diseases among trucking company workers in Kenya: Results of a behaviour risk-reduction programme. *AIDS* 1997; 11:903–909.

40. Alary M, Baganizi A, Guedeme A. Evaluation of clinical algorithms for the diagnosis of gonococcal and chlamydial infections among men with urethral discharge or dysuria and women with vaginal discharge in Benin. *Sexually Transmitted Infections* 1998; 74: S44–S49.

41. Hawkes S, Morison L, Foster S, et al. Reproductive-tract infections in women in low-income, low-prevalence situations: Assessment of syndromic management in Matlab, Bangladesh. *Lancet* 1999; 354:1776–1781.

42. Sweat M, Denison J. Reducing HIV incidence in developing countries with structural and environmental interventions. *AIDS* 1995; 9:S251–S257.

43. Tawil O, Verster A, O'Reilly K. Enabling approaches for HIV/AIDS prevention: Can we modify the environment and minimize the risk? *AIDS* 1995; 9:1299–1306.

44. Guerrero E, De Moya E, Rosario S. *Ongoing Impact of the Condom Use Promotion/Desensitization Program for Preventing AIDS in the Dominican Republic: Report for the Programa ETS/SIDA (PROCETS).* Geneva: World Health Organization, 1988.

45. Futures Group. *Contraceptive Social Marketing Database.* Washington, DC: Futures Group International, 1998.

46. Futures Group. The transition to the commercial sector: What happens to socially marketed products after graduating from USAID support? Washington, DC: Futures Group International, 1997.

47. Meekers D. The effectiveness of targeted social marketing to promote adolescent reproductive health: The case of Soweto, South Africa. *Journal of HIV/AIDS Prevention and Education for Adolescents and Children* (in press).

48. Van Rossem R, Meekers D. An evaluation of the effectiveness of targeted social market-

ing to promote adolescent and young adult reproductive health in Cameroon. *AIDS Education and Prevention* 2000; 12:383–404.

49. Meekers D. Going underground and going after women: Trends in sexual risk behaviors among gold miners in South Africa. *International Journal of STD & AIDS* 2000; 11:21–26.

50. Meekers D. Personal communication, 1998.

51. Robinson N, Hanenberg H. Condoms used during most commercial sex acts in Thailand. *AIDS* 1997; 11:1064–1065.

52. Hanenberg R, Rojanapithayakorn W, Kunasol P, Sokal D. Impact of Thailand's HIV-control programme as indicated by the decline of sexually transmitted diseases. *Lancet* 1994; 344:243–245.

53. Nelson K, Celentano D, Eiumtrakol S, et al. Changes in sexual behavior and a decline in HIV infection among young men in Thailand. *N Engl J Med* 1996; 335:297–303.

54. Celentano D, Nelson K, Lyles C, et al. Decreasing incidence of HIV and sexually transmitted diseases in young Thai men: Evidence for success of HIV/AIDS control and prevention program. *AIDS* 1998; 12:F29–36.

55. Bunnell R, Yanpaisarn S, Kilmarx P, et al. HIV-1 seroprevalence among childbearing women in northern Thailand: Monitoring a rapidly evolving epidemic. *AIDS* 1999; 13:509–515.

56. Asiimwe-Okiror G, Opio A, Musinguzi J, Madraa E, Tembo G, Carael M. Change in sexual behavior and decline in HIV infection among young pregnant women in urban Uganda. *AIDS* 1997; 11:1757–1763.

57. Kilian A, Gregson S, Ndyanabangi B, et al. Reductions in risk behaviour provide the most consistent explanation for declining HIV-1 prevalence in Uganda. *AIDS* 1999; 13:391–398.

58. Quigley M, Munguti K, Grosskurth H. Sexual behaviour patterns and other risk factors for HIV infection in rural Tanzania: A case-control study. *AIDS* 1997; 11:237–248.

59. Kwesigabo G, Killewo J, Makwaya C, et al. Decline in the prevalence and incidence of HIV-1 infection in population-based studies in Bukoba Urban, Kegara, Tanzania. Twelfth World AIDS Conference, Geneva, June 28–July 3, 1998.

60. Fylkesnes K, Carael M. HIV epidemics and behaviors: Evidence of favorable change in Zambia. Twelfth World AIDS Conference, Geneva, June 28–July 3, 1998.

61. Ndoye I, Delaporte E, Meda N, et al. HIV control program in Africa: A successful case study in Senegal. Twelfth World AIDS Conference, Geneva, June 28–July 3, 1998.

62. UNAIDS. *Senegal: Epidemiological Fact Sheet on HIV/AIDS and Sexually Transmitted Diseases.* Geneva: World Health Organization, 1998:1–12.

63. Porco T, Blower S. Designing HIV vaccination policies: Sub-types and cross-immunity. *Interfaces* 1998; 28:167–190.

64. World Bank. *World Development Report: Investing in Health.* New York: Oxford University Press, 1993, 99–106.

65. UNAIDS. *UNAIDS HIV Drug Initiative: Providing Wider Access to HIV-Related Drugs in Developing Countries.* Geneva: World Health Organization, 1997.

66. UNAIDS. AIDS Epidemic Update: December 1999. Geneva: World Health Organization, 1999.

Chapter 2 Implications of Economic Evaluations for National HIV Prevention Policy Makers

David R. Holtgrave and Steven D. Pinkerton

The course of HIV prevention programming in the United States is driven by policy makers at the local, state, and federal levels. But, unlike most public health programs in other disease areas, a formal mechanism—known as HIV prevention community planning—is available for HIV-infected and HIV-affected community members to participate in the HIV prevention decision making process by becoming members of their local community planning groups.[1,2] These groups are charged with analyzing the course of the epidemic in their jurisdiction; assessing and prioritizing prevention needs; and identifying science-based HIV prevention interventions to meet these needs. The HIV prevention community planning process is meant to ensure that the community voices are heard, that available HIV prevention resources closely follow epidemiologic impact and target unmet needs, and that specific prevention interventions are based on the latest science and public health practice. The community planning process is coordinated by the federal Centers for Disease Control and Prevention (CDC), which funds the vast majority of HIV prevention programming in the United States.

The multiplicity of policy makers involved in HIV prevention planning (including participants at the federal, state, local, and community levels) often makes it difficult to trace the decision making path for the establishment and evolution of any particular HIV prevention policy. The array of HIV prevention funding streams (which include governmental, nongovernmental, and sliding-scale fee-for-service revenue) ultimately blend together at the grassroots level, but this variety also contributes to the difficulty of tracking and describing HIV prevention policy making.

Policy makers at all levels require answers to key questions so that their decisions are based (even potentially based) on scientifically sound data and logical analysis.[3] In this chapter, we focus on several key questions that we have heard voiced by a variety of persons in the legislative and executive branches of the federal government, as well as national leaders employed by nongovernmental organizations (including academic and activist organizations). Thus, we focus on a relatively small set of the wide array of persons involved in HIV prevention policy making. The key national-level questions are as follows:

1. What do HIV prevention programs really cost?
2. Are HIV prevention programs worth the investment?
3. Which programs are the most cost-effective?
4. How can we estimate the impact of a national rollout of a program before it is actually implemented?
5. How can we rule out economically inefficient programs prior to implementation?
6. Does HIV prevention funding follow the epidemic and flow to areas in most need?
7. Short of obtaining perfection in HIV prevention programs, how can meaningful performance standards be set?
8. Is the national HIV prevention effort truly making a difference in stemming the epidemic?

We address these questions in turn, emphasizing the role that economic evaluation studies have in answering each. (Clearly, economic evaluation information is not the only type of information considered by or relevant to policy makers; factors such as equity and "the rule of rescue" play an important role, and we do not mean to diminish them by our emphasis on economic evaluation methodologies in this chapter.) Economic evaluation research relevant to each of these five areas has already been conducted and much of it already published.[4] We do not limit ourselves here to published sources, however; we also provide some analyses for the first time in printed form. We do not attempt to provide comprehensive, substantive answers to each question; rather, we illustrate how economic evaluation techniques can inform, and are informing, the policy questions. Hence, our purpose is to illustrate the value of various economic evaluation methodologies for informing key HIV prevention policy questions. We end the chapter with some further thoughts on increasing the relevance of economic evaluation research to HIV prevention policy makers.

WHAT DO HIV PREVENTION PROGRAMS REALLY COST?

Those responsible for funding HIV prevention programs need to know if they can afford each of the various types of interventions (e.g., HIV counseling and testing services, street outreach activities, small-group risk reduction interventions, public information campaigns, and so on). Simply put, they need to know if the resources required for specific types of interventions put them out of reach of the available budget. These funders must know what the programs truly cost (in terms of resources consumed), not just what those who field the programs "charge" for their delivery. Cost analysis can provide exactly this type of information.

Just a few years ago, there were essentially no published analyses that carefully estimated the costs of HIV prevention programs via scientifically sound methods of cost analysis. This situation has changed substantially in recent years. The economic evaluation published literature now includes cost information on the following HIV prevention intervention types (references given are illustrative, not exhaustive, and we reference review papers where possible): (a) HIV antibody testing and pre-/post-test counseling;[6,7] (b) street outreach services for drug injectors and other hard-to-reach populations;[8,9] (c) small-group risk reduction interventions that help clients change the sexual or drug-related behaviors that place them at risk for HIV infection;[10] (d) community-level interventions that attempt to alter the behaviors and behavioral norms of the community as a whole;[10] (e) needle and syringe exchange programs and other activities to increase drug injectors' access to sterile injection equipment;[8] (f) prophylaxis with antiretroviral medications following suspected occupational (e.g., in the health care setting)[11] and nonoccupational (e.g., sex- or injection-related) exposures to HIV;[12] (g) prevention of perinatal HIV transmission through the administration of zidovudine (AZT) or other antiretroviral medications to the mother, the infant, or both;[13] (h) prevention and treatment of other sexually transmitted diseases (STDs), viewed as an HIV prevention intervention;[14] and (i) counseling and referral services for the partners of HIV seropositive individuals.[15] As this list suggests, there is now at least one published study that contains rigorous cost-analytic information for most of the major types of HIV prevention interventions. One area in which additional cost-analytic work is clearly needed is the determination of economic resources consumed by public information campaigns and prevention marketing activities.

ARE HIV PREVENTION PROGRAMS
WORTH THE INVESTMENT?

In addition to knowing the cost of HIV prevention interventions, policy makers need information on the economic efficiency, or cost-effectiveness, of these interventions. For example, they might be interested in whether an intervention saves society money in the long run, or they might want to know how their investments in HIV prevention programs compare to investments in programs for preventing or curing other diseases (such as cancer or heart disease). More generally, most decision makers will want to know what approach to investing their resources will yield the maximum overall public health benefit.

The three main methods for evaluating the economic efficiency of an HIV prevention program (or other public health or medical care intervention) are cost-benefit analysis (CBA), cost-effectiveness analysis (CEA), and cost-utility analysis (CUA).[16] Cost-benefit analysis is especially well suited for answering the first type of question: Does the intervention yield overall, long-term savings? In a CBA of an HIV prevention intervention, all consequences, whether positive or negative, are converted to dollar equivalents.[16] Thus, for example, the *net value* of an intervention might be calculated by subtracting the cost of the intervention from the overall savings obtained by preventing people from becoming infected. According to one analysis published in 1997, the lifetime medical care cost of treating someone with HIV is approximately $154,000 (discounted at 3%).[17] If this figure is taken as an estimate of the "value" of preventing an HIV infection, then the net value of the intervention would be $154,000 · A − C, where A is the number of HIV infections prevented by the intervention and C is its cost. If the net value is positive—so that the cost of the intervention is more than offset by the savings in reduced medical care costs—then the intervention is considered to be "cost-saving." Cost-saving interventions are clearly good investments. Later in this section and in other sections of this chapter, we highlight a number of HIV prevention interventions that have been found to be "cost-saving" as defined here.

The economic benefits of preventing someone from becoming infected with HIV extend beyond simply averting future medical costs. From a societal perspective, one obvious additional benefit is the savings in economic productivity that would otherwise be lost to disability and death.[16] Studies conducted in the mid-1980s estimated the forgone earnings of an HIV-infected person at between $540,000 and $625,000,[18-20] or about $750,000 to $1,000,000 in 1998 dollars. (We note that (a) these forgone earnings estimates are dated, (b) research must be done to update them, (c) they would change over time as the socioeconomic characteristics of the epidemic change, and (d) dynamic changes in them have the potential for influencing the results of CBAs.) However, treatment options and effectiveness have changed radically since the time of these studies, when zidovudine was the only available antiretroviral medication. The introduction of combination therapies consisting of three or more antiretrovirals has led to remarkable improvements in the health of many HIV-infected individuals, some of whom have returned to work after extended health-related absences.[21] At present there is considerable uncertainty regarding the impact of combination antiretroviral therapies on HIV patients' longevity, long-term health, and economic productivity.[17] Studies are needed to better quantify both the short- and long-term economic costs associated with HIV disease and the mediational effects of various treatment regimens. The main point here is that when an HIV prevention intervention is found to avert more medical costs than the prevention program costs to deliver, it is "cost-saving" in a very conservative sense. That is, a number of potentially important benefits (e.g., benefits in productivity, certain psychological benefits of avoiding infection and transmission, and hard-to-quantify benefits such as overall benefits to society of reductions in HIV transmission) are omitted from these analyses, making them highly conservative.

In addition, several cost-effectiveness and cost-utility analyses of HIV prevention programs have found the cost per HIV infection averted by some intervention to be clearly less than the medical costs of treating HIV disease.[4] Although these studies are not strictly CBAs, they nevertheless indicate that the interventions under study are cost-saving to society, and are thus sound investments in the nation's health. (Note again that a number of benefits—indicated above—are not included in such analyses, making them highly conservative.)

An intervention need not be cost-saving to represent a good investment. However, it is difficult to compare the economic efficiency of different noncost-saving programs on the basis of net value alone (i.e., using CBA). Cost-effectiveness and cost-utility analyses are better suited to this purpose.[22] In CEA, health-related benefits are valued in natural units, such as HIV infections averted.[22] In CUA, health outcomes are generally measured in quality-adjusted life years (QALYs) saved.[22] Different prevention programs can then be compared on the basis of their cost-per-infection-averted or cost-per-QALY-saved ratio, depending on the analytic methodology adopted.

Cost-utility analysis is recommended for comparisons between HIV prevention programs and other health care or health promotion interventions for several main reasons.[22] First, unlike disease-specific measures, such as HIV infections averted or clients served (e.g., by a screening program), QALYs can be used for a wide range of health-related interventions, including those that primarily affect length of life, those that primarily affect quality of life, and those that have appreciable effects on both. (In the QALY framework, each year of life spent in a particular health state is associated with a numerical weight that indicates the quality of life in that health state. Weights range from 0 to 1, which correspond to death and perfect health, respectively.) As a reflection of the general applicability of CUA, the U.S. Panel on Cost-Effectiveness in Health and Medicine recommends that all economic efficiency analyses include a "reference case" CUA, regardless of the method used in the main analysis.[22] Because all referent case CUAS conducted in conformance with the panel's guidelines share a common methodology, they should be comparable.

Almost all the HIV prevention CUAS that currently exist have been published within the past few years. Cost-utility analyses have been performed for the following types of interventions: (a) small-group behavioral risk reduction interventions;[10] (b) community-level interventions that seek to change safer sex norms;[10] (c) hybrid interventions consisting of group risk reduction services, counseling and testing, and referral for other needed services;[23] and (d) occupational and nonoccupational post-exposure prophylaxis (PEP).[11,12] By and large, these studies have followed the panel's recommendations for the conduct of referent case CUAS.[22] This renders the results of these studies methodologically comparable to one another and to similarly conducted CUAS from other disease areas.

The several studies that examined behavioral interventions have all found the services examined either to be cost-saving (in the conservative sense of the medical costs averted by the intervention outweighing the cost of the intervention) or to have a cost-per-QALY saved ratio of under $10,000.[10] Most health services researchers would agree that interventions that cost less than $30,000 to $50,000 per QALY saved are generally accepted as being cost-effective.[24] In contrast to the behavioral interventions, PEP was not universally cost-effective.[12] Rather, whether or not PEP appeared economically attractive depended on the values of several risk-related parameters, such as HIV seroprevalence and the probability of transmission. Following some conditions (e.g., deep, percutaneous occupational exposure to HIV-infected blood or unprotected receptive anal intercourse with an HIV-infected partner), PEP is highly cost-effective. In other cases (such as low HIV seroprevalence or low transmissibility), PEP has an extremely unfavorable cost-utility ratio and appears to be a very poor use of fiscal resources.

WHICH PROGRAMS ARE THE MOST COST-EFFECTIVE?

Policy makers who fund various types of HIV prevention programs need to know how these programs compare to one another. Clearly, CUA can be used to provide such information. However, a popular type of economic evaluation technique for answering this type of "within-disease resource allocation" question is CEA with cost-per-HIV-infection-averted as the main outcome measure (stopping short of converting infections averted to QALYs saved).[25–27] Although CEA is useful for comparing HIV prevention programs to one another, this type of analysis has two major limitations. First, it requires additional work before the study results can be extrapolated to compare the HIV prevention intervention assessed to a program in any other disease area (unless the results indicate cost-savings to society). Second, it cannot be used fruitfully for any HIV-related services (such as social services) that might improve quality of life but not longevity. For these reasons, we recommend that both across-disease and within-disease analyses employ CUA methodologies.[28]

Despite these limitations, policy makers interested expressly in comparing HIV prevention interventions to one another would find such CEAs useful. The literature contains CEAs for a variety of HIV prevention interventions, in addition to those for which CUAs have been performed, including: (a) needle and syringe exchange;[8] (b) counseling and testing;[6,7] (c) partner notification;[15] (d) street outreach;[8] and (e) antiretroviral prophylaxis to prevent perinatal HIV transmission.[13]

Although this chapter focuses on national-level policy makers, it is worth noting that some key local policy makers are expressly interested in comparing different HIV prevention interventions to one another. These local decision makers are health departments partnering with local HIV prevention community planning groups.[29] Their purpose is to prioritize HIV prevention funding across populations, small geographic areas, and intervention types.[30] Kaplan has developed an economic evaluation modeling technique designed to take as input intervention cost information and empirical or subjective estimates of intervention effectiveness, and yield as output the cost per infection averted by various interventions.[31] The associated software goes further and even suggests optimal spending allocations across interventions so as to maximize the number of infections prevented at any given level of available funding. Several simpler intervention prioritization algorithms have also been proposed in the literature.[25-27]

HOW CAN WE ESTIMATE THE IMPACT
OF A NATIONAL ROLLOUT OF A PROGRAM
BEFORE IT IS IMPLEMENTED?

Even after an intervention has been subjected to efficacy and effectiveness trials (preferably including an economic evaluation component) and shown to be effective at reducing HIV transmission, policy makers may be reluctant to roll out the intervention on a national level. There may still be unanswered questions regarding the national cost of the program, and whether its marginal cost-effectiveness will continue to appear favorable at ever increasing levels of program intensity or whether there is an optimal program size that maximizes economic efficiency. Economic evaluation modeling can be used prior to the implementation of any such program to give a carefully estimated (albeit not empirically measured) sense of its national cost. This modeling can also be used to determine the theoretically optimal program size as indicated by the estimated marginal cost-effectiveness ratios. Although deciding whether or not to implement a program nationally, and at what intensity, is a situation of substantial uncertainty, economic evaluation modeling is designed to aid decision making under precisely these conditions.

As a recent example of such an exercise, Holtgrave and colleagues conducted an a priori economic evaluation modeling study of a nationwide needle and syringe distribution program.[32,33] The study was premised upon the following observations. First, programs to increase access to sterile syringe equipment have been found to be effective and cost-effective means for reducing HIV transmission among persons who inject drugs. These programs include needle and syringe exchange programs as well as pharmacy-based syringe purchase programs. Although current federal law prohibits federal funding of the delivery of these services, they continue to garner funding and support from other levels of government and from private funders. Indeed, such services are currently on the increase in the United States.[34] Therefore, questions about the cost and cost-effectiveness of a national implementation of a syringe provision program are scientifically meaningful, even if the policy option of national implementation with federal funds is currently outlawed.

Holtgrave and colleagues considered a national program that would provide sterile syringe equipment to persons who inject drugs at increasing levels of coverage (where coverage was defined as the percentage of all syringes needed, given current levels of drug injection in the United States).[32,33] The analysis assumed that there are currently 1 million active injection drug users in the United States and that each injects 868 times per year with nonsterile syringes, despite the syringe access programs that are already in place. The authors estimated that each needed syringe costs 44 cents (assuming a weighted average of 25% of needed syringes coming from syringe exchange programs and the rest coming from pharmacy syringe sales), and that there are 19,000 new HIV infections among injection drug users each year in the United States, 65% of which are caused by injection as opposed to sexual behaviors. Finally, they assumed that $108,469 is saved in averted HIV-related medical care costs each time HIV infection of an injection drug user is averted (this represents a very conservative adjustment of HIV-related costs of illness for lack of access to treatment among injection drug users).

The authors mapped coverage levels to HIV infections averted using a mathematical model of program effectiveness. The model was based on the behavioral assumption that if presented with two syringes—one sterile, one not—an injection drug user would choose the sterile one, and on the optimistic programmatic assumption that the drug user's one-year allotment of sterile syringes could be provided as needed. (We return to this point below.)

The results of the analysis indicated that if all syringes needed by injection drug users were provided, an estimated 12,350 HIV infections would be prevented at a gross societal cost of $423,336,522. This may seem like an enormous cost. However, the average cost-effectiveness ratio would be $34,278 per HIV infection averted—a figure well below the medical costs saved per infection prevented. Thus, the net cost of this program is negative, indicating that it would actually be cost-saving to society to implement this program.

The marginal CEAs, which compared one level of program coverage to the next lower level at increments of 10%, indicated that the program would be cost-saving at each increment, until just before the program coverage reached 90%. At a coverage threshold of 88.4% the marginal cost-effectiveness ratio (cost per HIV infection averted) equaled the present value of the medical costs saved when an infection is averted; the program would no longer be cost-saving at coverage levels in excess of this threshold.

The authors conducted numerous sensitivity analyses and found the main conclusions of the analysis to be highly robust to changes in parameter assumptions. They concluded that a national implementation of a program to increase access to sterile injection equipment would be cost-saving to society, especially up to a coverage level of approximately 88% of all needed syringes.

HOW CAN WE RULE OUT ECONOMICALLY INEFFICIENT PROGRAMS PRIOR TO IMPLEMENTATION?

This question is similar to the previous one, which also required an a priori estimate of program effectiveness prior to its actual implementation. The same caveats apply—namely, that there is always considerable uncertainty in analyses that rely on nonempirical, model-based estimates. Nevertheless, if it can be demonstrated that a program is clearly inefficient or, as above, clearly cost-saving under certain circumstances, then these observations can be used to guide program implementation.

As an illustration of the use of these techniques, consider the cost of a potential national program to make post-exposure prophylaxis (PEP) available, on demand, to individuals who believe they may have been exposed to HIV through sexual intercourse or as a result of sharing a needle or syringe with another drug user. The use of antiretroviral drugs such as zidovudine to prevent the establishment of infection in health care workers who were occupationally exposed to HIV-contaminated blood and other bodily fluids is a well-established prophylactic practice.[35,36] Several studies indicate that PEP is a cost-effective, as well as effective, method for preventing infection after high-risk occupational exposures (e.g., following a deep percutaneous exposure to blood that is known to be contaminated with HIV).[11,36] The effectiveness of PEP in the occupational setting has led some members of the HIV prevention community to advocate the use of PEP for nonoccupational exposures, such as following unprotected intercourse or needle/syringe sharing. Despite extremely limited information regarding the effectiveness of nonoccupational PEP, a number of doctors are already prescribing PEP for their patients.[37]

Previous economic evaluations have established that the cost-effectiveness of post-exposure prophylaxis following sexual or drug-related exposures critically depends upon the level of risk associated with the suspected exposure.[38] The limited cost-effectiveness of PEP is due, in large part, to the relatively high cost of this treatment, which can total $1100 for post-exposure prophylaxis with two antiretrovirals, and $1600 for three-drug PEP. The high cost of PEP also limits the usefulness of this strategy on a national level, as the following modeling exercise makes clear. In fiscal year 1997 (which spans portions of calendar years 1996 and 1997), the CDC's HIV prevention budget was $616,790,000.[24] Currently, federal policy considers nonoccupational PEP to be "treatment," and these prevention dollars are not used for treatment as such. However, suppose that a comparable amount of money were made available to fund a national PEP program. Simple calculations show that $600 million would be sufficient to pay for approximately 550,000 PEP treatments at a cost of $1092 for dual-combination PEP. Even assuming that PEP is highly effective (e.g., 80% effective in preventing infection) and that transmission would be very likely (1%) in the absence of this treatment, these 550,000 PEP treatments would prevent only 440 new infections in a population with a 10% existing prevalence of HIV. Thus, even if a sum of money comparable to the CDC's *entire* HIV prevention budget were used to fund PEP programs, these programs would avert only about 1% of the approximately 40,000 new HIV infections that are estimated to occur in the United States each year.[39] Further, such an intense focusing of the prevention budget on one type of intervention might be accompanied by increased transmission that might have otherwise been prevented by other extant programs.

This analysis suggests that PEP may be too expensive to be made available on a very large scale, and that if it were, its impact on the HIV epidemic would be comparatively small. Rather than providing a single person with PEP, the same $1042 could be used to provide him or her with an array of HIV prevention services, such as (a) HIV antibody testing and counseling; (b) an intensive, multi-session intervention based on cognitive-behavioral risk reduction skills development; (c) booster sessions of the small-group intervention; and (d) a one-year supply of condoms and sterile syringes.[12] Compared to other strategies for HIV prevention, PEP does not appear to represent an especially good "buy." Therefore, while it is important to provide persons who suffer accidental exposures to HIV with viable options, including PEP, the best strategy remains to prevent people from experiencing such exposures in the first place. We acknowledge, of course, that factors other than cost-effectiveness may come into play when someone is exposed to HIV and PEP is considered—the "rule of rescue" may come into play despite the results of economic analyses.

DOES HIV PREVENTION FUNDING TRULY FOLLOW THE EPIDEMIC AND FLOW TO AREAS IN MOST NEED?

Although it is important to know what HIV prevention interventions cost and whether they are cost-effective compared to other life-saving interventions, there remains the question of whether overall HIV prevention funding accurately tracks the epidemic. While there are public health arguments for such matching (to ensure that programs are conducted where the need is greatest), this matter of matching of funding to the epidemic is perhaps more of an equity and social justice issue than a cost-effectiveness one.

One major purpose of HIV prevention community planning was to allow grassroots input to determine where HIV prevention services would provide the greatest benefit and serve the most serious unmet needs. Since the inception of community planning, CDC has requested that health department grantees provide detailed information on how its prevention funds are utilized, categorized by race/ethnicity, risk group (e.g., injection drug users, men who have sex with men), and other descriptive variables. In the first published analyses of these "budget tracking" data, it was found that from 1993 (the last fiscal year before the implementation of community planning) to fiscal year 1997, community planning increased the funding to nongovernmental grassroots organizations (funded by health departments) by 74%.[1,40] It further increased the funding for health education and risk reduction efforts from 23% of the total budget (in 1993) to 39% (in 1997).[1,40] Taken together, these statistics indicate that in its first years, community planning had the effect of moving monies to more grassroots organizations and to more intensive types of risk reduction activities.

In 1998, CDC unveiled an even more intensive type of budget tracking analysis. CDC took the budgetary information on health education and risk reduction services reported by its health department grantees and compared it (on the basis of race/ethnicity and risk category) to cumulative AIDS case statistics and the most recent year of AIDS incidence statistics. CDC made similar comparisons for counseling, testing, referral, and partner notification (CTRPN) services funds; however, for these services, CDC has available to it data on the race/ethnicity and risk categorization of clients receiving services. Hence, for counseling and testing funds, the budgetary information can be compared to AIDS

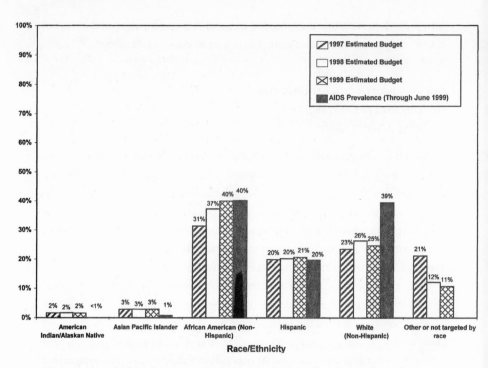

Figure 2.1. HIV health education and risk reduction budget allocations and prevalent AIDS cases by race/ethnicity. *Note:* AIDS not reported for other or not targeted by race.

statistics and to service delivery statistics. An example of this type of analysis (for health education and risk reduction activities) is portrayed in Figure 2.1.[1]

The figure shows that in fiscal year 1999 there was a very strong match between funding levels and AIDS prevalence for racial/ethnic minority communities. This figure shows that this was not always the case. The fiscal year 1997 funding in African American communities showed a substantial shortfall, which has now been remedied for this pool of funds.

There are clear limitations to this type of analysis. First, these analyses track only federal funding, as opposed to a more comprehensive approach of tracking federal, state, and private funding. Second, analyses such as these highlight the limitations of using (even recent) AIDS case statistics as an indicator of where the epidemic is going in a given locale. HIV statistics, or even risk behavior information, would better show where service activities are needed to *prevent* future HIV infections.

Third, these analyses are national-level calculations, which aggregate data over dozens of highly diverse jurisdictions. In 1997, CDC began to examine each state's detailed budgetary report separately. This approach appears promising because it yields specific, viable courses of action that CDC can take, should a grantee's uses of funds appear to be out of line with the local epidemic. Relying on a national analysis yields only national-level exhortation as a course of action to bring allocations more closely into alignment with the epidemic. Although the state-by-state approach to analysis appears promising, some policy makers still want the national analysis as a kind of "report card" of how community planning is performing overall. Therefore, ultimately, a combination of national-level analyses and state-by-state analyses will be needed to answer all information needs. Clearly, budget tracking and matching the information to unmet prevention needs is an area of urgent interest and one that is in need of further methodological development.

SHORT OF OBTAINING PERFECTION IN HIV PREVENTION PROGRAMS, HOW CAN MEANINGFUL PERFORMANCE STANDARDS BE SET?

Ideally, the goal of HIV prevention interventions and programs should be the total elimination of HIV transmission. All those involved in prevention programming aspire to the achievement of this worthy goal. However, simply hoping that transmission will completely stop, and making a real, viable plan for true disease elimination are two different things.[41] Indeed, disease elimination is a special area of public health study and programming. For a disease to be eliminated, the following are required, at a minimum: (a) an inexpensive vaccine, preventive agent, or cure that is extremely effective; (b) the ability to provide the vaccine, preventive agent, or cure to all infected or at-risk persons; (c) the individual will, ability, and empowerment of community members to engage in the preventative or curative activities; (d) the economic and other resources to implement the necessary public health programming; and (e) a political willingness to focus national attention on the disease and to commit sufficient resources to battle the disease until the goal of elimination is achieved.

Sadly, not all these conditions are currently met with regard to HIV elimination in the United States. While we must endeavor to rectify this situation so that all conditions are met, HIV transmission elimination seems to be a goal that is not achievable in the very near term. Therefore, it is meaningful to ask what performance standards, short of disease elimination, would constitute an important yet feasible level of achievement given current societal levels of investment in HIV prevention. Economic evaluation provides some guidance in this area.

In an initial attempt to address this question, Holtgrave and Pinkerton conducted a study to determine the number of HIV infections that would need to be prevented by CDC-funded HIV prevention programs in order to consider the CDC's national investment a cost-saving (or cost-effective) use of fiscal resources.[24] It is a major challenge to evaluate a national program, because one is essentially comparing the world as we know it, which includes the national efforts that are already in place, to a hypothetical world without the national program. The true level of effectiveness can never be known with certainty. Hence, methods for quantitative policy analysis (especially economic evaluation) under conditions of uncertainty are well-suited to this problem.

Threshold analysis is an especially appropriate technique for addressing this sort of question.[42] In threshold analysis, the known quantities (e.g., spending on HIV prevention programs) are combined with known target parameters (e.g., the cost of HIV-related medical care) to establish a threshold on the unknown quantity (e.g., the number of infections the national prevention program would need to avert in order to be cost-saving). This method has been used to set performance standards for an HIV surveillance program in England and Wales,[43] an HIV counseling and testing program in Wisconsin,[44] and a street outreach program for injection drug users in North Carolina.[9]

In the current application, we employed threshold analysis using a societal perspective and a 3% discount rate.[24] We focused on one fiscal year's HIV prevention budget for CDC, which was $616,790,000 in fiscal year 1997. The threshold analysis was performed as follows. First, we established a cost-saving threshold. In particular, we determined how many HIV infections would have to be prevented for the entire CDC HIV prevention program to be considered cost-saving. This was calculated by dividing the budget ($616,790,000) by the discounted, present-value medical care costs saved each time an HIV infection is prevented. This value for medical costs averted was previously conservatively estimated at $154,402 (also discounted at a 3% rate and expressed in dollars that match the fiscal budget year period).[17] Dividing these two values provides the result that in fiscal year 1997 3995 HIV infections would have had to be prevented by CDC-sponsored programs in order for the expenditure to be considered cost-saving. Compared to the estimated 40,000 new infections that occur each year in the United States, this threshold represents only about 9% of the annual HIV incidence.

As an alternative performance standard, we can ask how many HIV infections would have to be prevented for the entire CDC HIV prevention program to be considered cost-effective.[24] This can be determined in a manner similar to that used above for the cost-saving threshold. The fiscal year 1997 budget is simply divided by a valuation of each HIV infection prevented. In this case, however, that value is not simply the medical costs saved per prevented infection. Rather, it is medical costs saved plus the product of: (a) the number of quality-adjusted life years (QALYs) saved per prevented infection and (b) how much society would be willing to pay to save a single QALY. The discounted number of QALYs saved per HIV infection prevented was previously estimated to be 11.23. There is no one particular value at which the cost per QALY saved by a public health intervention is suddenly too large to be considered cost-effective. However, there does seem to be general agreement that an intervention that can save a QALY for $30,000 or less is definitely cost-effective in comparison with other life-saving interventions. Therefore, we selected $30,000 for this parameter. Performing the arithmetic needed to calculate the cost-effectiveness threshold yields the following result: if the CDC HIV prevention program can avert at least 1255 HIV infections per year (or about 3% of the annual incidence), it is clearly cost-effective, even by very conservative standards.

While these two performance standards seem readily achievable by the national prevention program, as we argued above, ultimately the actual number of HIV infections prevented by the national program is unknowable. However, we can look at some service delivery data in order to come close to answering the question "Does the program exceed the cost-saving threshold?" We examined data on the number of persons who receive publicly funded HIV counseling and testing services and adjusted for failure to return for test results and for previous knowledge of serostatus (i.e., previous testing history). This simple analysis indicated that the program exceeds the cost-saving threshold only if 22% of persons who learn that they are HIV-positive through the program go on to avoid transmitting the virus to at least one of their partners, even if the rest of the CDC program contributed nothing to the national prevention effort. (The corresponding value is 7% to reach the cost-effective threshold.) Given the literature on the effectiveness of HIV counseling and testing for persons testing HIV seropositive, we believe that this standard is attainable.

As this example illustrates, threshold analysis can be very useful for performance standard setting. The results of this analysis also appear to indicate that the thresholds for CDC's program are very attainable and likely are being attained. However, this is an analysis under conditions of uncertainty and should be taken as such. Further, it is important to remember that ultimately disease elimination will be the performance standard of choice once some key conditions are met that will enable zero new infections to be a meaningful and viable performance goal.

IS THE NATIONAL HIV PREVENTION EFFORT
TRULY MAKING A DIFFERENCE
IN STEMMING THE EPIDEMIC?

Even with all the effectiveness and cost-effectiveness information presented above, a number of policy makers still wish to directly, quantitatively address the question of how investment in HIV prevention programs has influenced the HIV epidemic curve over the course of the epidemic to date at a national level. This is a methodologically problematic question to address. As discussed in the previous section, determining the exact (or even the approximate) number of HIV infections prevented by the national program is a very difficult task. Also, there is a sense among some that only if the HIV incidence curve has gone down have the prevention programs made any difference, when, in fact, an incidence curve that is flat might reflect highly effective programs that have prevented a massive growth in the epidemic from occurring. In some ways, an incidence curve taken in isolation is best interpreted as the work remaining to be accomplished in addressing an epidemic. Further, calculating the timing and extent of investment in HIV prevention programs at a national level poses challenges if one wishes to include federal, state, local, and private resources. To answer directly the policy question (stated above) would require knowing and comparing the HIV incidence curves that would have occurred without—and did occur with—existing HIV prevention efforts in place (information that we will never have directly).

To answer this policy question in a less definitive way would require plotting the estimated HIV incidence curve and overlaying the best estimate of HIV prevention resources expended. The best available approximation of such an analysis is illustrated in Figure 2.2. It shows (without error bars) the HIV incidence curve estimated by back-calculation from AIDS statistics and published by Brookmeyer.[45] (Back-calculation is a mathematical technique for inferring the past distribution of HIV cases based on the currently observed distribution of AIDS cases, taking into account the variable period between HIV infection and diagnosis.) It is important to note that Brookmeyer's back-calculation estimates ended in April 1990; the curve is shown as flat thereafter because the federal government has never updated the estimate of very roughly 40,000 new HIV in-

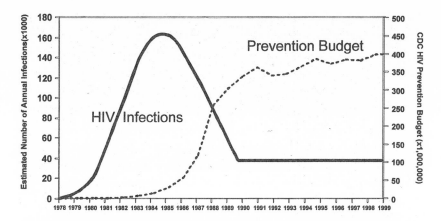

Figure 2.2. Extrapolation of Brookmeyer's 1978–1990 HIV incidence back-calculation curve and CDC's HIV prevention budget (adjusted for inflation and expressed as 1983 dollars) by year. *Source:* R. Brookmeyer, Reconstruction and future trends of the AIDS epidemic in the United States, *Science* 1991; 253:37–42. Copyright 1991 American Association for the Advancement of Science.

fections every year. Clearly, though, there is much uncertainty in the HIV incidence curve presented in Figure 2.2. In addition to HIV incidence estimates, the figure shows the CDC budget for HIV prevention programs adjusted for inflation. Of course, this ignores state, local, and private investments in HIV prevention.

The curves suggest (but certainly do not prove) an interesting correlation: as the investment in HIV prevention increased markedly, from about 1984 to 1990, the HIV infection rate appeared to decrease. When the investments flattened out, so too did the epidemic curve (again, note the uncertainty in the incidence estimates). Although the decrease in HIV incidence might have been due to a saturation effect or to some unknown cause, Figure 2.2 seems to imply some relationship between HIV infection and the national level of effort in prevention. Of course, an alternative explanation might be that private resources (especially in the form of voluntary, community-based HIV prevention efforts) preceded the federal investment, and that the federal resources followed the epidemic.

To provide further support for this argument, one would have to replicate this analysis for several jurisdictions (perhaps states and large cities) to see if the pattern held in multiple areas in which the epidemic peaked and flattened out at different times. A more comprehensive analysis would include state, local, and private funds in the analysis as well as CDC funds. And much more work in the estimation of HIV incidence remains to be done. Still, the relationship between the two curves is not easily ignored or dismissed. Further, the relationship hints that recent declines in AIDS incidence may be due to a combination of effective prevention efforts and improved clinical benefits of antiretroviral therapy—not just treatment effects, as some have speculated.

Finally, even if one believes that the content of Figure 2.2 does not provide a compelling causal argument, it must be recognized that this is currently the only available analysis attempting to directly address this particular policy question, and that much methodological work must be done to address this urgent policy question. Hence, the analysis shown in Figure 2.2 was presented both for its content and for the methodological challenges it raises.

FUTURE DIRECTIONS AND CONCLUSIONS

In addition to the methodological challenges raised just above, several important future directions in this field would benefit from immediate attention. First, broader use must be made of the economic evaluation techniques described above—especially as they relate to priority setting at the community planning group level. Although several economic resource allocation models exist, only a small number of planning groups have embraced them. This situation is partly a result of a reluctance to accept such quantitative models, but it is also a reflection of the need for the development of more user-friendly software packages that implement these methods and that can be widely disseminated and easily understood and used. The technology described here will never be adopted broadly without such steps to improve dissemination.

Second, it is critical that HIV prevention policy making in the United States be reconceptualized as a matter of decision making under conditions of uncertainty. Too often policy makers tend to look for absolute answers or measures of effectiveness. Given the national scope of the HIV prevention efforts, the local variants of implementation, and the extremely rapidly changing science of HIV/ AIDS, it is impossible to predict the best course of action for, say, the next decade. However, reasonable, scientifically sound steps can be taken to chart a course for prevention efforts, one step at a time, and thereby to manage this high level of uncertainty. Understanding HIV prevention policy making as decision making under uncertainty is a first step toward managing and accommodating the dynamic changes in the epidemic.

In addition, it is often noted that these economic evaluation techniques need further development to explicitly incorporate issues of equity of costs and consequences. Given the current national attention to racial and ethnic health disparities, it is critical and urgent that equity becomes a more central construct of economic evaluation of public health programs. This is true especially in the realm of HIV prevention policy. More generally, techniques must be developed to assist policy makers in weighing economic evaluation information with a myriad of other types of information that they may need to take into account in a given situation.

Despite these challenges and the need for further work in several critical areas, we conclude that HIV prevention policy questions can be informed by economic evaluation methods. Several illustrations of this point were provided in this chapter. As these policy questions regard matters of life and death, and given that these economic evaluation techniques can truly inform policy making, we believe that the analytic tools described in this chapter can be meaningfully used to improve public health.

ACKNOWLEDGMENT

The contributions of Seth Edlavitch and Craig Thomas to the analysis of HIV prevention community planning budget data are gratefully acknowledged.

REFERENCES

1. CDC. HIV prevention community planning: Shared decision making in action. Atlanta: CDC, 1998, 1–21.
2. Valdiserri RO, Aultman TV, Curran JW. Community planning: A national strategy to improve HIV prevention programs. *J Comm Health* 1995; 20:87–100.
3. Holtgrave DR. Preface. In DR Holtgrave (Ed.), *Handbook of Economic Evaluation of HIV Prevention Programs.* New York: Plenum Press, 1998, ix–xii.
4. Holtgrave DR. The cost-effectiveness of the components of a comprehensive HIV prevention program: A road map of the literature. In DR Holtgrave (Ed.), *Handbook of Economic Evaluation of HIV Prevention Programs.* New York: Plenum Press, 1998, 128–134.
5. Gorsky RD. A method to measure the costs of counseling for HIV prevention. *Public Health Rep* 1996; 111(Suppl. 1):115–122.
6. Owens DK. Economic evaluation of HIV screening interventions. In DR Holtgrave (Ed.), *Handbook of Economic Evaluation of HIV Prevention Programs.* New York: Plenum Press, 1998, 81–101.
7. Farnham PG. Economic evaluation of HIV counseling and testing programs: The influence of program goals on evaluation. In DR Holtgrave (Ed.), *Handbook of Economic Evaluation of HIV Prevention Programs.* New York: Plenum Press, 1998, 63–80.
8. Kahn JG. Economic evaluation of primary HIV prevention in injection drug users. In

DR Holtgrave (Ed.), *Handbook of Economic Evaluation of HIV Prevention Programs*. New York: Plenum Press, 1998, 45–62.

9. Norton EC, Martin RF, Wechsberg WM. Threshold analysis of AIDS outreach and intervention. In DR Holtgrave (Ed.), *Handbook of Economic Evaluation of HIV Prevention Programs*. New York: Plenum Press, 1998, 195–209.

10. Holtgrave DR, Pinkerton SD. The cost-effectiveness of small group and community-level interventions. In DR Holtgrave (Ed.), *Handbook of Economic Evaluation of HIV Prevention Programs*. New York: Plenum Press, 1998, 120–126.

11. Pinkerton SD, Holtgrave DR, Pinkerton HJ. Cost-effectiveness of chemoprophylaxis after occupational exposure to HIV. *Arch Int Med* 1997; 157:1972–1980.

12. Pinkerton SD, Holtgrave DR. Prophylaxis after sexual exposure to HIV. *Ann Int Med* 1998; 129–671.

13. Gorsky RD, Farnham PG, Straus WL, Caldwell B, Holtgrave DR, Simonds RJ, Rogers MF, Guinan ME. Preventing perinatal transmission of HIV—Costs and effectiveness of a recommended intervention. *Public Health Rep* 1996; 111:335–341.

14. Gilson L, Mkanje R, Grosskurth H, et al. Cost-effectiveness of improved STD treatment services as a preventive intervention against HIV in Mwanza region, Tanzania. Paper presented at the 11th International Conference on AIDS, Vancouver BC (abstract MoC444), July 1996.

15. Holtgrave DR, Qualls NL, Graham JD. Economic evaluation of HIV prevention programs. *Annu Rev Public Health* 1996; 17:467–488.

16. Drummond M, Stoddard G, Torrance G. *Methods for the Economic Evaluation of Health Care Programmes*. New York: Oxford University Press, 1987.

17. Holtgrave DR, Pinkerton SD. Updates of cost of illness and quality of life estimates for use in economic evaluations of HIV prevention programs. *J Acquir Immune Defic Syndr Hum Retrovirol* 1997; 16:54–62.

18. Bloom DE, Carliner G. The economic impact of AIDS in the United States. *Science* 1988; 239:604–610.

19. Hardy AM. Rauch K, Echenberg D, Morgan WM, Curran JW. The economic impact of the first 10,000 cases of acquired immunodeficiency syndrome in the United States. *JAMA* 1986; 255:209–211.

20. Scitovsky AA, Rice DP. The cost of AIDS. *Issues Sci Technol* 1987; 4:61–66.

21. Rabkin JG, Ferrando S. A "second life" agenda: Psychiatric research issues raised by protease inhibitor treatments for people with the human immunodeficiency virus or the acquired immune deficiency syndrome. *Arch Gen Psychiatry* 1997; 54:1049–1053.

22. Gold MR, Siegel JE, Russell LB, Weinstein MC (Eds.). *Cost-Effectiveness in Health and Medicine*. New York: Oxford University Press, 1996.

23. Tao G, Remafedi G. Economic evaluation of an HIV prevention intervention for gay and bisexual male adolescents. *J Acquir Immune Defic Syndr Hum Retrovirol* 1998; 17:83–90.

24. Holtgrave DR, Pinkerton S. Setting performance standards for a national HIV prevention program. International Conference on AIDS 1998; 12:944 (abstract no. 356/43500).

25. Bibus DP, Wood RW, Hartfield K, Hanrahan M, Wood C. A model for distributing HIV-prevention resources. *AIDS & Pub Pol J* 1994; 9:197–207.
26. Holtgrave DR. Setting priorities and community planning for HIV-prevention programs. *AIDS & Pub Pol J* 1994; 9:145–150.
27. Johnson-Masotti AP, Pinkerton SD, Holtgrave DR. Prioritization methods for HIV prevention community planning. *J Public Health Manage Prac,* in press.
28. Holtgrave DR, Pinkerton SD. Assessing the economic costs and benefits of behavioral interventions. In N Schneiderman, J Gentry, JM daSilva, M Speers, H Tomes (Eds.), *Integrating Behavioral and Social Sciences with Public Health.* Washington, DC: American Psychological Association, 2000; 249–265.
29. Pinkerton SD, Holtgrave DR, Willingham M, Goldstein E. Cost-effectiveness analysis and HIV prevention community planning. *AIDS & Pub Pol J* 1998; 13:115–127.
30. Johnson-Masotti AP, Pinkerton SD, Holtgrave DR, Valdiserri RO, Willingham M. Decision making in HIV prevention community planning: An integrative review. *J Community Health* 2000; 25:95–112.
31. Kaplan EH. Economic evaluation and HIV prevention community planning: A policy analyst's perspective. In DR Holtgrave (Ed.), *Handbook of Economic Evaluation of HIV Prevention Programs.* New York: Plenum Press, 1998, 177–193.
32. Holtgrave DR, Pinkerton SD, Jones TS, Lurie P, Vlahov D. Cost and cost-effectiveness of increasing access to sterile syringes and needles as an HIV prevention intervention in the United States. *J Acquir Immune Defic Syndr Hum Retrovirol* 1998; 18(Suppl. 1): S133–S138.
33. Holtgrave DR. Policy interventions. Paper presented at AIDS Behavioral Prevention Research and Service: A Symposium and Charette, San Francisco, CA, Aug. 13, 1998.
34. Paone D, Des Jarlais DC, Shi Q. Syringe exchange use and HIV risk reduction over time (letter). *AIDS* 1998; 12:121–123.
35. Gerberding JL. Management of occupational exposures to blood-borne viruses. *N Engl J Med* 1995; 322:444–451.
36. CDC. Update: Provisional Public Health Service recommendations for chemoprophylaxis after occupational exposure to HIV. *MMWR Morb Mortal Wkly Rep.* 1996; 45:468–472.
37. Katz MH, Gerberding JL. The care of persons with recent sexual exposure to HIV. *Ann Intern Med* 1998; 128:306–312.
38. Pinkerton SD, Holtgrave DR, Bloom FR. Cost-effectiveness of post-exposure prophylaxis following sexual exposure to HIV. *AIDS* 1998; 12:1067–1078.
39. Holmberg SD. The estimated prevalence and incidence of HIV in 96 large US metropolitan areas. *Am J Public Health* 1996; 86;642–654.
40. Valdiserri, RO, Robinson C, Lin L, West G, Holtgrave DR. Determining allocation for HIV prevention interventions: Assessing a change in federal funding policy. *AIDS & Pub Pol J* 1997; 12:138–148.
41. Cochi SL, Sutter RW, Strebel PM, Heningburg A-R, Keegan RA. Advantages and disadvantages of concurrent eradication programs. In WR Dowdle, DR Hopkins (Eds.), *The Eradication of Infectious Diseases.* New York: Wiley, 1998, 137–144.

42. Holtgrave DR, Qualls NL. Threshold analysis and programs for prevention of HIV infection. *Med Decis Making* 1995; 15:311–317.
43. Morris S, Gray A, Noone A, Wiseman M, Jathanna S. The costs and effectiveness of surveillance of communicable disease: A case study of HIV and AIDS in England and Wales. *J Public Health Med* 1996; 18:415–422.
44. Holtgrave DR, DiFranceisco W, Reiser W, et al. Setting standards for the Wisconsin HIV counseling and testing program: An application of threshold analysis. *J Public Health Manage Prac,* 1997; 3:42–49.
45. Brookmeyer R. Reconstruction and future trends of the AIDS epidemic in the United States. *Science* 1991; 253;37–42.

Chapter 3 Statistical Issues in HIV Prevention

Ron Brookmeyer

In the past two decades we have accumulated considerable knowledge about the pathogenesis of the human immunodeficiency virus (HIV) and treatment of the HIV-infected individual. Nevertheless, there remains considerable uncertainty about the type and characteristics of effective public health control programs to prevent new HIV infections from occurring. Indeed, new HIV infections continue to occur at an alarming rate, particularly in developing countries. Furthermore, no phase III vaccine trial has yet been completed. This chapter is concerned with some of the statistical issues that arise in the quantitative evaluation of HIV prevention programs. The objective is to review statistical issues in the design and analysis of studies of HIV prevention.

HIV prevention can refer to a broad range of interventions including vaccines, needle exchange programs, counseling and testing programs, blood screening programs, sexually transmitted disease (STD) control programs, therapies to reduce maternal-infant transmission, and various behavioral interventions. Much of what we have learned about HIV prevention has come from observational studies, in sharp contrast to AIDS/HIV therapeutics where most advances in knowledge have come from randomized controlled trials. Although observational studies have been the cornerstone of HIV prevention evaluation, there have been some important examples of the use of randomized controlled trials, including studies to evaluate the impact of STD control programs and prophylactic regimens to reduce maternal-infant transmission rates.

The goal of this chapter is to review some of the statistical issues in the design and analysis of HIV prevention studies. The strengths and limitations of different study designs and sources of data for drawing reliable inferences about HIV prevention efficacy are discussed, and examples are drawn from other areas of public health. In the next section we discuss various study designs including the randomized trial, natural experiments and observational studies. Following this, we discuss the use of HIV/AIDS surveillance data for drawing inferences about HIV prevention. The final section highlights some statistical and analytical issues in the evaluation of HIV prevention programs.

STUDY DESIGNS

Randomized Trials of HIV Prevention

There have been several important examples of the use of randomized trials in HIV prevention. For example, AIDS Clinical Trial Group (ACTG) Protocol 076 evaluated the efficacy of AZT to reduce maternal-infant transmission.[1] This study consisted of mothers who were individually randomized to receive either a placebo or AZT beginning at about 36 weeks gestation. This important study showed that the perinatal transmission rate could be reduced by almost two-thirds, from approximately 25% to 8%.

In another study in Tanzania, communities were randomized to receive a special program of STD case management or a control program.[2] The hypothesis of this study was that sexually transmitted diseases could be a cofactor for transmission and acquisition of HIV infection, and thus reduction of the prevalence of STDs could reduce HIV incidence rates. In a related study in Uganda, communities were randomized to receive a mass-treatment intervention to reduce STD prevalence.[3] The unit of randomization was the community in the studies in both Tanzania and Uganda. In contrast, the unit of randomization was the individual (pregnant woman) in the AIDS Clinical Trial Group Protocol 076 on perinatal transmission.

There are several reasons why randomized trials are preferable to observational studies for evaluating HIV prevention programs (see Chapter 4).[4,5] First, and perhaps most important, randomization avoids "self-selection." Self-selection refers to bias that arises when individuals selectively choose one treatment over another. Those individuals who choose a particular treatment may be at a different risk of HIV infection than the individuals who choose another treatment. Second, randomization avoids "investigator selection," whereby investigators systematically assign certain types of individuals to one treatment or another. Third, randomization helps achieve balance between the treatment groups with respect to risk factors for HIV infection that are either difficult to measure or unknown. For example, suppose certain genetic or nutritional factors protect one from acquiring HIV infection but exactly which factors they are is unknown or these factors are very different to measure. Randomization of a large trial ensures that it is highly probable that these genetic or nutritional factors would be approximately balanced among the treatment groups.

How important is it to have a randomized comparison group in studies of disease prevention? The debate goes back to Karl Pearson and the issue of prevention of typhoid.[6] In a discussion of the need for a control group for typhoid prevention in the 1930s, Pearson said, "Controls cannot be considered as true controls until it is demonstrated that the men who are most anxious and particular about their health, the men who are most likely to be cautious and run no risk, are not the very men who will volunteer to be inoculated; thus a spurious correlation may be produced between disease and absence of inoculation."[7]

However, Major Greenwood took a different position and argued that Pearson's objection "would be fatal . . . if there were evidence that volunteers for immunization were more careful than the uninoculated in their personal hygiene, for example, if typhoid were water borne and careful individuals boiled their drinking water, but if typhoid were conveyed by food fouled by flies or carriers, no individual action could have affected the issue. Karl Pearson's objection seems to me less formidable than it would appear."[7]

Of course, AIDS is not typhoid. One could easily argue that in a study of voluntary vaccinees, those who choose to be vaccinated might have behaviors that place them at higher (or perhaps lower) risk of HIV infection than those who choose not to be vaccinated. In such situations, one often tries to rely on statistical adjustments in the analysis to account for imbalances between the treatment groups. Ideally, one would like the probabilities of exposure to HIV to be equal in the treatment groups. Unfortunately, these probabilities are typically unknown, and randomization helps assure that the average probability of exposure to HIV for an individual is approximately equal among treatment groups.

In the absence of randomization, we must rely on surrogate variables such as reported frequency of high-risk behaviors (e.g., certain sexual practices or needle
sharing among intravenous drug users) to determine if the individuals in the
two treatment groups have equal likelihood of exposure to HIV. However, these
variables are only surrogates for exposure to HIV and are often self-reported and
are thus measured with error. Furthermore, even if the numbers of self-
reported behaviors were perfectly accurate, they still may not be a good predic-
tor of the probability of HIV exposure. For example, if an individual has a high
number of sexual contacts but all those contacts are with an uninfected partner,
then the individual would not have been exposed to HIV. Randomization
avoids these problems because in a large trial it helps to ensure that the probability of exposure to HIV is approximately equal among the treatment groups.
Randomized trials offer the best protection against bias.

The dangers of self-selection can be seen from a study of coronary artery disease.[8] In this study, 1103 patients were randomized to one treatment group,
the clofibrate group, and 2789 patients were randomized to the placebo group.
The 5-year mortality rates in the clofibrate and placebo groups were 20% and
21%, respectively, and were not statistically different ($p > 0.10$). The comparison of the two groups (treatment [clofibrate] versus placebo) based on the initial randomization is commonly called the "intent to treat analysis." The intent
to treat analysis did not reveal any treatment effects. However, when the two
groups were decomposed into the compliers (those who took at least 80% of
the assigned medication) and the noncompliers (those who did not take at least
80% of the assigned medication) a startling result was obtained (Table 3.1).
The 5-year mortality rates among the compliers and noncompliers among
those initially randomized to clofibrate were 15% and 25%, respectively ($p <
0.01$). A naive interpretation of these results is that there is a significant effect
of clofibrate on reducing mortality because those patients who took clofibrate
(the compliers) had a lower mortality rate than those patients who did not take
the drug (the noncompliers). However, when the placebo group was also decomposed, the 5-year mortality rates among the compliers and noncompliers
were 15% and 28%, respectively ($p < 0.01$). Thus, the apparent difference between compliers and noncompliers observed among those randomized to clofibrate was also observed among those randomized to placebo, and this strongly
suggested that individuals who self-select and comply were different than noncompliers with respect to mortality risks. Attempts were made to explain away
the complier effect by trying to identify a covariate that was associated with
both compliance and mortality. However, no such variable could be identified.

Table 3.1. Illustration of the Effects of Self-Selection (or the "Complier Effect") from the Coronary Research Group

Treatment	5-Year Mortality (%)
Clofibrate (All)	20%
Compliers	15%
Noncompliers	25%
Placebo (All)	21%
Compliers	15%
Noncompliers	28%

Source: P. Rosenbaum, Observational Studies (New York: Springer-Verlag, 1995).

This study highlights the dangers of drawing causal inferences about the efficacy of a treatment in studies where patients self-select into treatment groups.[9] Fortunately this study was randomized and comparison of the mortality rates between the two treatment groups using the intent to treat analysis left little doubt that there was no clinically significant treatment effect.

However, randomized studies are not perfect. For example, differential drop-out rates could bias results even if the trial is randomized. To illustrate this, suppose a randomized prevention trial is performed to evaluate the efficacy of a certain counseling program versus a control program to reduce high-risk behaviors. If the counseling program requires more effort to attend on the part of the participant, it is plausible that individuals who are more motivated may be more likely to return for follow-up appointments while the individuals who are less motivated may be more likely to drop out. If the more motivated participants are also the participants at lower (or perhaps higher risk) of HIV infection, then it could appear that the counseling program is more effective than the control program because "person-years" of observation are coming primarily from the motivated participants. The two randomized groups will grow increasingly imbalanced (with respect to risk of HIV) over time. Randomization helps protect against bias by making it likely that the groups are balanced *at baseline* with respect to key risk factors, but randomization does not necessarily ensure that the treatment groups will remain balanced *after* baseline.

Another complication arises in community randomized prevention trials. In such studies, communities are randomized to one of several treatments; however, there may be contamination or spillover effects between the randomized units. For example, one community may be randomized to intervention A and a geographically adjacent community may be randomized to intervention B. Residents in the two communities may travel between the two communities and commingle. The observations from these two communities are no longer statistically independent. One would expect that the effect of this statistical dependence between the communities would be to attenuate the estimated efficacy of the intervention. Further, even two geographically adjacent communities randomized to the same intervention could cause complications because if the inhabitants commingle there would be a lack of statistical independence between the randomized units (i.e., the communities). For example, in the Tanzania study of the Mwanza region, 5 pairs of communities were randomized.[2] Each community within a pair was geographically close. One approach that has been suggested to deal with spillover or contamination between randomized units was to randomize a large cluster of communities that are close geographically rather than randomizing individual communities. The assumption of this approach is that individuals within such a large cluster will mingle or associate only with other individuals within the same cluster of communities. This was the approach taken in the community trial of intensive sexually transmitted disease treatment control using mass treatment in the Rakai district of Uganda.[3] However, there is also an important disadvantage with randomizing clusters of communities rather than individual communities. The trade-off is that if several communities are grouped into a single cluster and if the cluster is being randomized rather than the community, then fewer units are actually randomized. Generally the statistical power of the study to detect treatment effects decreases as the number of independent randomized units (the sample size) decreases. Indeed, in the extreme case when only two clusters of communities are randomized, a single chance occurrence in one cluster, such as a syphilis epidemic or a flood or the construction of a new road, would be completely confounded with the treatment effects.

Natural Experiments

Unfortunately, we do not always have the luxury of randomized experiments. Sometimes, though, we are fortunate to have a "natural" experiment. In a natural experiment, treatment assignment is not based on formal randomization algorithms, but rather fortuitous reasons that are unrelated to the outcome and thus make selection biases implausible.[6]

A leading example of the use of natural experiments in public health is the investigation into the causes of cholera in the mid-nineteenth century. A water

Table 3.2 Cholera Mortality Rates per 1000 Person-Years in London in the 1800s

| | Water Company | |
	Lambeth	Southwark & Vauxhall
Before water law of 1852	12.5	11.8
After water law of 1852	3.7	13.0

Mortality rates before and after the water law of 1852 refer to the cholera epidemics in London in 1848–1849 and 1853–1854, respectively. *Source:* J. M. Eyler, *Victorian Social Medicine: The Ideas and Methods of William Farr.* Baltimore: Johns Hopkins University Press, 1979.

law was passed in London in 1852 that required that only unpolluted parts of the Thames River be used as a source for drinking water.[10] Unfortunately, only one water company, the Lambeth Waterworks Company, complied with the law. Lambeth had formerly supplied some of the most polluted water, but now it was supplying some of the best. No differences could be discerned other than water quality between the customers of the different water companies. Indeed, the Lambeth company competed directly, street by street, house by house with other water companies.[10] This created a natural experiment. Table 3.2 compares the mortality rates by water company before and after Lambeth changed its source of water. Before the change, mortality rates among Lambeth customers were similar to rates of other customers. But after the change, Lambeth rates were less than one-fourth the rates of other customers. This was powerful evidence that cholera was transmitted through contaminated water. Obviously, one could never have done a formal randomized trial in which persons were randomized to receive either polluted or unpolluted water.

An example of a natural experiment in HIV concerns some of the original studies of HIV etiology among hemophiliacs. The problem facing early researchers who were studying the cause of AIDS was that there was no completely satisfactory animal model for HIV to perform the necessary experiments to prove causation. For years, there was a persistent small minority of scientists who questioned whether HIV was the cause of AIDS, and they suggested instead that it was a simple case of confounding with lifestyle factors such as drug use. Subsequently an analysis was published on the complete cohort of more than 6000 hemophiliacs in the United Kingdom that was essentially a natural experiment.[11] Now there is essentially no drug use among hemophiliacs, so that the issue that HIV is confounded with drug use does not arise. Table 3.3 shows

Table 3.3. Mortality Rates per 1000 Person-Years Among HIV-Infected and
Uninfected Hemophiliacs in the United Kingdom

	Severe Hemophilia		Moderate/Mild Hemophilia	
	Uninfected	Infected	Uninfected	Infected
1985–1992	8.1	49.1	3.5	45.2
	(5.4–10.9)	(43.7–54.4)	(2.3–4.6)	(33.7–56.7)
1977–1984	7.9		3.7	
	(6.4–9.4)		(3.0–4.5)	

The 95% confidence intervals are given in parentheses. *Source:* S. C. Darby, D. W. Ewart, P. L. F. Giangrande, et al., Mortality before and after HIV infection in the complete United Kingdom population of haemophiliacs, *Nature* 1995; 377:79–82.

the mortality rates for uninfected and HIV-infected hemophiliacs after 1985, when testing for HIV became available, stratified by the severity of the hemophilia. The post-1985 mortality rates among the infected were over 10 times that of uninfected hemophiliacs. This can be considered a natural experiment because a random subset of hemophiliacs became infected from the bad luck of getting contaminated blood products. It would not have been ethical in any sense to perform a formal randomized trial. The occurrence of this natural experiment provided additional sufficient proof for many researchers that HIV infection leads to AIDS.[11]

The criteria for a "natural" experiment is that the probability of being in one treatment or another does not depend on any variables that are related to the risk of the outcome such as mortality or HIV infection. In the cholera and hemophiliac examples discussed above it is very plausible that this criterion is satisfied, yet there are examples in HIV prevention where it is less clear that the condition for a natural experiment has been satisfied. For example, in a study of AIDS education, suppose some morning college courses were assigned to receive one type of intervention and some afternoon college courses received a second type of intervention.[4] If students who enroll in morning classes are systematically different than students who enroll in afternoon courses with respect to risk of HIV, then the criterion for a natural experiment would not be satisfied. Another example concerns the evaluation of the Baltimore Needle Exchange Program.[12] The Baltimore Needle Exchange Program was intended to provide clean needles to residents of Baltimore City. One could compare HIV incidence rates in Baltimore City with incidence rates in the surrounding area (Baltimore County). Is this a "natural" experiment? One would need to assume that city residents are comparable to county residents with respect to risk of HIV which is a tenuous assumption at best because HIV incidence rates were higher in Baltimore City even before initiation of the Needle Exchange Program in 1994. Alternatively, one could compare the *change* in the HIV incidence rates before and after initiation of the Needle Exchange Program (1994) in Baltimore City and the corresponding change in Baltimore County. However, even this comparison of changes in rates is suspect for the following reason. The change in HIV incidence in a community depends on the current prevalence of HIV infection, or in other words, the stage of the epidemic as predicted by simple mathematical models of the growth of epidemics.[13] For example, one community could be in the early exponential growth phase, while another could be reaching saturation. If the epidemic in Baltimore County was in a different stage of maturation than the epidemic in Baltimore City then one would have observed different *changes* in incidence even in the absence of any intervention.

Observational Studies

In the absence of a controlled randomized trial or natural experiment, one must rely on observational studies to evaluate HIV prevention programs. The two main study designs for an observational study are the cohort study and the case-control study. The key issue that must be addressed in an observational cohort or case-control study is whether or not those individuals who choose to participate in a prevention program (the treated) are systematically different than those individuals who choose not to participate in the program (the controls) with respect to risk of HIV. If there are differences, then statistical adjustment using stratification or regression analyses could be performed on variables that are *known* to be related to those risks of HIV, provided those variables have been measured on all individuals. There is no satisfactory adjustment for variables that are unknown to the investigator.

One example of the use of the case-control study in HIV concerned the hypotheses that "poppers" (or amyl nitrites), a recreational drug, was related to the development of AIDS. A case-control study performed in the early 1980s matched AIDS cases to controls and found a positive association between amyl nitrites and AIDS. The unadjusted odds ratio of AIDS associated with amyl nitrite use was 8.6, which suggested a strong effect of amyl nitrites. A multiple logistic regression analysis that controlled for number of sexual partners, a potential confounding variable, still suggested that the amyl nitrite association was very strong, with an adjusted odds ratio of 12.3. These results were obtained in 1982, before HIV was discovered. However, the authors of that case-control study cautiously warned that "amyl nitrite use may have been a surrogate for another causal variable . . . such as exposure to a sexually transmitted oncogenic virus."[14] Indeed, subsequent larger studies showed that after adjustment for more detailed information about sexual behavior, amyl nitrites were no longer associated with significant increased risks, suggesting that the original association between AIDS and amyl nitrites was an artifact that resulted from multicollinearity between certain sexual practices and recreational drug use. Multicollinearity makes interpretations difficult, and establishment of a biological mechanism to corroborate such associations is important. However, such mechanisms sometimes seem to be suggested all too quickly, after the association is observed, and one must wonder how biologically plausible the proposed mechanism really is.[15] For example, in 1982 the *New England Journal of Medicine* published a paper suggesting a biochemical mechanism for amyl nitrites to cause AIDS.[16] However, after HIV was isolated in 1983, this amyl nitrite hypothesis all but disappeared.

A second example of the use of observational studies in evaluation of an HIV prevention program concerns needle exchange programs. A simple although naive evaluation of a needle exchange program would involve the comparison of HIV incidence rates of those who *voluntarily* participated and attended needle exchange programs compared to suitable controls. The key issue is the identification of a suitable control group. Ideally, the controls would consist of individuals of comparable risk of HIV infection as those who joined the needle exchange program. Unfortunately, individuals who voluntarily join a needle exchange program are not a randomly selected subset of the population but rather are self-selected, and their risk of HIV may well be different than non-participants. How should one choose comparable controls? Obviously, the control group should be limited to individuals who are currently using intravenous drugs. Even so, those who participate in needle exchange programs may well use or share needles more frequently (or perhaps less frequently) than those who do not choose to participate.

Studies in New York and Montreal have attempted to compare HIV incidence rates among intravenous drug users who did and did not join the needle exchange programs in the cities.[17,18] Because participants of the program may be systematically different than non-participants, it becomes critical to adjust for potential confounding variables such as frequency of injection drug use or age. Table 3.4 shows the adjusted hazard ratio (relative risks) for acquiring HIV infection associated with being a needle exchange program participant versus a non-participant in Montreal and New York, and the results from the two cities

Table 3.4. Adjusted Hazard Ratios for Incident HIV Infection Associated with Participation in a Needle Exchange Program in Montreal and New York City

	Hazard Ratio	95% Confidence Interval
Montreal[a]		
Non-participants	1.0	—
Users < 50% time	0.9	0.3–2.7
Users ≥ 50% time	2.6	0.1–6.7
Consistent users	10.2	0.1–31.5
New York City[b]		
Non-users	1.0	—
Continued users	0.3	0.1 –0.7

Source: [a]J. Brunean, F. Lamothe, E. Franco, N. Lachance, M. Desy, J. Soto, and J. Vincelette, High rates of HIV infection among injection drug users participating in needle exchange programs in Montreal: Results of a cohort study, *Am J Epidemiol* 1997; 146:994–1002. Adjusted for IV drug use since last visit, number of time IV drugs used in previous month, borrowed IV equipment since last visit, number of times new IV equipment used in previous month, and practice of disinfection; matched on gender, age, language (French vs. other), and year of enrollment. Consistent users defined as those who reported participation at all follow-up visits. Results based on conditional logistic regression.
[b]D. C. Des Jarlais, M. Marmor, D. Paone, S. Titus, S. Qiuhu, T. Perlis, J. Benny, and S. Friedman, HIV incidence among injecting drug users in the New York City Syringe-Exchange Programs, *Lancet* 1996; 348:987–991. Adjusted for age, gender, race, and frequency of infection. Continued users defined as those who reported use of exchanges at all interviews. Results based on Cox proportional hazards regression.

are strikingly different. The Montreal study showed a higher risk of HIV infection associated with "consistent use" of the needle exchange (hazard ratio of 10.2), while the New York study showed a significant protective effect of needle exchange (hazard ratio of 0.30). The authors of both studies cautiously warned that these are observational studies and that statistical adjustment for potential confounders does not guarantee the elimination of bias.[17–19] Bruneau and colleagues noted, "it is possible that despite the exhaustive data driven process to identify confounders, some had been left unaccounted for."[17] Des Jarlais and colleagues commented that "none of the studies reported was a randomized clinical trial, so a causal link cannot be inferred. . . . We could not control for whatever factors led some subjects to use the syringe exchanges (potential self-selection bias)."[18] In an attempt to explain the discrepant finding in Montreal and New York, Lurie wrote that "the likely explanation is that powerful selection forces attracted the most risky intravenous drug users (IDU) in Montreal. The major Montreal Needle Exchange Program (NEP) was open only from 9PM to 4AM. . . . NEP was likely to be disproportionately utilized by IDUs who were out in the streets in the very early hours of the morning and who had difficulty obtaining or affording purchases of syringes through pharmacies. It is not surprising that these individuals would be at greater risk of HIV."[20] Whether or not that is the explanation for the discrepant findings between Montreal and New York is not entirely clear. Were there also selection biases in the New York study that should also be considered? One must be careful to be equally vigilant in looking for selection biases in studies that give results that are inconsistent with prior beliefs as well as those studies that give results consistent with prior beliefs. In any event, the discrepant findings based on observational data from the two cities are unsettling.

An alternative to the simple empirical analysis of cohort studies is the use of modeling, such as circulation theory, to explain the effects of needle exchange programs on risk of HIV infection.[21-23] Such an approach can be an important tool and may provide insight and help reconcile the occasionally conflicting results obtained from simple empirical analyses of observational cohort studies.

TRENDS IN SURVEILLANCE DATA

Trends in AIDS or HIV surveillance data have also been used to help evaluate AIDS prevention efforts. Surveillance data may refer to reported AIDS cases over time in a community or community-based HIV prevalence surveys. The hope is that the effects of HIV prevention efforts will ultimately be reflected in reductions in disease burden as measured by disease surveillance data in the community. The strength of this approach is that the evaluation is based on measures of disease burden in the community rather than among participants in a study. Demonstrating that an intervention is effective in a controlled setting or among trial participants is quite different from demonstrating that the intervention applied at the community or country level is an effective public health intervention for decreasing disease burden. For example, an educational or counseling intervention might be effective when implemented in a controlled setting and on a small scale; when implemented on a large scale, in contrast, it may be considerably less effective. There are, however, important disadvantages and limitations with the use of surveillance data for evaluation of HIV prevention efforts. The main disadvantage is the lack of adequate control or comparison surveillance data. Ideally, one would like measures of disease burden in the community if there had not been any intervention. If disease burden appears to be decreasing after an intervention is begun, the conclusion that the decrease is *causally* related to the intervention is tenuous at best because the decrease could have occurred even in the absence of the intervention.

An additional concern is that surveillance data on reported AIDS cases, which in most developed countries is fairly complete, temporally lags behind the occurrence of HIV infections. Decreases in the number of newly occurring HIV infections that might result from effective public health interventions would not be seen in terms of AIDS cases for many years because of the long and variable incubation period. Nevertheless, attempts have been made to learn about HIV incidence rates from trends in AIDS cases using the method of back-calculation.[24–26] AIDS cases and HIV incidence are linked by the deconvolution relationship,

$$A(t) = \int_0^t g(s)F(t - s|s)ds$$

where $A(t)$ are the cumulative numbers of AIDS cases diagnosed prior to calendar time t, $g(s)$ is the infection rates at calendar time s (i.e., the number of new infections per unit time at time s) and $F(t|s)$ is the incubation period distribution for an individual infected at calendar time s. The incubation period distribution is the probability the incubation period is shorter than time t. The basic idea is to use trends in AIDS incidence data $A(t)$ (counts of AIDS cases over time) to infer something about trends in HIV incidence $g(s)$ (number of new infections over time).

We will give two examples of the use of back-calculation of AIDS surveillance data to glean information about AIDS prevention efforts. Gail, Rosenberg, and Goedert used back-calculation to investigate the effect of treatments such as AZT on lengthening the incubation period and delaying the progression to AIDS among HIV infected individuals.[27] While clinical trials had previously demonstrated that AZT and other treatments were therapeutically effective, there had been no population-based studies that showed that such treatments were in fact having an impact in the broad community of HIV-infected persons.[28] Gail, Rosenberg, and Goedert used back-calculation methods to analyze AIDS incidence data in San Francisco, Los Angeles and New York.[27] Their calculations were first based on a stable or stationary incubation period distribution (i.e., one that was not lengthening), and those calculations overpredicted the numbers of observed AIDS cases beginning in July 1987. Back-calculation suggested that there was an unexplained fall-off in the growth in AIDS incidence. However, Gail and colleagues showed that a non-stationary incubation period that allowed for lengthening incubation periods beginning in 1987 could explain the decreasing trends in numbers of newly diagnosed AIDS cases.[27] Yet decreases in HIV incidence rates could not explain the falloff in AIDS cases. Indeed, as part of a sensitivity analysis, it was shown that even if the HIV incidence rates were assumed to be effectively zero in and after 1983, the falloff in AIDS cases still could not be explained except by allowing the incubation period to lengthen. This was one of the first studies to indicate that the therapies for AIDS were indeed having a significant public health effect and were lengthening the incubation period. Nevertheless, there are a number of key uncertainties with back-calculation approaches including changes in the AIDS surveillance definition, the incubation distribution, parameterization of the HIV incidence curve, and underreporting and reporting delays in AIDS incidence data.[26]

A second example off the use of back-calculation and surveillance data concerns evaluation of efforts to reduce maternal-infant transmission. Figure 3.1 shows the numbers of perinatally acquired AIDS cases in the United States by calendar quarter of diagnosis.[29,30] There was a marked decline in new cases beginning around 1994. While Figure 3.1 indicates striking reductions in perinatally acquired AIDS, it doesn't explain why. Is the reason a lengthening incubation period of pediatric AIDS, or decreasing HIV prevalence rates among childbearing women, or perhaps decreasing maternal-infant transmission rates? AIDS Clinical Trial Group Protocol 076 had demonstrated that AZT given to a pregnant woman could reduce maternal-child HIV transmission rates by as much as two-thirds,[1] and so prophylactic use of AZT is a plausible hypothesis to explain the declines in pediatric AIDS in the United States.

Byers and colleagues used surveillance data (of the type illustrated in Figure 3.1) and back-calculation methods to estimate the number of children born with HIV infection over time.[31] In addition, they estimated the number of new mothers with prevalent HIV infection in the United States using the *Survey of Child Bearing Women,* and then were able to calculate the maternal-infant transmission rate by dividing the number of children born with HIV infection by the number of new mothers with prevalent HIV infection. They found that the estimated transmission rate was about 23% in 1988, and then the transmission rate fell steadily to about 17% in 1994. What can we infer from these analyses? The analyses suggest that the declines in perinatally acquired AIDS shown in Figure 3.1 reflect decreasing maternal-child transmission rates that are most likely the result of prophylactic use of AZT as demonstrated by ACTG Protocol 076.[1,30,31] However, additional explanations for the declining transmission rates such as changes in breastfeeding practices cannot be completely ruled out based only on these data and analyses.

In some cases, naive interpretations of HIV surveillance trends can be mis-

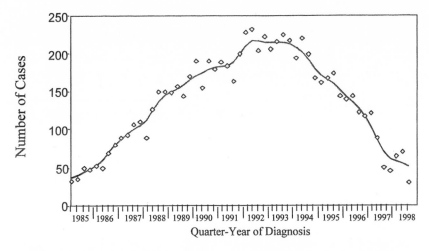

Figure 3.1. Number of perinatally acquired AIDS cases in the U.S. by quarter of diagnosis, 1985–1998. Based on cases reported through March 1999 and adjusted for reporting delays. *Sources:* M. Stoto, D. Almario, and M. McCormick, eds., *Reducing the Odds: Preventing Perinatal Transmission of HIV in the United States* (Washington, D.C.: National Academy Press, 1999); R. H. Byers, M. B. Caldwell, S. Davis, M. Gwinn, and M. Lindegren, Projections of AIDS and HIV incidence among children born infected with HIV, *Statistics in Medicine* 1998; 17:169–181; Centers for Disease Control (http://www.cdc .gov/hiv/graphics/pediatri.htm).

leading, as demonstrated by Brookmeyer and colleagues in their analysis of trends in HIV-1 incidence and prevalence rates among patients attending sexually transmitted disease clinics in Pune, India, from May 1993 to April 1995.[32] Table 3.5 shows that HIV prevalence was constant or perhaps decreasing during this time period, whereas HIV incidence rates were very high—in excess of 10% per year. Falling or stable HIV prevalence does not imply that no new HIV infections are occurring. Indeed, in a steady state where losses from HIV morbidity and mortality in a population are equal to the number of newly occurring HIV infections, HIV prevalence will remain constant even though the HIV incidence rate could be high. Thus, one should not naively interpret constant or falling HIV prevalence as evidence that the epidemic is under control or that HIV prevention efforts are successful.[32]

As discussed above, gleaning information about the effectiveness of HIV prevention programs in reducing HIV incidence rates from surveillance data on AIDS cases or HIV prevalence surveys has important limitations and is fraught with pitfalls in interpretation. In contrast, population-based HIV incidence rates can provide invaluable direct information about whether prevention ef-

Table 3.5. Trends in HIV-1 Seroincidence and Seroprevalence Among Patients Attending Sexually Transmitted Disease Clinics in Pune, India, May 1993 to April 1995

	HIV Seroprevalence			HIV Seroincidence	
	Tested (n)	Positive (%)	Person-years	Seroconverters (n)	Rate (%/year)
May 1993–Oct 1993	1466	23.3	87.0	8	9.2
Nov 1993–April 1994	806	20.0	195.6	29	14.8
May 1994–Oct 1994	1165	19.8	232.8	20	8.9
Nov 1994–April 1995	911	18.0	207.6	19	9.2
Total (May 1993–April 1995)	4348	20.6	722.9	76	10.5

Source: R. Brookmeyer, S. M. Mehendale, R. K. Plez, M. E. Shepherd, T. Quinn, J. J. Rodrigues, R. C. Bollinger, Estimating the rate of occurrence of new HIV infections using serial prevalence surveys: The epidemic in India. *AIDS* 1996; 8:924–925.

forts are working to decrease numbers of newly occurring infections. Unfortunately, HIV incidence rates are extremely difficult to obtain. One reason is that HIV incidence is typically estimated from a longitudinal cohort study that requires enrollment of uninfected study participants who are then followed and monitored for the occurrence of HIV infection. Those individuals who enroll in the study may be different than those individuals who do not enroll with respects to their risks of HIV infection. In addition, even among those who enroll in the study, there may be a considerable number of drop-outs and the follow-up rate may be low. Furthermore, those individuals who return for follow-up visits may be very different from those who drop out; we call this phenomenon follow-up bias. New methods have been developed to overcome some of the limitations with traditional cohort studies for estimation of HIV incidence rates such as low follow-up rates and follow-up bias. In particular, snapshot estimators of HIV incidence based on early markers of HIV infection have been proposed that require only a single cross-sectional study[33,34] and the theoretical properties have been developed.[35,36] The basic idea is to test individuals in a population for presence or absence of a biological marker of early infection to identify recently infected individuals. The methodology uses only a single cross-sectional study or "snapshot" and does not require longitudinal follow-up and thus the methods are not subject to low follow-up rates or follow-up bias. One problem with the first attempt at this approach was that the marker of recent infection, such as p24 antigen, was very short and thus the statistical precision of the resulting estimates was low. Satten and colleagues (Chapter 14, this volume) discuss a snapshot estimator based on a dual antibody test[37] that increases the duration of the biological marker and thus represents a considerable advance in the technology.

ANALYTIC ISSUES

Quantifying Efficacy

The statistical analysis of an HIV prevention study often involves a hypothesis test and the production of a p-value. While the limitations of p-values have been discussed by many others in other contexts, it is worthwhile to emphasize again shortcomings of p-values for evaluation of the public health significance of an HIV prevention program. We want to know not just whether a particular intervention reduced HIV incidence rates but also by how much. A measure of the effectiveness is desired. However, there are different ways of measuring efficacy. One of the most popular measures is simply the relative risk (or hazard ratio) of HIV infection. Various functions of the relative risk such as the vaccine efficacy have also been used. The hazard or incidence rate of HIV is the risk per unit time of an uninfected person becoming infected. The hazard ratio is the hazard of HIV incidence among those exposed to an HIV prevention program divided by the hazard of HIV incidence among those not exposed to the HIV prevention program. For example, the New York Needle Exchange Program found that a hazard ratio of 0.3 among consistent users of the program relative to nonusers, suggesting that needle exchange programs could potentially reduce HIV incidence rates by as much as two-thirds. However, such an interpretation should be tempered because of the potential for selection bias, as described earlier.

The issue of selection bias aside, quantifying efficacy based on relative risks has limitations. Relative risks say nothing about the absolute number of infections that could be avoided with the HIV prevention program. For example, if the intervention targets one route of transmission (e.g., needle sharing among intravenous drug users) and that route makes up only a small component of the epidemic in a community, the intervention may be relatively ineffective in reducing a significant percentage of the total number of new HIV infections in a community even if the relative risk based on studies in drug users suggests a strong effect. In contrast, an intervention with a less impressive relative risk that targets a transmission route that makes up a large component of the epidemic in a community will have a considerably larger public health impact in terms of total numbers of infections avoided. Furthermore, a simple relative risk does not account for both direct and indirect effects. For example, the prevention of an infection in a male intravenous drug user may indirectly prevent an infection in the injecting drug user's female sexual partner (resulting from sexual transmission), and that in turn may prevent an infection in an infant born to that female sexual partner. Thus, prevention of one infection can prevent a cascade of other infections. Ideally, one would want to know the total number of infections that could be avoided both directly and indirectly from an HIV prevention program. Longini, Halloran, and colleagues (Chapter 12, this volume)[38] have emphasized the importance of accounting for both direct and indirect effects in vaccine evaluation.

The HIV/AIDS epidemic is propagated through a mix of multiple routes of transmission. This creates additional ambiguities in the interpretation of a relative risk and application to populations with a mix that is different than the study population used to calculate the relative risk. For example, consider the case of the evaluation of a bleach intervention to clean injecting drug needles. An uninfected drug user is at risk of HIV infection either from sexual contact or from exposure to a contaminated needle. Suppose the incidence rate of HIV infection from sexual contact is I_S, and the incidence rate of HIV infection from drug use is I_D. Suppose further that the effect of bleach intervention is to reduce the risk of infection from injecting drugs from I_D to $(R_0 \times I_D)$, where R_0 is the relative risk associated with the bleach intervention. Then the total HIV incidence rate in the absence of the bleach intervention, I_I, is

$$I_I = I_S + I_D.$$

The total HIV incidence rate with the bleach intervention is

$$I_2 = I_S + R_0 \times I_D$$

The ratio of incidence rates with and without the intervention is

$$R = R_0 \times P_D + (1 - P_D)$$

where $P_D = I_D / (I_D + I_S)$ and represents the proportion of total infections that result from sharing needles among intravenous drug users. Thus, a simple cohort analysis that divides the HIV incidence rate among bleach users by the rates among non-bleach users would estimate the effect of bleach as R rather than R_0. What are the consequences of this? If $R_0 < 1$, then $R_0 < R < 1$; in other words R is attenuated toward 1. Furthermore, as P_D approaches zero, R approaches 1. The value of R depends on the proportion of infections that arise from transmission through needle sharing, namely P_D. Two communities could have different values for R, even though R_0 is the same in the two communities. One could naively attribute observed differences in R between two communities to differences in the operational characteristics of the bleach distribution programs when in fact it is due to different values of P_D in the two communities. The point is that the relative risk parameter (R) from two communities may not be directly comparable because of differences in the epidemics—in one community the epidemic may be propagating predominantly through sexual transmission while in the other community the epidemic may be propagating predominately through needle sharing among drug users. Nevertheless, the interventions could be equally effective in the two communities with respect to the particular targeted route of transmission.

An example can help clarify the distinction between R and R_0. Consider a community where 50% of all infections result from sharing of contaminated needles among drug users and the other 50% result from sexual transmission, thus $P_D = 0.5$; and suppose the bleach relative risk is $R_0 = 0.5$, that is, bleach can reduce the risk of transmission through needle sharing by 50%. Then it follows that $R = 0.75$. If we use the parameter R to describe the efficacy of bleach we might state that bleach reduces HIV incidence by 25%. If instead we use the parameter R_0 we might state that bleach reduces HIV incidence by 50%. Obviously both statements cannot be correct. It is more accurate to state that the bleach intervention is associated with a 25% reduction in *total* HIV incidence rates and a 50% reduction in HIV incidence that result from *needle sharing*. To avoid confusion, the parameter R could be referred to as the total relative risk associated with the intervention, and R_0 is the transmission route-specific relative risk. One would expect the total relative risk R to vary among communities.

The Unit of Analysis

An important consideration in the analysis of intervention trials is the unit of analysis. Sometimes individuals are randomized and sometimes communities or clusters are randomized. For example, ACTG Protocol 076 to reduce perinatal transmission involved the randomization of pregnant women, while the studies in Tanzania and Uganda to evaluate the impact of sexually transmitted disease control on HIV incidence involved the randomization of communities or villages.[1-3]

If the unit of randomization is the individual, standard person-time analyses could be performed to compare incidence rates in two groups. For example, suppose the number of observed incident infections (seroconversions) in group 1 and group 2 are X_1 and X_2, respectively; and the total person-times of follow-up in group 1 and group 2 are T_1 and T_2, respectively. Then, a simple statistical analysis is to assume X_1 has a Poisson distribution with mean $I_1 \times T_1$ where I_1 is the true incidence rate in group 1, and X_2 has a Poisson distribution with mean $I_2 \times T_2$. A test of the null hypothesis that $I_1 = I_2$ is derived by conditioning on the total number of observed incident infections $(X_1 + X_2)$. P-values are obtained by referring X_1 to a binomial distribution with sample size $(X_1 + X_2)$ and "success" probability equal to $T_1/(T_1 + T_2)$.[39]

If the unit of randomization was the community, the analysis proceeds somewhat differently. For example, the trial in Tanzania involved 6 matched pairs of communities. Within each pair, one community was randomized to the control group and the other to the intervention. This study involved over 4000 subjects in both the intervention and control groups. It would be inappropriate to conduct a naive person-time analysis as described above with total person-time simply aggregated for each of the two groups comprised of over 4000 individuals. This is because the responses of individuals within a community are not independent. Individuals who live within the same defined geographic community share common characteristics. For example, in the Uganda or Tanzania studies, the construction of new roads or trucking routes or the opening of new commercial sex establishments in a particular community could increase the risk of infection for all individuals living in that community. Furthermore, epidemics may occur in one community and not another simply because of chance. Thus, for example, if an epidemic of syphilis occurred in one community during the course of the study, it could increase the risk for all individuals living in the affected community. The more appropriate analyses to perform on the 6 pairs are either a paired t-test, a permutation test, or perhaps a sign test. There is considerable literature on the analysis of community randomized trials. For example, Donner and Klar studied statistical methodology for cluster designs with dichotomous outcomes.[40-42] Gail, Mark, Carroll, Green, and Pee reported the results of detailed simulations of randomization-based approaches.[43] Brookmeyer and Chen evaluated statistical methods for cohort analysis of community intervention using person-years specifically when the numbers of randomized communities are small.[44]

Careful consideration of the unit of analysis is also important in determining design and sample size. In community randomized trials, the number of communities that must be randomized will depend crucially on the variability in incidence rates between communities. The more variability there is between communities, the larger the sample (number of communities to be randomized) required to achieve a specified power. Sample size calculations for community randomized trials have been considered by a number of authors. Hays and colleagues have considered sample size issues for community randomized trials specifically in connection with HIV prevention trials.[45]

DISCUSSION

The objective of this chapter was to review some of the statistical issues in the design and analysis of studies of HIV prevention. Randomized trials offer the best protection against bias. Nevertheless, randomized trials are not perfect. Furthermore, in some circumstances it may be neither ethical nor feasible to randomize. In the absence of a formal randomized trial, natural experiments can provide unique opportunities for evaluation. One should take advantage of natural experiments when the opportunities arise.

In the absence of a randomized trial or a natural experiment, all too frequently one must rely on observational studies to evaluate HIV prevention efforts. The main concern with observational studies is self-selection. Researchers can never be sure if the observed effect that they attribute to the intervention is due to differences between those individuals who voluntarily join and those individuals who do not join the intervention program.

AIDS and HIV surveillance data have also been used to try to draw inferences about the efficacy of HIV prevention activities. A strength of this approach is it is based on community-wide measures of disease burden rather than outcomes among participants in a very controlled setting. However, in most cases the use of surveillance data is a rather blunt tool for drawing reliable inferences about the efficacy of HIV prevention efforts.

The design of trials must consider carefully the strengths and weaknesses of randomizing at the community or individual level. In either case, both sample size calculations and the statistical analysis must account for the unit of randomization and, more generally, correlation among observations. Finally, special care is needed in choosing and interpreting summary statistical measures of the efficacy of an HIV prevention program. It must be clearly communicated whether such measures account for direct and indirect effects and under what conditions measures observed in one community should be applicable to other communities.

REFERENCES

1. Connor EM, Sperling RS, Gelber R, Kiselev P, Scott G, O'Sullivan MJ, VanDyke R, Bey M, Shearer N, Jacobson RL, Jimenez E, O'Neill E, Bazin B, Del fraissy JF, Culnane M, Coombs R, Elkins M, Moye J, Stratton P, Balsley J. Reduction of maternal-infant transmission of HIV type 1 with zidovudine treatment: Pediatric AIDS Clinical Trials Group Protocol 076 Study Group. *N Engl J Med* 1994; 331:1173–1180.
2. Grosskurth H, Mosha F, Todd J, Mwijarubi E, Klokke A, Senkoro K, Mayand P, Changalucha J, Nicholl A, Ka-Gina G, Newell J, Mugeye K, Mabey D, Hayes R. Impact of improved treatment of sexually transmitted diseases on HIV infection in rural Tanzania: A randomized control trial. *Lancet* 1995; 346:530–536.
3. Gray RJ, Wawer MJ, Sewan Kambo NK, et al. Issues in sampling and study design for a community-based trial of STD control for AIDS prevention, in Rakai District, Uganda. International Society for STD Research, New Orleans, abstract 078, p. 61 (1995).
4. Coyle S, Borsch R, Turner C, editors. *Evaluating AIDS Prevention Programs.* Washington, DC: National Academy Press, 1991.
5. Piantadosi S. *Clinical Trials: A Methodologic Perspective.* New York: John Wiley, 1997.
6. Brookmeyer R. AIDS, epidemics and statistics. *Biometrics,* 1996; 52:781–796.
7. Greenwood, M. *Epidemics and Crowd Diseases: An Introduction to the Study of Epidemics.* New York: Macmillan, 1935.
8. Coronary Drug Project Research Group. Influence of adherence to treatment and response of cholesterol and mortality in the coronary drug project. *N Engl J Med* 1980; 303:1038–1041.
9. Rosenbaum P. *Observational Studies.* New York: Springer-Verlag, 1995.
10. Eyler JM. *Victorian Social Medicine: The Ideas and Methods of William Farr.* Baltimore, MD: Johns Hopkins University Press, 1979.
11. Darby SC, Ewart DW, Giangrande PLF, et al. Mortality before and after HIV infection in the complete United Kingdom population of haemophiliacs. *Nature* 1995; 377:79–82.
12. Vlahov D, Junge B, Brookmeyer R, et al. Reductions in high-risk drug use behaviors among participants in the Baltimore Needle Exchange Program. *J Acquir Immune Defic Syndr Hum Retrovirol* 1997; 16:400–406.
13. May RM, Anderson RM. Transmission dynamics of HIV infection. *Nature* 1987; 326: 137–142.
14. Marmor M, Friedman-Kien A, Laubenstein L, et al. Risk factors for Kaposi's sarcoma in homosexual men. *Lancet* 1992; 1:1083–1086.
15. Vandenbroucke JP, Pardoel V. An autopsy of epidemiological methods: The case of poppers in the early epidemic of the acquired immunodeficiency syndrome (AIDS). *Am J Epidemiol* 1989; 129:455–457.

16. Jorgenson KA, and Lawesson SO. Amyl nitrite and Kaposi's sarcoma in homosexual men. *N Engl J Med* 1982; 307:893–894.

17. Bruneau J, Lamothe F, Franco E, Lachance N, Desy M, Soto J, and Vincelette J. High rates of HIV infection among injection drug users participating in needle exchange programs in Montreal: Results of a cohort study. *Am J Epidemiol* 1997; 146:994–1002.

18. Des Jarlais DC, Marmor M, Paone D, Titus S, Qiuhu S, Perlis T, Benny J, Friedman S. HIV incidence among injecting drug users in New York City Syringe-Exchange Programs. *Lancet* 1996; 348:987–991.

19. Bruneau J, Franco E, Lamothe F. Assessing harm reduction strategies: The dilemma of observational studies. *Am J Epidemiol* 1997; 146:1007–1010.

20. Lurie P. Invited commentary: Le mystère de Montreal. *Am J Epidemiol* 1997; 146: 1003–1006.

21. Kaplan EH, O'Keefe E. Let the needles do the talking. *Evaluating the New Haven Needle Exchange Interfaces* 1993; 23:7–26.

22. Kaplan EH, Heimer R. A circulation theory of needle exchange. *AIDS* 1994; 8:1083–1086.

23. Kaplan EH. A method for evaluating needle exchange programs. *Statistics in Medicine* 1994; 13:2179–2187.

24. Brookmeyer R, Gail MH. Minimum size of the acquired immunodeficiency syndrome (AIDS) epidemic in the United States. *Lancet* 1986; 2:1320–1322.

25. Brookmeyer R. Reconstruction and future trends of the AIDS epidemic in the United States. *Science* 1991; 253:37–42.

26. Brookmeyer R, Gail MH. *AIDS Epidemiology: A Quantitative Approach.* New York: Oxford University Press, 1994.

27. Gail MH, Rosenberg PS, Goedert JJ. Therapy may explain recent deficits in AIDS incidence. *J Acquir Immune Defic Syndr* 1990; 3:296–306.

28. Gail MH. Use of observational data, including surveillance studies for evaluating AIDS therapies. *Statistics in Medicine* 1996; 15:2273–2288.

29. Centers for Disease Control. Downloaded from *http://www.cdc.gov/hiv/graphics/pediatri.htm* on June 27, 2000.

30. Stoto M, Almario D, McCormick M, editors. *Reducing the Odds: Preventing Perinatal Transmission of HIV in the United States.* Washington, DC: National Academy Press, 1999.

31. Byers RH, Caldwell MB, Davis S, Gwinn M, Lindegren M. Projections of AIDS and HIV incidence among children born infected with HIV. *Statistics in Medicine* 1998; 17:169–181.

32. Brookmeyer R, Mehendale SM, Plez RK, Shepherd ME, Quinn T, Rodrigues JJ, Bollinger RC. Estimating the rate of occurrence of new HIV infections using serial prevalence surveys: The epidemic in India. *AIDS* 1996; 8:924–925.

33. Brookmeyer R, Quinn T. Estimation of current HIV incidence rates from a cross-sectional survey using early diagnostic tests. *Am J Epidemiol* 1995; 141:167–172.

34. Brookmeyer R, Quinn T, Shepherd M, et al. The AIDS epidemic in India: A new method for estimating current HIV incidence rates. *Am J Epidemiol* 1995; 142:709–713.

35. Brookmeyer R. Accounting for follow-up bias in estimation of HIV incidence rates. *Journal of the Royal Statistical Society* (A) 1997; 160:127–140.

36. Kaplan E, Brookmeyer R. Snapshot estimators of recent HIV incidence rates. *Operations Research* 1999; 47:29–37.

37. Janssen RS, Satten G, Stramer SL, et al. New testing strategy to detect early HIV-1 infection for use in incidence estimates and for clinical prevention purposes. *JAMA* 1998; 280:42–48.

38. Haloran ME, Haber M, Longini IM Jr, Struchiner CJ. Direct and indirect effects in vaccine efficacy and effectiveness. *Am J Epidemiol* 1991; 133(4):323–331.

39. Breslow NE, Day NE. *Statistical Methods in Cancer Research*, Vol. 2. *Design and Analysis of Cohort Studies*. Lyon, France: International Agency for Research on Cancer, 1987.

40. Donner A, Klar N. Cluster randomization trials in epidemiology: Theory and application. *Journal of Statistical Planning and Inference* 1994; 42:37–56.

41. Donner A, Klar N. Methods for comparing event rates in intervention studies when the unit of allocation is a cluster. *Am J Epidemiol* 1994; 140:279–289.

42. Donner A, Klar N. Statistical considerations in the design and analysis of community intervention trials. *Journal of Clinical Epidemiology,* 1996; 49:435–439.

43. Gail MH, Mark SD, Carroll RJ, Green SB, Pee D. On design considerations and randomization-based inference for community intervention trials. *Statistics in Medicine* 1996; 15:1069–1092.

44. Brookmeyer R, Chen YQ. Person-time analysis of paired community intervention trials when the number of communities is small. *Statistics in Medicine* 1998; 17:2121–2132.

45. Hayes R, Mosha F, Nicoll A, Grosskurth H, Jewell N, Todd J, Killewo J, Rugemalila J, Mabey D. A community trial of the impact of improved sexually transmitted disease treatment on the HIV epidemic in rural Tanzania: Design. *AIDS* 1995; 9:919–926.

Chapter 4 Epidemiological Issues in the Evaluation of HIV Prevention Programs

Nancy S. Padian and Stephen C. Shiboski

In this chapter, we discuss the contribution of epidemiological methods to the development of HIV prevention strategies and policy. First, we consider the importance of study design and the precedence of randomized controlled trials (RCTs) in influencing policy makers. The limitations of this study design are discussed, specifically with reference to practical considerations in implementation of RCTs and the urgency of critical public health concerns, the importance of compliance to the intervention or treatment being evaluated in the RCTs, the importance of measurement of compliance, and finally, the ability to generalize results from RCTs to the larger community. Next, in addition to design, we consider causal criteria. The implication is that causal associations, where the exposure (or intervention) is causally related to the outcome (acquisition of HIV), merit implementation at a policy level. We conclude by stressing the importance of continued study even after policy decisions are made. The objective should be a rigorous epidemiological basis on which to base the implementation of an intervention, and the integration of epidemiological data with data from other disciplines, which also helps to shape public health policy. Working toward this goal rarely ends after policy makers implement particular intervention strategies. Time and scientific progress alone require constant vigilance and reassessment of what we currently believe to be state-of-the-art prevention strategies.

STUDY DESIGN

The most important contribution of epidemiological methods to the development of HIV prevention programs is to determine how and when the results of epidemiological studies can be translated into the development of interventions and strategies of prevention. These questions apply for basic epidemiologic studies that identify predictors where the objective is to identify the modifiable risk factors and to intervention studies where the question is whether or not the intervention should be implemented as part of a sustained program. The U.S. Preventive Services Task Force had to confront similar issues: when to perform a preventive clinical service depending on evidence accrued from previous studies.[1] The consensus was that interventions that have proved effective in well-designed studies (RCTs are inherently considered as better designed than observational studies) or that have demonstrated consistent benefits in a large number of studies of weaker design were considered worthy of implementation.

In fact, scientific evidence, as determined by study design, is the fundamental criterion for the Preventive Services Task Force for establishing whether a particular clinical practice should be executed. The current trend toward implementation of "evidence-based" clinical medicine,[2,3] and the ascendancy of RCTs provide the strongest evidence in support of clinical practice, and some have suggested that the same principles be applied to epidemiologic studies.

RANDOMIZED CONTROLLED
TRIALS—GENERAL PRINCIPLES

The concern is that the results of observational studies are correlative rather than causative and must therefore be verified through use of experimental designs. Before definitive conclusions can be drawn and the results disseminated and implemented as part of public health strategies, it is recommended that randomized controlled trials (RCTs) be conducted. The use of RCTs, where the exposure is controlled by random allocation to experimental and control groups, minimizes the possible biases that might occur when subjects are allowed to choose the exposure of interest (e.g., a cohort or longitudinal design where some women choose a particular method of contraception that might also protect against acquisition of sexually transmitted diseases or HIV, and others do not). In the observational design, it is possible that those who choose the exposure or intervention might differ from those who do not, in ways that are associated with the outcome (those who choose the method might be at greater or lesser risk of disease than those who do not). Thus, the preferred design to evaluate the efficacy of a particular intervention is usually an RCT where the possibility that the results can be attributed to anything other than the intervention or exposure is minimized. (These issues are discussed in detail in Chapter 3.)

However, whether one ideal RCT is sufficient to evaluate a prevention strategy once and for all, and whether results from one such study would be stronger than results from studies with other designs, is not always obvious. As knowledge is likely to change over time, implementation of an experiment at one point in time, in one sample, does not necessarily confer results that imply causality. As Mainland, a statistician closely associated with work on clinical trials, said in 1960: "The only way to learn something about the safety of our numerical findings is by more extensive exploration under other conditions, in other places, and at other times."[4] Conducting numerous RCTs is one solution to this limitation; however, there are other limitations to this study design. Below we discuss practical concerns in implementation, the issue of compliance with the treatment of interest (including measurement of compliance), and the generalizability of results from the sample in the trial to the larger community.

PRACTICAL CONSIDERATIONS IN RCTS

The costs associated with an RCT and the time associated with its implementation are often far greater than the costs associated with execution of other study designs. Setting up the experiment, standardizing the exposure, randomizing the sample, and implementing the study can incur greater costs and take more time than an observational study or natural experiment where the exposure is not imposed by the researcher. Some argue that in the face of an urgent public health problem, as is the case with HIV/AIDS, public health officials must consider the minimum level of evidence necessary to move from research to policy. This is based in part on reliance on the precautionary principle,[5] which states that when there is a threat to human health, public health actions should be taken in the absence of 100% certainty or proof of cause and effect. Both the cost and the time involved in conducting a large-scale RCT may not be justified

Table 4.1. Criteria for Evaluating Existing Data from Prevention/Intervention
Studies

	Intervention	
Criterion	Abstinence/Delay Age of Sexual Onset	New Microbicide
Side effects	Minimal	Unknown
Observational data	Strong	Varies
Biological plausibility	Strong	Moderate

when data are available from studies with inherently less rigorous designs. Nevertheless, establishing the threshold for what constitutes minimally sufficient evidence is not trivial. Table 4.1 compares criteria for determining whether available data are adequate and whether additional studies, particularly an RCT, should be conducted before programs are implemented as part of public health policy.

In this table, evaluation of sexual abstinence and delaying age of onset of sexual activity are contrasted with evaluation of a new microbicide. In the former, complying with the intervention has no side effects, and there exist convincing supporting data from numerous observational studies as well as corresponding biological plausibility (see criteria, discussed below), the criterion that supports causal association because the association makes sense from a biological perspective. Obviously, delaying or abstaining from sexual activity should reduce risk of STDs and HIV. Here one might argue that policy should be implemented and these strategies should become standard public health practice with no additional study. In contrast, the evaluation of a new microbicide with unknown side effects, few observational studies, and moderate (not strong) biological plausibility might be best conducted in an RCT. Even so, RCTs do not always offer the clear-cut results for which one might hope.

THE IMPORTANCE OF COMPLIANCE WITH THE
STUDY PROTOCOL (INTENTION-TO-TREAT
PRINCIPLE IN RCTS)

In an RCT, randomization balances confounding factors between treatment groups.[4] The intention-to-treat (ITT) principle, typically applied in RCTs, states that all subjects should be analyzed according to the treatment group to which they were randomized. Thus, compliance with the protocol, use of the study product, or participation in the intervention as designed is irrelevant. However, because adherence is inextricably bound up with the results of the study in an ITT analysis, it is possible to measure only effectiveness (efficacy as determined in real-world settings where compliance is as important as randomization)[6], rather than efficacy (effect in an ideal setting). In its most extreme case, if no one in either treatment arm adhered to the study protocol, obviously there would be no association between the treatment and any outcome of interest.

Although maintaining randomization in the analysis minimizes bias and preserves the balance of known and unknown confounding factors[4] in the presence of nonadherence, the associated ITT analysis does not estimate the true biologic efficacy of the intervention. As a result, the utility of the intervention may be underestimated. Moreover, it seems intuitive that we should know the full potential of the intervention as manifest among those individuals who complied with the study protocol. Following is one example of potential pitfalls of an ITT analysis in evaluating an intervention to prevent HIV acquisition among sex industry workers.

In a recent randomized placebo-controlled clinical trial among commercial sex workers in Cameroon, which used 70 mg nonoxynol-9 (N-9) film, no statistically significant difference in HIV incidence was observed between women who used the treatment and those who received the placebo.[7] Incomplete diffusion of the N-9 film and/or the low concentration of the product (70 mg) were possible explanations for the lack of significant effect on HIV acquisition in the Cameroon study. More specific focus on the results of this trial is merited because of the strength of its design and the rigor with which it was implemented.

The overall results of the trial are presented in Table 4.2. Because women in both arms of the trial were counseled to use condoms (and in fact, this counseling was quite effective: overall condom use was reported for over 90% of vaginal sexual acts), the placebo arm is, in effect, an evaluation of the efficacy of condoms, whereas the experimental arm is an examination of the efficacy of N-9 in conjunction with condoms.

The rate ratio of 1.01 indicates no added protection by the use of N-9. However, another equally valid interpretation is that male condoms are also ineffective, as the same number of events occurred among those randomized to placebo. Condoms and N-9 appear equally effective (and ineffective) in preventing HIV. Similar results were found with regard to gonorrhea, chlamydia, and genital ulcers. The authors were very clear about the importance of analyz-

Table 4.2 Measure of N-9 Effect on HIV Transmission

	Number of Women	Woman-Years	Number of Events	Event Rate
Placebo	575	697	46	6.6
N-9	595	720	48	6.7

Rate ratio = 1.01; 95% confidence interval = 0.68–1.52.

ing their data using an ITT analysis, where the comparison is made according to the group at randomization.

Feinstein and Horwitz point out that intent-to-treat analyses do not consider critical post-randomization events such as whether the intervention is something that is accepted and can be used.[8] For these reasons they suggest that such analyses might be inappropriate when the intervention is prophylactic or when the results of comparative efficacy are equivocal, as they are here. In fact, Feinstein and Horwitz propose that RCTs themselves may not be appropriate for prophylactic trials (as would be the case for intervention studies conducted to assess prevention strategies) where behaviors associated with use and compliance may be more critical than in a treatment trial, and where participants have already chosen to enter the health care system and receive a treatment, regardless of its effect.

MEASUREMENT OF COMPLIANCE

Still, accounting for compliance is not simple. Equivocal results can also arise from measurement error, regardless of study design. Measurement of contraceptive compliance hinges on self-report of a behavior that is socially desirable, as is obvious from the counseling session that stressed the importance of condom use. If participants are not accurately reporting their use (or lack of use) of condoms, their reports on the use of the study product, which they have also been counseled to use at each sex act, may also be unreliable. Such nondifferential misclassification (equal measurement error regardless of the study arm) would bias the measure of effect for the study product towards the null hypothesis of no effect.

Further examination of compliance with condom use in the same study indicates additional information. Table 4.3 shows the effect of 100% condom use on acquisition of HIV among those randomized to the treatment arm and to those in the placebo arm. Condoms seem effective when used in conjunction

Table 4.3. Condom Use Among Women in the Study

Treatment (N-9) Arm

Condom Use	HIV+	HIV−
100%	10	202
<100%	22	158
Odds ratio = 0.35 (0.15–0.81), p = 0.01		

Placebo Arm

Condom Use	HIV+	HIV−
100%	12	169
<100%	18	191
Odds ratio = 0.75 (0.33–1.7), p = 0.5		

with N-9, but are ineffective when used alone, a result that is not consistent with the protective effect of condoms that is widely accepted. These results may instead be an indication that reports of their use may have been inaccurate, and as discussed above, if reports of condom use are inaccurate, reports of use of the study product may be inaccurate as well. This may also account for high incidence of STDs and HIV in spite of high levels of condom use.

One solution to sorting out results that reflect efficacy versus those that reflect noncompliance is, in addition to the ITT analyses, to conduct a per-protocol analysis focusing on individuals who adhered to the protocol, or to employ statistical methods that adjust the measure of effect derived from an ITT analysis by compliance factors.[9] This should be the standard in a phase I or II clinical trial where safety and the biological mechanism of action are key, but even in a phase III trial, such as that described above, comparing the results between both types of analyses can help interpret the results, particularly results that indicate no difference between treatment arms.

Results from this study have been widely touted as the death knell for research on N-9 film, even though male condoms continue to be recommended as the best protection against HIV infection among heterosexuals, and counseling to promote them is still required for all microbicide trials. Regardless of the appropriate explanation, generalizations based on isolated studies should neither propel an intervention to the level of policy nor be interpreted to mean that a negative finding means no additional research is necessary.

GENERALIZATIONS FROM THE RCT
TO THE COMMUNITY

Rather than rigidly adhering to studies with an individualized random design as the only gold standard, some have suggested that RCTs accomplish different objectives than do observational studies. Feinstein pointed out that, owing to strict eligibility criteria for participation in most RCTs, although RCTs may provide the best means to show the efficacy of a treatment for an "average" patient, they cannot reveal information about efficacy for particular subgroups where disease severity or other contextual issues may restrict use of the study product.[8] Clinical trial participants may be different from those members of the community from which the trial sample was recruited. For example, they may be more motivated to use the product or to participate in the intervention. Furthermore, they may be more informed than other community members of additional options to participate in an observational study where choice, and not randomization, is permitted. As a result, Stein and Susser propose that in order to evaluate the effect of physical barrier forms of contraception in protecting against STDs and HIV, we ought to intentionally evaluate real use, observational data, and the behavior of participants as part of effectiveness.[10] In addition, by focusing on the average participant results from observational studies and/or analyses of RCT studies, which include compliance with the study product in the analysis of effect, these may be more easily generalized to larger, more diverse populations.

CAUSAL CRITERIA

In addition to the limitations with RCTs discussed above, other factors contribute to choice of epidemiologic study designs that are not experimental. Human behavior simply cannot be controlled in the same way as laboratory science. Some hypotheses do not lend themselves to an experimental design: for example, assessment of an exposure that might be associated with a deleterious health outcome such as smoking and cancer. Thus, criteria for assessing causality from epidemiologic studies have evolved. The following list, derived from the criteria suggested by Bradford Hill for the first Surgeon General's Report on Smoking and Health,[11] summarizes these criteria:

• strength of association
• consistency of observed association

- specificity of association
- temporal sequence of events
- dose-response relationship
- biological plausibility of observed association
- experimental evidence

Strength of association refers specifically to the measure of effect or association, odds ratio, relative risk, and so on. The larger the effect, the more likely the association is causal. The consistency of the association means that similar results should be found in multiple studies and using different samples. The specificity of the association conveys that causality is more likely if the association between the exposure or intervention and the outcome is unique. This is less important in an intervention study when the intervention of interest might have an effect on multiple outcomes, such as an intervention to reduce high-risk sexual behavior. The temporal sequence of the events is confirmed by ensuring that the exposure precedes the outcome; this would occur by definition in an intervention study. Dose response means more of the exposure results in greater likelihood of the outcome (e.g., more counseling results in more behavior change), although this also may not hold for an intervention such as spermicide use, where more use could have deleterious effects. Biological plausibility implies confirmation that the association can be explained through a biological or behavioral mechanism of action, and experimental evidence means that results observed in observational studies are confirmed in experimental designs, including laboratory and animal studies.

No one of these criteria is sufficient, and not all may apply to intervention studies. However, in addition to the study design, consideration of these factors provides a framework by which to judge whether findings merit implementation of a prevention strategy. For example, it is noteworthy that experimental evidence (RCTs) is only one criterion. Another critical consequence of consideration of these criteria is the inadequacy of judging the significance of an association based on findings from only one study. In order to assess the criteria of consistency and specificity, examination of multiple studies is required. Two statisticians who are both revered for their contribution to current methodology (including the importance of clinical trials), recognized this. In 1934, R. A. Fisher said that in order to assert that a natural phenomenon is experimentally demonstrated, we need a reliable method of procedure, not an isolated record.[4] Similarly, as stated above, in 1960, Mainland stated that the only way to learn something about the safety of our numerical findings is by more extensive exploration under other conditions, in other places, and at other times.[4]

REVIEW OF EXISTING PREVENTION STRATEGIES

Although one might be able to cite criteria for causality to weigh scientific evidence, some epidemiologists contend that whether or not findings are implemented, a part of policy is determined more by politics than by scientific evidence. "The process of policy choice may be studied as a scientific endeavor, but policies are set by a political balancing (or unbalancing) that uses science without being beholden to it."[12] In fact, if one reviews those interventions now widely accepted to be part of our armamentarium for prevention of HIV, a variety of studies and designs were implemented; no consistent criteria emerge that determined whether study evidence is sufficiently compelling to warrant implementation as part of prevention policy. Table 4.4 reviews several accepted HIV prevention strategies and the study designs that were used to propel study findings to policy.

Treating STDs as a means to prevent HIV has proved promising based on observational studies as well as in an experimental design. *Chlamydia trichomatis* infection has been associated with HIV infection in numerous studies,[13-17] but studies also support the importance of a range of STDs as cofactors for HIV transmission by increasing infectiousness in the HIV-infected individual and susceptibility in the uninfected partners.[13,16,18-21] Thus, primary prevention of STDs can have a major effect on preventing the sexual transmission of HIV.[19,20,22] The importance of STD control as a means to reduce the spread of HIV was emphasized in a 1997 Institute of Medicine report.[23] Mathematical modeling has supported these claims, and Boily and Brunham developed a model which shows that HIV infection via heterosexual transmission could not become established in a community in the absence of significant prevalence of bacterial STDs.[24]

A large prospective, randomized controlled trial in Tanzania found that the incidence of HIV infection was 42% lower in communities with improved management of syndromic STDs after two years when compared with control communities.[25] However, results from a later randomized controlled trial in Uganda called these results into question.[26] Here the design was again a randomized trial using the community as the target (in this case it was clusters of villages), but the intervention consisted of mass treatment. Although STDs such

Table 4.4. Design Determines Policy/Intervention

	Observational	Experimental
STD treatment for HIV	+	+
Primary HIV	0	0
Female condom	0	0
Male condoms	+	0
N-9 for STD/HIV	+	−

Key: + = Design implemented with positive results; − = design implemented with negative results; 0 = design not implemented.

as syphilis and trichomoniasis decreased, a concomitant decrease in HIV incidence was not observed. Based on these results, STD interventions to prevent HIV have now been questioned despite the fact that there were many differences in design between the two studies. Such differences include the maturity of the HIV epidemic in each target area, as well as the target population in each study (individuals with syndromic STDs in one study, and the general population regardless of risk or infection in the other). The more prudent strategy would be to take the two studies as separate pieces of evidence, both of which need replication. Neither RCT was the "definitive" study.

Targeting primary infection has been suggested as an efficacious strategy for preventing spread of HIV (e.g., identifying individuals with recent infection and then directing counseling efforts at such people, or promoting condom use more strongly with new partners than among partners of long duration).[27] Nevertheless, other than mathematical models that support this hypothesis,[28,29] little direct evidence supports this claim. Measurement error, variations in susceptibility, and the exhaustion of susceptible individuals[30] may account for what seems to be an effect of targeting infection early in the natural history of disease. Individuals *not* enrolled in the study may be sicker or more susceptible, and thus exit the pool of potential eligible subjects, leaving a cohort of relatively healthy individuals who may not be representative of the entire spectrum of disease. These may all equally account for what looks to be a decrease in infectiousness over time. No observational or experimental studies have confirmed this assumption. Nevertheless, publicity surrounding the findings of a modeling exercise has spawned a number of prevention programs where the significance of transmission among recently infected partners (insofar as they can be identified) has been emphasized.

The female condom is widely promoted through social marketing strategies in southern Africa and other places throughout the world. To date only two studies have examined the effect of the female condom with regard to prevention of STDs and HIV.[31,32] In the observational study of women treated for trichomoniasis, none of the women who used the female condom consistently and correctly at every act of intercourse became reinfected with trichomoniasis, compared to 14.7% of those who used it inconsistently and 14% who did not use it at all. In the second study,[32] a community intervention in Kenya where intervention sites received male and female condoms whereas control sites only received male condoms, no additonal benefit in reduction of STDs was observed in communities that had access to female condoms.

The female condom is being promoted largely based on biological plausibility. So much physical coverage should provide protection; in fact, owing to a greater area of coverage and based on a similar mechanism of action, the female condom ought to provide more protection than the male condom. Yet this has yet to be demonstrated through epidemiologic studies. Similarly, male condoms have proved efficacious only in observational designs.[33] It is the biological plausibility afforded through coverage of the cervix and vaginal vault combined with consistent findings from a number of observational studies that has promoted the male condom as the gold standard method for HIV and STD prevention.

Nonoxynol-9 products with doses ranging from 52.5 mg to 150 mg are available over the counter in the United States as spermicides. These products have been used for over thirty years as contraceptive agents and are regulated by the U.S. Food and Drug Administration under the over-the-counter review process. A review of the effect of N-9 on sexually transmitted infections identified 12 studies, 6 of which were clinical trials.[34] Overall, the authors concluded that N-9 had a protective effect against bacterial STDs. In contrast, HIV prevention studies have yielded mixed results and the ability of N-9 products to reduce HIV transmission remains uncertain. The most recently reported study[39] showed enhanced HIV transmission in the women using N-9, possibly due to detergent compromise of the epithelial barrier after intensive use.

CONCLUSIONS

Bradford Hill made the following observation: "All scientific work is incomplete whether it be observational or experimental. All scientific work is liable to be upset or modified by advancing knowledge. That does not confer upon us a freedom to ignore the knowledge we already have, or to postpone the action that it appears to demand at a given time."[11] The role of advocacy in epidemiology is still debated.[40] In the face of an urgent pandemic, we side with those who contend that as public health practitioners, we have an obligation to advocate policies through public health recommendations.[41] Even so, the impact of such recommendations may remain uncertain. Can epidemiologic evidence at best provide supporting background when other factors, such as politics, drive the ultimate decision as to whether an intervention is implemented? As scientists we are always faced with the reality that preconceived notions (difficulty in accepting unexpected findings, such as that male condoms may not work in all circumstances) as well as politics drive implementation of prevention strategies. Perhaps the greatest weakness in policy decisions is basing prevention strategies on findings from one study. Still, as Hill pointed out above, we must not be reduced to inactivity while we continue to improve the rigor of the data.

In addition to causal criteria as developed by Hill, we suggest adding the following factors that have more practical significance before moving from research to policy. In this world of scarce resources, attention must be paid to the risk-benefit ratio. This can be determined based on cost and determined by cost-benefit analyses and issues such as short-term benefits compared to long-term risks. For example, an intervention aimed at treatment of STDs to prevent HIV might in the short run reduce HIV transmission, but in the long term may be responsible for evolution of resistant strains of infection, which could then facilitate future spread of HIV. Closely related to the strength of the association is calculation of the attributable risk (the proportion of the disease that would be eliminated by a particular intervention); some interventions will have more impact than others. Finally, sustainability (if effective, can the intervention be maintained?) is another critical criterion. For many interventions, this means that researchers must consider steps toward sustainability at the inception of their research. For example, working with industry to lower the cost of the product and creating clinics and laboratories that will exist beyond the length of the study both contribute to sustainability. Such measures require involving the community at the outset of research, the results of which might be used to implement ongoing prevention strategies.

Findings from epidemiologic studies must be combined with results from other disciplines[41] with similar aims (e.g., biological sciences that elucidate the mechanism of transmission and acquisition, policy studies that evaluate cost-benefit ratios and sustainability, sociological studies that assess the needs and desires of the community at risk). The results from one study or one modeling exercise should not be considered in isolation. Given an epidemic of this magnitude, the zeal to report a positive result with potential promise in the absence of supporting data is strong, and the balance between prudence and unnecessary delay of action is difficult to maintain. In those instances where rash or unfounded strategies have been adopted, policy can be changed, even after implementation. Continued study can help to support or redirect existing policy as well as to shape future directions. The objective is to strive for a rigorous epidemiological and scientific basis for the implementation of an intervention. Working toward this goal rarely ends after policy makers implement particular strategies. The passage of time and scientific progress may alter priorities; even what is believed to be the state-of-the-art prevention requires constant vigilance and reassessment.

REFERENCES

1. *Guide to Clinical Preventive Services: Report of the U.S. Preventive Services Task Force.* Baltimore: Williams & Wilkins, 1996.
2. Sackett DL, Rosenberg WM. The need for evidence-based medicine. *J R Soc Med* 1995; 88:620–624.
3. Evidence-Based Medicine. A new approach to teaching the practice of medicine: Evidence-Based Medicine Working Group. *JAMA* 1992; 268:2420–25.
4. Mainland D. The use and misuse of statistics in medical publications. *Clinical Pharmaceutical Therapeutics* 1960; 1:411–22.
5. Weed DL. Principles and the practice of precautionary public health. *J Medicine and Philosophy* (2000) (in press).
6. Cochrane L. *Effectiveness and Efficiency: Random Reflections on Health Services.* London: Nuffield Provincial Hospitals Trust, 1972.
7. Roddy RE, Zekeng L, Ryan KA, et al. A controlled trial of N-9 film to reduce male-to-female transmission of sexually transmitted diseases. *N Eng J Med* 1998, 339:504–510.
8. Feinstein AR, Horwitz RI. Problems in the "evidence" of "evidence-based medicine." *American Journal of Medicine* 1997; 103:529–535.
9. Sheiner LB, Rubin DB. Intention-to-treat analysis and the goals of clinical trials. *Clin Pharmacol Ther* 1995; 57:6–15.
10. Stein Z, Susser M. Annotation: prevention of HIV, other sexually transmitted diseases, and unwanted pregnancy—testing physical barriers available to women. *American Journal of Public Health* 1998; 88:872–874.
11. Hill B. The environment and disease: Association or causation? *Proc R Soc Med* 1965; 58:295–300.

12. Rothman KJ, Poole C. Science and policy making [editorial]. *American Journal of Public Health* 1985; 75:340–41.

13. Ghys PD, Fransen K, Diallo MO, et al. The associations between cervico-vaginal HIV-1 shedding and sexually transmitted diseases, immunosuppression, and serum HIV-1 viral load in female sex workers in Abidjan, Cote D'Ivoire. Eleventh International Conference on AIDS. Vancouver, Canada, 1996.

14. Hayes RJ, Schulz KF, Plummer FA. The cofactor effect of genital ulcers on the per-exposure risk of HIV transmission in sub-Saharan Africa. *Journal of Tropical Medicine and Hygiene* 1995; 98:1–8.

15. St. Louis ME, Wasserheit JN, Gayle HD. Janus considers the HIV pandemic—harnessing recent advances to enhance AIDS prevention [editorial]. *American Journal of Public Health* 1997; 87:10–12.

16. Wasserheit JN. Epidemiological synergy. Interrelationships between human immunodeficiency virus infection and other sexually transmitted diseases. *Sexually Transmitted Diseases* 1992; 19:61–77.

17. Westrom L, Svensson L, Wolner-Hansen P, Mardh PA. Chlamydial and gonococcal infections in a defined population of women. *Scandinavian Journal of Infectious Diseases.* Supplementum 1982; 32:157–62.

18. Kreiss J, Willerford DM, Hensel M, et al. Association between cervical inflammation and cervical shedding of human immunodeficiency virus DNA. *Journal of Infectious Diseases* 1994; 170:1597–601.

19. Moss GB, Overbaugh J, Welch M, et al. Human immunodeficiency virus DNA in urethral secretions in men: association with gonococcal urethritis and CD4 cell depletion. *Journal of Infectious Diseases* 1995; 172:1469–74.

20. Hoffman I, Maida M, Royce R, et al. Effects of urethritis therapy on the concentration of HIV-1 in seminal plasma. XI International Conference on AIDS. Vancouver, Canada, 1996.

21. Deschamps MM, Pape JW, Hafner A, Johnson WD, Jr. Heterosexual transmission of HIV in Haiti. Annals of Internal Medicine 1996; 125:324–30.

22. Laga M, Manoka A, Kivuvu M, et al. Non-ulcerative sexually transmitted diseases as risk factor for HIV-1 transmission in women results from a cohort study. *AIDS* (Philadelphia) 1993; 7:95–102.

23. Eng TR, Butler WT. *The Hidden Epidemic: Confronting Sexually Transmitted Diseases.* Washington, DC: National Academy Press, 1997.

24. Boily MC, Brunham RC. The impact of HIV and other STDs on human populations. Are predictions possible? *Infectious Disease Clinics of North America* 1993; 7:771–92. [Published erratum appears in *Infect Dis Clin North Am* 1994 Jun; 8 (2):xi–xii].

25. Grosskurth H, Mosha F, Todd J, et al. Impact of improved treatment of sexually transmitted diseases on HIV infection in rural Tanzania: Randomized controlled trial. *Lancet* 1995; 346:530–536.

26. Wawer MJ, Sewankambo NK, Serwadda D, Quinn TC, Paxton LA, Kiwanuka N, Wabwire-Mangen F, Li C, Lutalo T, Nalugoda F, Gaydos CA, Moulton LH, Meehan MO, Ahmed S, Gray R. Control of sexually transmitted diseases for AIDS prevention

in Uganda: A randomized community trial. Rakai Project Study Group. *Lancet* 1999; 353(9152):525–35.

27. Cates W, Jr, Chesney MA, Cohen MS. Primary HIV infection—A public health opportunity. *American Journal of Public Health* 1997; 87:1928–30.

28. Jacquez JA, Koopman JS, Simon CP, Longini IM Jr. Role of the primary infection in epidemics of HIV infection in gay cohorts. *J Acquir Immune Defic Syndr* 1994; 7:1169–84.

29. Koopman JS, Jacquez JA, Welch GW, et al. The role of early HIV infection in the spread of HIV through populations. *J Acquir Immune Defic Syndr Hum Retrovirol* 1997; 14: 249–58.

30. Shiboski SC, Padian NS. Epidemiological evidence for time variation in HIV infectivity. *J AIDS* 1998; 19:627–35.

31. Soper DE, Shoupe D, Shangold GA, Shangold MM, Gutmann J, Mercer L. Prevention of vaginal trichomoniasis by compliant use of the female condom. *Sexually Transmitted Diseases* 1993; 20:137–39.

32. Feldblum P, Kuyoh M, Bwayo J, Omari M, Wong E, Tweedy K, Welsh M. Female condom introduction and sexually transmitted infection prevalence: results of a community intervention trial in Kenya. *AIDS* 2001; 15:1037–1044.

33. Cates W Jr, Stone KM. Family planning, sexually transmitted diseases and contraceptive choice: a literature update—Part II. *Family Planning Perspectives* 1992; 24:122–28.

34. Cook RL, Rosenberg MJ. Do spermicides containing N-9 prevent sexually transmitted infections? A meta-analysis. *Sexually Transmitted Diseases* 1998; 25:144–50.

35. Kreiss J, Ngugi E, Holmes K, et al. Efficacy of nonoxynol 9 contraceptive sponge use in preventing heterosexual acquisition of HIV in Nairobi prostitutes. *JAMA* 1992; 268: 477–82.

36. Niruthisard S, Roddy RE, Chutivongse S. Use of nonoxynol-9 and reduction in rate of gonococcal and chlamydial cervical infections. *Lancet* 1992; 339:1371–1375.

37. Wier S, Roddy R, Zekeng L, Feldblum PJ: Nonoxynol-9 use, genital ulcers, and HIV infection in a cohort of sex workers. *Genitourin Med* 1995; 71:78–81.

38. Zekeng L, Feldblum PJ, Oliver RM, Kaptue L: Barrier contraceptive use and HIV infection among high-risk women in Cameroon. *AIDS* 1993; 7:725–731.

39. Van Damme, L. Advances in Topical Microbicides, *UNAIDS*. *XIII International AIDS Conference*. Durban. July 2000, [abstract P104, 2000].

40. Weed DL. Science, ethics, guidelines, and advocacy in epidemiology. *Ann Epidemiology* 1994; 4 (2):166–71.

41. Taubes G. Epidemiology faces its limits. *Science* 1995; 269:164–69.

Part Two Cost-Effectiveness and Resource Allocation

Chapter 5 Difficult Choices, Urgent Needs: Optimal Investment in HIV Prevention Programs

Margaret L. Brandeau

Recent advances in treatment for human immunodeficiency virus (HIV) have significantly reduced the death rate from acquired immunodeficiency syndrome (AIDS) in the United States.[1] However, HIV prevention continues to be a significant problem. The estimated number of incident HIV cases in the United States has remained constant at about 40,000 cases per year for the past several years.[2] Fewer new cases are occurring among white homosexual men, but more new cases are occurring among women, injection drug users, and minorities.

Although millions of dollars are spent annually on HIV prevention in the United States and other industrialized nations, resources for HIV prevention are limited. Policy makers must choose which prevention programs to invest in, how much to spend on each program, and which population risk groups to target. Prevention resources can be invested in a wide range of programs, such as educational programs, screening and counseling programs, partner notification programs, condom availability programs, clean needle programs, needle exchange programs, and drug abuse treatment programs. Prevention programs can be aimed at the general population or targeted to population subgroups such as injection drug users, gay men, pregnant women, or other groups.

Decisions about allocating HIV prevention funds are often contentious. In 1987, a federal HIV prevention program with the theme "Anyone Can Get AIDS" was implemented, and since then a significant share of HIV prevention resources in the United States has been targeted to the general population or to relatively low-risk groups (such as non-drug-using heterosexuals). Recently, many policy makers have expressed concern that the same HIV prevention dollars would avert more HIV cases if they were instead targeted primarily to high-risk groups (particularly injection drug users and male homosexuals).[3] Needle exchange programs, which have been shown to be an effective means of slowing the spread of HIV, are funded by some states and cities,[4,5] but not by the federal government. The mayor of New York City has suggested discontinuing publicly funded methadone maintenance programs,[6] whereas the federal government has pledged to increase its funding for methadone maintenance programs.[7]

Determining the best way to invest limited HIV prevention resources is difficult for several reasons. First, epidemics of infectious disease are inherently nonlinear, so that saving one person from getting infected today could result in scores of people avoiding infection in the future. For the same reason, targeting all available HIV prevention resources to the subpopulation with the greatest HIV incidence may not lead to the greatest number of cases of HIV averted; failure to invest prevention funds in a lower-risk population may result in significant epidemic growth in that population. Second, investing a certain sum in incremental funds in a prevention program may not reduce HIV transmission by the same amount as the previous identical sum invested in that program. Although little empirical work has been done to examine the relationship between resources expended on various HIV prevention programs and the resulting transmission rate reduction,[8-10] it is likely that the relationship is not linear for many HIV prevention programs. Third, the allocation of HIV prevention resources that averts the greatest number of HIV infections (or leads to the largest gain in life years or quality-adjusted life years [QALYs]) may be unacceptable for political, social, or ethical reasons. Such concerns are often critical in decisions about allocating HIV prevention resources.

This chapter presents models for two problems of allocating resources for HIV prevention. The *resource allocation problem* is to determine how best to allocate limited HIV prevention resources among multiple interventions and populations. The *optimal investment problem,* a special case of the resource allocation problem, is to determine the optimal level of investment in a single HIV prevention program targeted to a single population. Our approach to solving these problems is based on analytical models that capture the spread of HIV over time and that explicitly incorporate "production functions" that link expenditures on prevention with reductions in HIV transmission. We discuss the development of exact and heuristic solutions to the models, and the use of those solutions to develop practical guidelines and insights for decision makers.

Before presenting our modeling framework, we discuss previous work on these and related problems.

BACKGROUND

Optimal Investment Problem

Little work has been done to analyze the optimal level of investment in single HIV prevention programs. Some authors have evaluated the cost effectiveness of specific HIV prevention programs retrospectively,[10-13] but have not attempted to make optimal spending recommendations. Kaplan[9] considered optimal funding for needle exchange programs assuming a short time horizon and decreasing returns to scale of the programs. Paltiel[14] considered when in the HIV epidemic different types of interventions can have the greatest effect.

Some researchers have used control theory to determine the optimal application over time of a single epidemic control program (e.g., vaccination of susceptible individuals) targeted to a single population. A typical objective might be to minimize the cost of control (e.g., immunization cost plus the fixed cost of establishing the immunization program) plus the cost associated with the number of individuals who become infected. With the exception of the fixed cost of establishing a control program, costs are usually assumed to be linear: the cost of control is a constant multiplied by the affected parameter, and the cost of disease is a constant multiplied by the number of individuals who become infected. Surveys of such models can be found in Wickwire[15] and Greenhalgh.[16] Our work on the optimal investment problem differs in that we allow for a general relationship between expenditure on a prevention program and reductions in the transmission rate; we assume that the prevention program is applied at the beginning of the time horizon; and we aim to determine the level of expenditure at which the benefits of the program are commensurate with the costs.

Resource Allocation Problem

The resource allocation problem is the broader problem of optimally allocating disease prevention resources among multiple interventions and populations. Most work on this problem has assumed that one intervention per population is available.

One stream of research on the resource allocation problem considers the goal of disease eradication, which is equivalent to reducing the disease equilibrium to zero. This approach has been applied to analyze general vaccine programs[17] and programs for controlling the spread of gonorrhea.[18,19] A drawback to this approach is that epidemic equilibrium may not occur for tens or hundreds of years. Such a long time horizon may not be useful for planning the allocation of HIV prevention funds.

Another approach to the resource allocation problem uses numerical analysis of more sophisticated epidemic models over a finite time horizon. Such models have been applied to evaluate policies for controlling tuberculosis[20,21] and to determine the optimal distribution of Influenza A vaccine among different age groups.[22] Tan and Yakowitz[23] proposed the application of a machine-learning algorithm for a Markov decision process to determine the optimal policy for control of a general epidemic. Researchers have used numerical analyses to evaluate the cost-effectiveness of targeting specific HIV prevention programs to different population risk groups[24] and to evaluate the relative effectiveness of different HIV prevention programs targeted to a single population group.[25,26] Numerical analyses of this type are useful for analyzing specific problems, but may not lead to insights for broader problems of resource allocation for HIV prevention.

Kahn[27] considered the impact of targeting HIV prevention resources to non-interacting populations. He considered an aggregate intervention with a fixed cost per person that reduces HIV incidence by a fixed percentage. He evaluated the impact of spending the entire budget on each single population. This approach implicitly assumes linear epidemic growth and a linear relationship between expenditure and reductions in HIV incidence and considers only all-or-nothing solutions.

Finally, Kaplan[28] has proposed a heuristic approach for community planners who must allocate HIV prevention resources. He suggests that decision makers subjectively construct functions that estimate the number of new HIV infections that would occur in a particular population group if a fixed amount of incremental funds were spent on a given HIV prevention program targeted to that group. Then the problem of allocating a fixed budget among prevention programs and populations so as to minimize new HIV cases becomes a mathematical programming problem that can be solved in a straightforward manner.

In the following subsections we introduce notation and assumptions underlying our models. Then we formulate and discuss the optimal investment problem and the resource allocation problem. We conclude with discussion.

NOTATION AND ASSUMPTIONS

Consider a single population in which HIV is spreading and a single HIV prevention program can be targeted to that population. We assume that the effects of HIV prevention in the population are measured over a finite time horizon T, indexed by t ($0 \leq t \leq T$). We assume that the spread of HIV in the population is modeled by a compartmental epidemic model with J compartments, indexed by j ($j = 1, \ldots, J$). We denote the HIV sufficient contact rate by λ. We let $f(\lambda,t)$ denote the HIV incidence in the population at time t given sufficient contact rate λ, and let $x_j(\lambda,t)$ denote the number of individuals in compartment j at time t given sufficient contact rate λ. We do not limit ourselves to any specific compartmental epidemic model; we assume only that $f(\lambda,t)$ is nonnegative and continuous for all λ, $t \geq 0$.

We assume that resources invested in HIV prevention reduce the sufficient contact rate λ. This may occur if the prevention program induces individuals to have fewer risky contacts and/or to reduce the riskiness of the contacts they do have. We assume that, before any incremental investment in HIV prevention is made, the sufficient contact rate is λ_0. We let $\lambda(c)$ denote the sufficient contact rate that is achieved if an amount c is invested in the prevention program; we refer to $\lambda(c)$ as the prevention program's *production function*. We assume that investment is made at time zero, and that the change in the sufficient contact rate is instantaneous and lasts throughout the time horizon. We assume that a budget B is available, so $0 \leq c \leq B$. We do not make any assumptions about the specific form of $\lambda(c)$, but we do assume that it is a continuous nonincreasing function of c with $\lambda(0) = \lambda_0$; we exclude prevention programs that increase the sufficient contact rate.

The use of a production function allows us to model the effectiveness of a prevention program in reducing risky behavior as a function of the amount invested in the program. In general, the relationship between resources expended and the reduction in the HIV sufficient contact rate may not be linear. For example, a minimum investment in the prevention program may be necessary before any behavior change occurs. This may reflect program startup costs or some minimum expenditure that is required to deliver the prevention program (e.g., the cost of an HIV screening test for each person screened). At a high enough level of expenditure, additional investment may have no further effect on reducing the HIV sufficient contact rate. This may occur because of characteristics of the epidemic, such as inherent infectivity of HIV, or because of limits on the attainable amount of behavior change. As another example, a prevention program's production function might exhibit decreasing returns to scale, with the sufficient contact rate changing less with each incremental dollar invested in the prevention program. This might occur if individuals who are reached first by the prevention program (i.e., those reached when a small amount of money is expended) are more willing to reduce their risky behavior than individuals reached when a greater investment is made in the program.

The use of production functions also allows us to model the relative effectiveness of prevention programs when targeted to different populations. The same investment in a given prevention program may induce different levels of behavior change when the program is targeted to different population groups. For example, investment of a fixed amount in an HIV screening and counseling program may induce greater behavior change in a population of gay men than in a population of injection drug users.

We assume that the benefit of a prevention program is measured in terms of HIV infections averted, life years gained, quality-adjusted life years (QALYs) gained, or a related health outcome. We allow for discounting at rate r, $r \geq 0$. Using the above notation, the number of (discounted) HIV cases averted over the time horizon T for an expenditure of c is given by

$$IA(c) = \int_0^T [f(\lambda_0, t) - f(\lambda(c), t)] e^{-rt} dt.$$

Letting q_j denote the quality adjustment associated with a year of life in compartment $j (q_j \leq 1)$, the number of (discounted, quality-adjusted) life years gained over the time horizon T for an expenditure of c is given by

$$QALY(c) = \sum_{j=1}^{J} q_j \int_0^T [x_j(\lambda(c), t) - x_j(\lambda_0, t)] e^{-rt} dt.$$

When $q_j = 1$ for all $j = 1, \ldots, J$, the function QALY(c) measures life years gained.

OPTIMAL INVESTMENT PROBLEM

The optimal investment problem was introduced and analyzed by Friedrich and Brandeau.[29] This section summarizes their findings.

Consider a single HIV prevention program targeted to a single population. The goal of the optimal investment problem is to determine the optimal level of investment in the prevention program. More specifically, we wish to answer the following question: at what level of investment is the prevention program's benefit greater than or equal to its cost? We assume that alternative HIV prevention programs or other public health programs exist, so that funds not invested in the given HIV prevention program can be invested in an alternative program.

We assume for the purpose of discussion that the benefit of the prevention program is measured in terms of HIV infections averted. For each level of expenditure on the prevention program, we consider the cost per HIV infection averted. One could also measure the program's benefit in life years or QALYs gained, and consider the program's cost per life year or QALY gained; the discussion below applies accordingly.

We assume that there exists some threshold cost per HIV infection averted (or cost per life year or QALY gained) above which a prevention program is considered not cost-effective and below which the program is considered cost-effective. In practice, no such well-defined threshold exists, although there do exist values below which programs are generally considered to be cost-effective and above which programs are generally considered to not be cost-effective.[30,31] Use of a single threshold value allows us to select the single "optimal" level of investment in a prevention program. If we instead selected lower and upper limits for the cost-effectiveness threshold, our analysis could be used to determine a range of optimal investment levels.

Suppose that, for each additional dollar invested in the program, the number of incremental HIV infections averted increases. In this case, the marginal cost per HIV infection averted is decreasing, as is the average cost per HIV infection averted. When this is the case, it is optimal to spend as much money as possible on the program if the resulting average cost per HIV infection averted is less than the threshold value, and to spend nothing otherwise. If the marginal cost per HIV infection averted is constant, the same criterion applies. Friedrich and Brandeau[29] point out that the case of increasing infections averted per dollar invested is analogous to the case of a firm that faces increasing returns to scale: if it is profitable to produce even one unit, the firm will produce as much as it can.

Conversely, suppose that, for each additional dollar invested in the program, the number of incremental HIV infections averted decreases. In this case, the marginal cost per HIV infection averted is increasing, as is the average cost per HIV infection averted. Thus, it is optimal to spend up to the point at which the marginal cost per infection averted equals the threshold cost-effectiveness value. The case of decreasing infections averted per dollar invested is analogous to the case of a firm that faces decreasing returns to scale: the firm produces up to the point at which marginal revenue equals marginal cost.

It is also possible that incremental expenditure can yield decreasing marginal cost per HIV infection averted (IA) for some levels of expenditure, and increasing marginal cost per HIV infection averted for other levels of expenditure. In this case, the above criteria for determining the optimal expenditure must be applied appropriately to different regions of the $IA(c)$ curve.

The second derivative of the infections-averted function can be written as[29]

$$\frac{\partial^2 IA}{\partial c^2} = \frac{\partial^2 IA}{\partial \lambda^2} \cdot \left(\frac{d\lambda}{dc}\right)^2 + \frac{d^2 \lambda}{dc^2} \cdot \frac{\partial IA}{\partial \lambda}.$$

The term $(d\lambda/dc)^2$ is strictly positive, and the term $\partial IA/\partial \lambda$ is negative, so the sign of the derivative is given by

$$\frac{\partial^2 IA}{\partial \lambda^2} \cdot (\text{positive quantity}) + \frac{d^2 \lambda}{dc^2} \cdot (\text{negative quantity}).$$

This expression shows explicitly how the "returns-to-scale" properties of the function $IA(\cdot)$ in c depend on both the growth of the epidemic (via the derivative $\partial^2 IA/\partial \lambda^2$) and the prevention program's production function (via the derivative $d^2 \lambda/dc^2$). Friedrich and Brandeau[29] developed examples for simple epidemic models showing that the function $IA(\cdot)$ can be concave, convex, or s-shaped in λ (concave for small values of λ and convex for larger values of λ); thus, in general, the derivative $\partial^2 IA/\partial \lambda^2$ can have any sign. The derivative $d^2 \lambda/dc^2$ can also have any sign, depending on the prevention program's production function.

From the above expression, it is clear that when $IA(\cdot)$ is a convex function of λ (i.e., when incremental reductions in the HIV sufficient contact rate lead to incrementally increasing numbers of HIV infections averted) and when the prevention program's production function $\lambda(c)$ is a concave function of c (i.e., when incremental expenditure leads to incrementally increasing reductions in the HIV sufficient contact rate), then if it is optimal to invest any money in the prevention program, it is optimal to invest as much as possible (that is, spend the entire budget). Similarly, when $IA(\cdot)$ is a concave function of λ (i.e., when incremental reductions in the HIV sufficient contact rate lead to incrementally decreasing numbers of HIV infections averted) and when the prevention program's production function $\lambda(c)$ is a convex function of c (i.e., when incremental expenditure leads to incrementally decreasing reductions in the HIV sufficient contact rate), then it is optimal to invest in the prevention program up to the point at which the marginal cost per HIV infection averted equals the threshold value (or up to the point at which the budget is spent, whichever occurs first).

Using numerical analysis of a simple susceptible/infective (SI) epidemic model with replacement,[32] Friedrich and Brandeau[29] showed that the function $IA(\cdot)$ tends to be convex in λ for rapidly growing epidemics and concave in λ for slowly growing or shrinking epidemics. They suggest the following rules of thumb for decision makers:

- For a population in which the HIV epidemic is growing rapidly and a prevention program that has increasing returns to scale, the decision maker should invest as much as possible in the prevention program.
- For a population in which the HIV epidemic is either growing slowly or shrinking, and a prevention program that has decreasing returns to scale, the decision maker should invest only up to the point at which the marginal cost per HIV infection averted reaches the threshold cost-effectiveness value.
- In other cases, further analysis of the relationship between expenditures on the prevention program and HIV infections averted is needed before one can determine the appropriate level of investment in the prevention program.

Friedrich and Brandeau[29] showed that the function $IA(c)$ is nondecreasing in T; the further out one measures the benefit of the prevention program, the greater the measured benefit for a given level of investment. Consequently, for any given prevention program, the optimal level of expenditure is a nondecreasing function of the time horizon considered. This implies that decision makers must choose the time horizon of analysis carefully. Use of a very short time horizon may fail to capture nonlinear epidemic effects associated with a prevention program and may understate the program's value. Use of too long a time horizon may overestimate the lasting effect of a prevention program and may ignore the possibilities of important treatment or behavioral changes in the future.

RESOURCE ALLOCATION PROBLEM

We now consider the problem of allocating HIV prevention resources across populations and prevention programs. We first consider a simplified version of the problem as analyzed by Richter et al.,[33] and then a more general version that has been developed and analyzed by Zaric and Brandeau.[34]

Consider the case of M populations indexed by i ($i = 1, \ldots, M$). We assume that there exists one HIV prevention program for each population and, as before, we assume that the prevention programs reduce the HIV sufficient contact rate. We assume that the populations do not mix (i.e., disease transmission occurs within but not across populations) and that a prevention program targeted to a given population will reduce the HIV sufficient contact rate in that population but will have no effect on the HIV sufficient contact rate in the other populations. We denote by λ_{0i} the initial HIV sufficient contact rate in population i (given no incremental investment in a prevention program targeted to population i), and let $\lambda_i(c_i)$ denote the sufficient contact rate that is achieved in population i with an investment of c_i in the prevention program targeted to population i. We define $IA_i(c_i)$ and $\text{QALY}_i(c_i)$ analogously to $IA(c)$ and $\text{QALY}(c)$ as the number of HIV infections averted and QALYs gained in population i, respectively, when an amount c_i is invested in the prevention program targeted to population i. We let $\mathbf{c}$ denote the vector $(c_1, \ldots, c_M)$.

The resource allocation problem considered by Richter et al.[33] can be written as

$$\underset{\mathbf{c}}{Max} \sum_{i=1}^{M} IA_i(c_i)$$

$$s.t. \sum_{i=1}^{M} c_i \leq B$$

$$a_i \leq \lambda_i(c_i) \leq \lambda_{0i} \qquad i = 1, \ldots, M$$

where a_i represents a lower limit on the attainable sufficient contact rate in population i. Such a limit could represent the minimum achievable level of risky behavior in the population or could arise from characteristics of the epidemic, such as the inherent infectivity of HIV.

Richter et al.[33] analyzed the above resource allocation problem for the case when the HIV epidemic in each population is described by an SI model with replacement. They showed that, even when the production functions $\lambda_i(c_i)$ are all linear, the objective function is not necessarily convex nor concave in $\mathbf{c}$. However, they proved that, for a sufficiently long time horizon, the function $IA_i(c_i)$

is concave and nondecreasing in λ_i for a shrinking epidemic (when the sufficient contact rate λ_i is less than the replacement rate) and is convex and nondecreasing in λ_i for a growing epidemic (when the sufficient contact rate λ_i is greater than the replacement rate). Furthermore, they showed that when the production function $\lambda_i(c_i)$ is concave in c_i and the infections-averted function $IA_i(c_i)$ is convex in λ_i, then $IA_i(c_i)$ is convex in c_i; and when the production function $\lambda_i(c_i)$ is convex in c_i and the infections-averted function $IA_i(c_i)$ is concave in λ_i, then $IA_i(c_i)$ is concave in c_i.

This leads to the following intuitive observations.

• For a sufficiently long time horizon, a shrinking epidemic in each population, and prevention programs with decreasing returns to scale (that is, convex production functions), it is likely that resources will be shared among prevention programs and populations; and if the lower limits on transmission (a_i) are zero (or nonbinding), the optimal solution to the resource allocation problem is such that the marginal cost per HIV infection averted is the same across all populations.

• For a sufficiently long time horizon, a growing epidemic in each population, and prevention programs with increasing returns to scale (that is, concave production functions), the optimal solution will be an all-or-nothing solution, with the investment in prevention for any population being either zero or the maximum allowable amount.

In later analysis of the problem, Zaric[35] showed that the QALYs-gained objective function leads to the same optimal resource allocation as the infections-averted objective function when the time horizon T is sufficiently long and certain weak conditions hold (e.g., when the relative quality adjustment between susceptible and infected compartments is the same for all populations i). He also showed that, when the time horizon T is sufficiently long, and some of the populations have growing HIV epidemics and some have shrinking HIV epidemics, it is never optimal to invest prevention funds in those populations with shrinking epidemics.

Richter et al.[36] applied their model to a problem of resource allocation for HIV prevention at a local Veterans Affairs (VA) hospital. They considered two population subgroups: injection drug users (IDUs) and all other patients (non-IDUs). They modeled the HIV epidemic in each population using a simple epidemic model.

They considered several prevention programs that could be targeted to each population, but represented the effects of the prevention programs using a single production function for each population, as follows. They assumed that, for a certain amount of money, non-IDUs could receive HIV testing combined with a routine counseling program; and, for a larger amount of money, non-IDUs could receive HIV testing combined with a more intensive counseling program. Similarly, they assumed that, for a relatively small expenditure, IDUs could receive testing and routine counseling; for a larger expenditure, IDUs could receive testing and intensive counseling; and, for an even larger expenditure, IDUs could be enrolled in methadone maintenance. They estimated the production functions using some of the few empirical studies that have examined the relationship between resources expended on HIV prevention programs and the resulting reduction in risky behavior.[8,10]

For different available budgets, Richter et al.[36] used numerical analysis to determine the optimal allocation of HIV prevention resources between the IDU and non-IDU populations, and to determine the cost-effectiveness of incremental HIV prevention funds. The work is notable because it is one of the first studies of resource allocation for HIV prevention that estimates the production functions associated with various HIV prevention programs and incorporates such functions into a dynamic HIV transmission model.

Zaric and Brandeau[34] considered a more general version of the resource allocation problem. As in the model of Richter et al.,[33] there are assumed to be M interventions. Now however, rather than assuming M independent subpopulations, it is assumed that the spread of the epidemic in the overall population is modeled by a compartmental model with J compartments; such a framework includes the special case of M independent subpopulations, but also allows for a more general definition of compartments and more general mixing patterns. The model is described by a set of P parameters (for example, sufficient contact rates between individuals in different compartments, mortality rates, and disease progression rates). The set of initial parameter values (before any incremental investment in HIV prevention) is given by $\mathbf{u} = (u_1, \ldots, u_P)$.

Let $\mathbf{c} = (c_1, \ldots, c_M)$ denote the investment in the M interventions and let $\mathbf{w}(\mathbf{c}) = (w_1(\mathbf{c}), \ldots, w_P(\mathbf{c}))$ denote the resulting parameter values given the investment $\mathbf{c}$. Each function $w_k(\mathbf{c})$ is a production function that expresses the relationship between the overall investment pattern $\mathbf{c}$ and the value of the kth parameter. As before, it is assumed that investment is made at time zero, that the change in the parameters is instantaneous, and that the changed parameter values remain constant throughout the time horizon $[0, T]$.

Let $x_j(\mathbf{u}, t)$ denote the number of individuals in compartment j at time t given parameter set $\mathbf{u}$ (i.e., in the absence of any incremental investment in prevention) and let $x_j(\mathbf{w}(\mathbf{c}),t)$ denote the number of individuals in compartment j at time t given investment $\mathbf{c}$; these are analogous to the terms $x_j(\lambda_0,t)$ and $x_j(\lambda(c),t)$ defined earlier. Analogously to $f(\lambda_0,t)$ and $f(\lambda(c),t)$ defined earlier, we define $f_j(\mathbf{u},t)$ and $f_j(\mathbf{w}(\mathbf{c}),t)$ as the number of newly infected individuals in compartment j at time t given no incremental investment in prevention and given investment $\mathbf{c}$, respectively. The number of HIV infections averted and the number of QALYs gained given investment $\mathbf{c}$ can be written as

$$IA(\mathbf{c}) = \sum_{j=1}^{J} \int_0^T [f_j(\mathbf{u},t) - f_j(\mathbf{w}(\mathbf{c}),t)]e^{-rt}dt,$$

$$QALY(\mathbf{c}) = \sum_{j=1}^{J} q_j \int_0^T [x_j(\mathbf{w}(\mathbf{c}),t) - x_j(\mathbf{u},t)]e^{-rt}dt.$$

The resource allocation model considered by Zaric and Brandeau[34] can be written as

$$\underset{\mathbf{c}}{Max} \quad IA(\mathbf{c}) \quad or \quad QALY(\mathbf{c})$$

$$s.t. \quad \sum_{i=1}^{M} c_i \leq B$$

$$\mathbf{c} \in \mathbf{C},$$

where the $\mathbf{C}$ is the set of feasible values for $\mathbf{c}$. The constraint $\mathbf{c} \in \mathbf{C}$ is analogous to, but more general than, the lower and upper limits on transmission considered in the previous formulations of the problem.

This resource allocation problem is a nonlinear optimization problem with a convex, linear constraint set. For most epidemic models, closed-form analytical solutions are not known, so it is not possible to write exact analytical expressions for $IA(\mathbf{c})$ and $QALY(\mathbf{c})$. Closed-form analytical solutions are known for very simple epidemic models, such as the SI model and its variants,[32] but even then the resulting objective functions ($IA(\mathbf{c})$ and $QALY(\mathbf{c})$) are nonlinear functions involving ratios of exponential terms. For the special case of M independent subpopulations, each modeled with an epidemic model that has a closed-form solution, and interventions that are each targeted to a single subpopulation, Kaplan[28] has suggested solving the resource allocation problem by discretizing the range of available funds and solving the resulting problem using dynamic programming. Because the budget can be discretized into arbitrarily small increments, this special version of the problem can be solved to within an arbitrary degree of optimality, although the computation time may become quite long.

For the general resource allocation problem, Zaric and Brandeau[34] developed a procedure to approximate the epidemic equations that leads to approximate but manageable expressions for the functions $IA(\mathbf{c})$ and $QALY(\mathbf{c})$. The procedure develops approximate expressions for epidemic growth over time, and may lead to relatively accurate approximations when the time horizon T is short. The approximation may be reasonable in many situations because policy makers typically make HIV prevention resource allocation decisions based on relatively limited time horizons (e.g., ten years or less).

Zaric and Brandeau[34] used a kth-order Taylor series expansion to approximate the functions $x_j(\cdot,t)$, expanded around $t = 0$. Substituting these approximations into the differential equations describing the epidemic yields derivative expressions that are quadratic functions of t. Appropriate terms from these derivative expressions are then integrated over the time horizon T to obtain approximate expressions for the functions $IA(\mathbf{c})$ and $QALY(\mathbf{c})$.

Zaric and Brandeau[34] applied the approximation procedure to the resource allocation problem considered by Richter et al.,[33] assuming that the production functions $\lambda_i(c_i)$ are linear and defined by $\lambda_i(c_i) = \lambda_{0i} - \alpha_i c_i$ and assuming no discounting. Use of a first-order approximation yields expressions for $IA_i(c_i)$ and $QALY_i(c_i)$ that are linear in c_i, so the resource allocation problem reduces to a linear program of the form

$$\underset{\mathbf{c}}{Max} \ \sum_{i=1}^{M} d_i c_i$$

$$s.t. \ \sum_{i=1}^{M} c_i \leq B$$

$$\mathbf{c} \in \mathbf{C} \quad .$$

We now specify the terms d_i. We let N_i represent the total number of individuals in population i (this value is constant in the SI model with replacement) and let δ_i denote the replacement rate in population i (a parameter from the SI epidemic model). The SI model comprises two compartments, susceptible and infected individuals. We will deviate slightly from our defined notation and let $x_{i1}(\lambda,t)$ denote the fraction of population i that is susceptible at time t and $x_{i2}(\lambda,t)$ the fraction of population i that is HIV infected at time t. Similarly, we will let q_{i1} denote the quality adjustment for years of life lived in the susceptible compartment in population i, and q_{i2} the quality adjustment for years of life lived in the infected compartment in population i. Using this notation, the terms d_i are given by

$$d_i \equiv a_i N_i x_{i2}(\lambda_{i0},0)[1 - x_{i2}(\lambda_{i0},0)]\left[T + \delta_i \frac{T^2}{2}\right]$$

for the infections-averted objective function, and as

$$d_i \equiv a_i(q_{i1} - q_{i2})N_i x_{i2}(\lambda_{i0},0)[1 - x_{i2}(\lambda_{i0},0)]\frac{T^2}{2}$$

for the QALYs-gained objective function.

The optimal solution to the linear program is a greedy solution: resources are allocated to populations (and corresponding interventions) in nonincreasing order of d_i until the budget is spent. The intuitive meaning of this solution can be inferred from the above definitions of the objective function coefficients. For the infections-averted objective function, the coefficient d_i is an approximate linear expression for the number of HIV infections averted per unit expenditure (c_i) on the prevention program targeted to that population: it is the product of the rate α_i at which λ_i changes per unit change in c_i multiplied by an approximate expression for the number of new infections that will occur in population i up to time T. Similarly, for the QALYs-gained objective function, the coefficient d_i is an approximate linear expression for the number of QALYs gained per unit expenditure (c_i) on the prevention program targeted to that population: it is the product of the rate α_i at which λ_i changes per unit change in c_i multiplied by the difference in the quality-of-life multipliers for uninfected and infected compartments (when an infection is averted, an individual's quality of life is higher by this amount) multiplied by an approximate expression for the cumulative HIV incidence in population i by time T. The solution to the linear program funds those prevention programs first which have the largest values of d_i—and these are the programs that yield the greatest return in infections averted or QALYs gained per dollar spent.

The above linear programming formulation assumed linear production functions for the prevention programs. A linear programming formulation also occurs when first-order approximations are used for the compartment size functions, and when each production function is convex and is approximated by a set of linear functions. For the case of linear production functions or convex production functions approximated by linear functions, the resource allocation problem becomes a quadratic program when second-order approximations are used for the compartment size functions. In numerical tests,[34] the first-order approximation led to optimal solutions for the resource allocation problem when the time horizon was two years or less, while the second-order approximation was accurate for time horizons of up to five years.

Zaric and Brandeau[34] illustrated the application of the approximation procedure to several more general versions of the resource allocation problem. They considered an epidemic model with two subpopulations (high risk and low risk), two disease states, and mixing between subpopulations. They considered interventions that reduce the HIV sufficient contact rate in each population and an intervention that causes high-risk individuals to change their behavior and migrate to the low-risk population. They characterized the optimal solution to the problem for the QALYs-gained objective with a second-order approximation and for the infections-averted objective with a first-order approximation.

Zaric and Brandeau[34,37] also illustrated the use of the approximation procedure to solve problems in which the prevention programs are not independent. Interaction between interventions may occur when an HIV prevention program targeted to one risk group leads to reduced HIV risk in another group: for example, a general AIDS awareness campaign may increase the effectiveness of specific HIV risk-reduction programs. Such effects may be important to include when determining the appropriate allocation of HIV prevention resources.

Zaric and Brandeau[38] extended the static resource allocation model to a dynamic framework in which funds for HIV prevention are allocated over multiple time periods. For a special case with two time periods, independent populations, and linear production functions, they showed that the optimal solution is to allocate either as much as possible or nothing to each population in each time period. They also presented several algorithms for solving the multiperiod resource allocation problem and showed that good resource allocation decisions can be made based on some fairly simple heuristics.

The resource allocation problem described above has the goal of maximizing QALYs gained or infections averted, subject to a budget constraint and constraints on values of parameters in the epidemic model. Other formulations of the resource allocation problem are possible. For example, if changes in health care costs due to investment in HIV prevention programs are realized by the decision maker (e.g., if the decision maker is a health maintenance organization), then they could be included in the budget constraint. As another example, the problem could be formulated as one of minimizing cost subject to a minimum acceptable level of health benefit, or minimizing the average cost-effectiveness ratio (total cost divided by total health benefit). Further discussion of alternative formulations can be found in Zaric and Brandeau.[34]

DISCUSSION

We have described a stream of research on the problem of resource allocation for HIV prevention, and its special case, the optimal investment problem. Our models differ from existing work in that they explicitly link the production functions of prevention programs with dynamic models of HIV transmission. The production functions capture the reductions in HIV sufficient contact rates (or changes in other epidemic model parameters) brought about by different levels of investment in HIV prevention programs, and the use of a dynamic HIV transmission model captures the effects on the HIV epidemic (in particular, HIV infections averted and QALYs gained) due to changes in HIV sufficient contact rates (or changes in other epidemic model parameters).

We have used an analytical approach in order to develop general insights into how prevention program production functions and epidemic growth affect optimal resource allocation decisions. Although we have analyzed the resource allocation problems using only relatively simple epidemic models, we can draw some limited conclusions.

Our analyses underscore the importance of considering not only epidemic growth but also the prevention programs' production functions when making decisions about allocating HIV prevention resources. The shape of a prevention program's production function is a key factor in determining the appropriate level of investment in the program. Little empirical work has been done to estimate the production functions associated with HIV prevention programs, but information about these functions is critical to making decisions about how to allocate HIV prevention resources most effectively.

Our analyses suggest that for populations in which the HIV epidemic is growing rapidly and prevention programs that reduce the HIV sufficient contact rate and have increasing returns to scale, it is optimal to invest as much as possible in the prevention programs. For a population in which the HIV epidemic is either growing slowly or shrinking, and a prevention program that reduces the HIV sufficient contact rate and has decreasing returns to scale, it is cost-effective to invest only up to the point at which the marginal cost per HIV infection averted reaches the threshold cost-effectiveness value. When there are multiple populations with slowly growing or shrinking epidemics, and prevention programs with decreasing returns to scale, it is likely that resources will be shared among prevention programs and populations; and if the lower limits on transmission are zero (or non-binding), then the optimal solution to the resource allocation program is such that the marginal cost per HIV infection averted is the same across all populations.

When the time horizon is short, a first-order approximation procedure applied to the epidemic model equations may provide reasonably good estimates of the number of HIV infections averted and QALYs gained over the time horizon. When the production functions are linear, the optimal solution to the approximated resource allocation problem funds those prevention programs first that yield the greatest return in infections averted or QALYs gained per dollar spent; and these health benefits can be well approximated using expressions based on initial HIV prevalence in each population and the coefficient expressing the (linear) reduction in the HIV sufficient contact rate per dollar invested in a prevention program.

For both the optimal investment problem and the resource allocation problem, the analyses suggest that decision makers must choose the time horizon of analysis carefully. A time horizon that is too short may fail to capture nonlinear epidemic effects associated with a prevention program and may understate the program's value. A time horizon that is too long may overestimate the lasting effect of a prevention program and may ignore the possibilities of important treatment or behavioral changes in the future.

An important goal of further work is to use the models to develop practical insights for decision makers. Our theoretical analyses are based on models of the HIV epidemic and production functions for HIV prevention programs. However, decision makers may not have complete information about the growth of the epidemic in various subpopulations, nor about the production functions for HIV prevention programs. Further analysis of the optimal investment problem and the resource allocation problem, perhaps using more sophisticated epidemic models and empirical data regarding production functions, is needed in order to develop heuristic rules for decision makers. Such rules could help decision makers best allocate HIV prevention resources in the absence of complete information.

HIV prevention funds are allocated through a complex political process. Decisions about allocating HIV prevention resources are made at federal, state, and local levels. Hundreds of millions of dollars in federal HIV prevention funds are allocated in the United States each year by local community planning groups.[39,40] Although policy makers must consider issues such as equity, fairness, and ethics when making decisions about allocating HIV prevention funds, the ultimate goal in allocating such funds is to prevent HIV transmission. By determining the allocation of prevention resources that will provide the greatest health benefit per dollar spent, and by determining the health consequences of different allocations of funds, our models can provide important input to policy makers as they address the difficult problem of determining how best to allocate scarce HIV prevention resources.

ACKNOWLEDGMENT

This work was supported by the Societal Institute of the Mathematical Sciences (SIMS) through a grant from the National Institute on Drug Abuse (NIDA), National Institutes of Health (NIH) (Grant #DA R-01-09531-01A2).

REFERENCES

1. National Center for Health Statistics. *Births and Deaths: United States, 1997.* Washington, DC: Public Health Service, 1997.
2. United States Department of Health and Human Services. AIDS falls from top ten causes of death; Teen births, infant mortality, homicide all decline. HHS News, at website *http://www.hhs.gov.* US Department of Health and Human Services, NCHS Press Office, 1998.
3. Bennett A, Sharpe A. Health hazard; AIDS fight is skewed by federal campaign that exaggerated risks; most heterosexuals face scant peril but receive large portion of funds; less goes to gays, addicts. *Wall Street Journal.* May 1, 1996:A1.
4. Lurie PG, Reingold AL. *The Public Health Impact of Needle Exchange Programs in the United States and Abroad.* San Francisco, CA: Institute for Health Policy Studies, University of California, 1993.
5. Kaplan EH, O'Keefe E. Let the needles do the talking! Evaluating the New Haven legal needle exchange. *Interfaces* 1993; 23:7–26.
6. Swarns RL. Mayor wants to abolish use of methadone. *New York Times.* July 21, 1998: B1.
7. Wren CS. Federal proposal would provide methadone to more drug addicts. *New York Times.* September 29, 1998:A1.
8. Kahn JG, Washington AE, Showstack JA, Berlin M, Phillips K, Watson S. *Updated Estimates of the Impact and Cost of HIV Prevention in Injection Drug Users. Report Prepared for Centers for Disease Control and Prevention.* San Francisco, CA: Institute for Health Policy Studies, University of California, 1992.
9. Kaplan EH. Economic analysis of needle exchange. *AIDS* 1995; 9:1113–1119.
10. Owens DK, Nease RF, Harris RA. Cost-effectiveness of HIV screening in acute care settings. *Arch Intern Med* 1996; 156:394–404.
11. Holtgrave DR, Kelly JA. Preventing HIV/AIDS among high-risk urban women: The cost-effectiveness of a behavioral group intervention. *Am J Public Health* 1996; 86: 1442–1445.
12. Holtgrave DM, Reiser WJ, Di Franceisco W. The evaluation of HIV counseling-and-

testing services: Making the most of limited resources. *AIDS Educ Prev* 1997; 9:105–118.

13. Pinkerton SD, Holtgrave DR, Valdiserri RO. Cost-effectiveness of HIV-prevention skills training for men who have sex with men. *AIDS* 1997; 11.

14. Paltiel AD. Timing is the essence: Matching AIDS policy to the epidemic life cycle. In: Kaplan EH, Brandeau ML, eds. *Modeling the AIDS Epidemic: Planning, Policy, and Prediction.* New York: Raven Press, 1994:53–72.

15. Wickwire K. Mathematical models for the control of pests and infectious diseases: A survey. *Theoretical Popu Bio* 1977; 11:182–238.

16. Greenhalgh D. Control of an epidemic spreading in a heterogeneously mixing population. *Math Biosci* 1986; 80:23–45.

17. May RM, Anderson RM. Spatial heterogeneity and the design of immunization programs. *Math Biosci* 1984; 72:83–111.

18. Hethcote HW. Gonorrhea modeling: A comparison of control methods. *Math Biosci* 1982; 58:93–109.

19. Hethcote HW, Yorke JA. Gonorrhea transmission dynamics and control. *Lect Notes Biomath* 1984; 56.

20. ReVelle C, Feldmann F, Lynn W. An optimization model of tuberculosis epidemiology. *Manage Sci* 1969; 16:B190–B211.

21. ReVelle C, Male J. A mathematical model for determining case finding and treatment activities in tuberculosis control programs. *Am Rev Resp Dis* 1970; 102:403–411.

22. Longini IM, Ackerman E, Elveback LR. An optimization model for influenza A epidemics. *Math Biosci* 1978; 38:141–157.

23. Tan W-Y, Yakowitz S. Machine learning for Markov decision processes with application to an AIDS allocation program. Tucson, AZ: Systems and Industrial Engineering Department, University of Arizona, 1996.

24. Brandeau ML, Owens DK, Sox CH, Wachter RM. Screening women of childbearing age for human immunodeficiency virus: A cost-benefit analysis. *Arch Intern Med* 1992; 152:2229–2237.

25. Hethcote HW. Modeling AIDS prevention programs in a population of homosexual men. In: Kaplan EH, Brandeau ML, eds. *Modeling the AIDS Epidemic: Planning, Policy, and Prediction.* New York: Raven Press, 1994:91–108.

26. Richter AR, Brandeau ML, Owens DK. Policy analysis of preventive HIV interventions targeted to adolescents: An application of STELLA. In: Anderson JG, Katzper M, eds. *Simulation in the Medical Sciences Conference: Proceedings of the 1996 Western Multiconference.* San Diego, CA: Society for Computer Simulation, 1996:55–63.

27. Kahn JG. The cost-effectiveness of HIV prevention targeting: How much more bang for the buck? *Am J Public Health* 1996; 86:1709–1712.

28. Kaplan EH. Economic evaluation and HIV prevention community planning: A policy analyst's perspective. In: Holtgrave DR, ed. *Handbook of Economic Evaluation of HIV Prevention Programs.* New York: Plenum Press, 1998:177–193.

29. Friedrich CM, Brandeau ML. What's the program worth? Analysis of optimal investment in HIV prevention programs. Technical Report. Stanford, CA: Department of Management Science and Engineering. Stanford University, 2000.

30. Owens DK. Interpretation of cost-effectiveness analyses [Editorial]. *J Gen Intern Med* 1998; 13:716–717.

31. Owens DK. Economic evaluation of HIV screening interventions. In: Holtgrave DR, ed. *Handbook of Economic Evaluation of HIV Prevention Programs.* New York: Plenum Press, 1998:81–102.

32. Bailey NT Jr. *The Mathematical Theory of Infectious Diseases and Its Applications.* New York: Hafner Press, 1975.

33. Richter A, Brandeau ML, Zaric GS. Optimal resource allocation for epidemic control among multiple independent populations. Technical Report. Stanford, CA: Department of Industrial Engineering and Engineering Management, Stanford University, 1999.

34. Zaric GS, Brandeau ML. Resource allocation for epidemic control over short time horizons. *Math Biosci* 2001; 171:33–58.

35. Zaric GS. Resource allocation for control of epidemics. PhD Dissertation. Stanford, CA: Department of Industrial Engineering and Engineering Management, Stanford University, 2000.

36. Richter A, Brandeau ML, Owens DK. An analysis of optimal resource allocation for HIV prevention among injection drug users and nonusers. *Med Decis Making* 1999; 19:167–179.

37. Zaric GS, Brandeau ML. Optimal investment in a portfolio of HIV prevention programs. *Med Decis Making.* In press.

38. Zaric GS, Brandeau ML. Dynamic resource allocation for epidemic control in multiple populations. Technical Report. Stanford, CA: Department of Management Science and Engineering, Stanford University, 2000.

39. Kaplan EH, Pollack H. Allocating HIV prevention resources. *Socio-Econ Planning Sci* 1998; 32:257–263.

40. Hoffman C, de Paomo FB, Greabill L. *HIV Prevention Priorities: How Community Planning Groups Decide.* Washington, DC: Academy for Educational Development and the National Alliance of State and Territorial AIDS Directors, 1996.

Chapter 6 Methadone Treatment as HIV Prevention: Cost-Effectiveness Analysis

Harold Pollack

As AIDS enters its third decade of public consciousness, domestic HIV prevention has changed from a crisis response to a frightening outbreak to a mature set of programs that compete for scarce public funds. In such an environment, practitioners face new pressure to critically evaluate ongoing HIV prevention efforts. More openly than in the past, sympathetic policy makers demand rigorous evaluation to allocate resources across competing interventions, and even between HIV prevention and other public health concerns.

The transformation of AIDS policy presents dangers, but the passage of time provides welcome opportunity to document the costs and benefits of HIV-prevention efforts. Such analysis allows more effective deployment of scarce HIV prevention resources. At the same time, careful analysis shows that needle exchange and other HIV prevention interventions compare favorably in efficacy and cost-effectiveness to other interventions that Americans value to extend human life. The most prominent cost-effectiveness analysis of needle exchange finds a cost per averted HIV infection of less than $100,000.[1,2] Properly implemented behavioral interventions for high-risk women appear similar in cost per averted HIV infection among program recipients.[3]

Given the high probability of mortality and morbidity, the large treatment costs associated with HIV, and the possibility of downstream infection, HIV prevention efforts appear cost-effective when compared with less controversial interventions in other policy domains. For example, a widely cited study of prenatal care and neonatal services finds that subsidized insurance coverage reduced infant mortality at an approximate cost of $4.2 million per life saved.[4] Tengs and colleagues[5] summarize 500 life-prolonging interventions ranging from auto safety seats to pollution abatement. The median cost per *life-year* was $42,000.

This chapter contributes to the policy debate by examining one of the most visible, costly, and intensive weapons in the prevention arsenal: methadone treatment for injection drug users (IDUS). A voluminous literature already documents the impact of methadone on health care costs, crime, and social performance of drug users. In contrast to existing research, this chapter evaluates methadone treatment solely as a mechanism to reduce the spread of HIV. Using highly simplified though empirically reasonable epidemiological models, this chapter analyzes the cost-effectiveness of a representative methadone program. In IDU populations with high rates of random sharing in shooting galleries and similar venues, methadone treatment appears to be an efficient use of public resources. In particular, the baseline case posits an 80% relapse rate, with no postprogram risk reduction among treatment participants who return to injection drug use. This estimate is intended to represent typical performance of feasible interventions targeting IDUS at greatest disease risk.[6–8]

Despite such pessimistic assumptions, widespread methadone treatment is found to reduce HIV incidence and prevalence at an average cost of between $100,000 and $300,000 per infection averted. These results are robust to most parameter changes in the simulation model. In some cases, treatment regimes that target high-risk individuals may be even more cost-effective, though data limitations preclude informed estimates of the magnitude of these effects.

Aside from exploring the overall cost-effectiveness of methadone treatment, this chapter uses epidemiological models to offer five tentative insights into the design, targeting, and evaluation of treatment efforts.

• There are important economies of scale in drug treatment. Limited results from oversubscribed treatment regimes do not fairly describe potential benefits associated with widespread treatment.

- Sufficient supply of drug treatment can drive steady-state HIV prevalence close to zero. Imperfect programs with high relapse rates can have a large impact on steady-state prevalence.
- By itself, the effect of methadone on the treated group understates the benefits associated with treatment by ignoring significant reductions in downstream infection. Applied to a sufficiently large fraction of active IDUs, drug treatment reduces population HIV incidence and prevalence, even among IDUs who do not obtain treatment.
- Post-treatment relapse rates are more important than in-treatment adherence in determining cost-effectiveness of treatment. Nonadherence raises the optimal number of treatment slots. However, this has a small impact on costs per averted infection.
- Methadone was more cost-effective during the early 1980s than it is today, because the prevalence of random needle-sharing has declined over the course of the HIV epidemic.

THE KNOWN IMPACT
OF METHADONE TREATMENT

A voluminous literature examines the impact of drug treatment on the well-being and social performance of injection drug users. Properly implemented methadone treatment has been shown to significantly reduce opiate use in many studies. In-treatment IDUs often relapse or attend a sequence of treatment interventions over a drug-using career. Even if relapse eventually occurs, methadone is associated with significant periods of halted or reduced drug use. Some policy analysts examine the effectiveness of treatment in terms of "drug-free days" to highlight the insight that spells of reduced drug use bring important benefits even when clients eventually return to previous levels of injection drug use.[9]

The efficacy of methadone treatment depends upon many factors: adequate dosage,[6] sociodemographic characteristics,[10] and risk factors such as poly-drug abuse and mental illness.[11] The quality of treatment administrators and clinicians is important, though difficult to capture in empirical studies.[6,12]

Two strands of the existing literature are especially pertinent to this chapter. Several studies document that methadone treatment is cost-effective and perhaps even cost-saving. Hubbard and colleagues and related work examine the impact of methadone on crime, health care costs, and other dimensions of social performance.[13–15] McGlothlin and Anglin[16] present an especially persuasive analysis of the criminal justice and welfare costs associated with the closure of methadone maintenance facilities. Despite methodological concerns and data limitations in specific studies, most published research finds that methadone compares favorably with other treatment modalities, and that methadone is more cost-effective than incarceration in reducing criminal activity, welfare dependence, and other social harms stemming from drug use.[14,17]

A second strand of the literature examines behavioral risk reduction and HIV seroconversion within treatment groups, examining HIV prevention as a component of drug treatment.[18,19] Treatment clients are less likely than out-of-treatment IDUs to share needles and to practice other high-risk behaviors.[20] Treatment clients inject drugs less frequently, thereby reducing accompanying risk.

Most dramatic, Metzger and colleagues found a sixfold difference in HIV seroconversion rates between steady methadone clients and an out-of-treatment group.[21] These results must be cautiously interpreted due to the likelihood of selection effects. In-treatment clients were less likely to report prior needle-sharing and may have been more motivated to avoid HIV risk. Other studies find that involvement in methadone treatment has a smaller protective effect.[6] It is notable, however, that controls for prior reported needle-sharing had only a small impact on the estimated treatment effect.

One unresolved question concerns the value of complementary services such as psychiatric treatment or job counseling in reducing HIV risk. Methadone clients with dual-diagnosis psychiatric disorders, unmarried young men, those with intense criminal justice involvement, and poly-drug users are more likely to engage in risky behavior.[22] The same characteristics are correlated with non-adherence and dropout from treatment.[10] Supplementary services may therefore improve outcomes for high-risk individuals. Yet these services are also costly and administratively complex, and therefore may not be cost-effective in the broader context of severely constrained treatment resources.

Kraft and colleagues[8] provide one of the most complete cost-effectiveness analyses of supplementary services. These authors report median costs per abstinent client-year of $11,887 for methadone treatment with minimum services, $7,932 for methadone plus intensive psychological counseling, and $9,471 for a more fully enhanced service model. Enhanced services produced slightly higher abstinence rates than the intermediate model; however, these superior outcomes did not justify the additional costs. Enhanced services demonstrated the highest level of abstinence over the full study period. It is therefore possible that enhanced services might appear superior when evaluated by other measures such as total drug use. These authors did not examine HIV-specific risk. Enhanced services might therefore prove cost-effective if they (temporarily) reduce needle-sharing or sexual risks among those at greatest risk.

Despite the wealth of studies on various aspects of drug treatment, the link with HIV epidemiology remains obscure. Explicit analytic models have been used to analyze policy issues in needle exchange.[1,2,23] A recent cost-effectiveness analysis by Barnett uses a Markov mortality model to explore the impact of methadone on mortality.[24]

Comparable tools are not available for the analysis of treatment interventions. The variety of drug-using behaviors, HIV incidence, and treatment interventions poses powerful obstacles in the development of relevant analytic models. Individuals vary greatly in the manner, frequency, and social context of their injection drug use. Because injection is a covert behavior, sharing patterns and even the overall number of drug users are unknown despite innovative methods now in development to study these questions.[25,26]

These behavioral uncertainties are especially central in the analysis of drug treatment. Needle exchange programs can be credibly analyzed through study of the needles themselves. For analytic purposes, exchanges are posited to have little effect on underlying behaviors. Such an approach is not appropriate to methadone maintenance, whose main impact on HIV transmission occurs through reduced drug use.

Basic uncertainties also remain concerning HIV epidemiology. Transmission through needle-sharing may depend upon viral load and other complex characteristics of infected and uninfected persons. Existing research on sexual transmission suggests that such matters have important implications for the targeting of prevention efforts.[27]

Perhaps most important, drug treatment itself is not a specific uniform product delivered to uniform consumers. The content and quality of methadone treatment varies greatly. The success of such efforts varies significantly by client population.[10] Some of these differences can be explicitly modeled; many cannot. Previous analyses of drug treatment[28] and needle exchange[29] provide guidance. However, published accounts do not explicitly model disease risk or the impact of treatment to prevent "downstream" infections.

A recent cost-effectiveness analysis by Barnett employs a two-state Markov mortality model to find that methadone is highly cost-effective.[24] However, Barnett does not explicitly consider methadone's impact on subsequent disease spread.

While this chapter was in press, two important analyses were performed by

Zaric and collaborators that consider the cost-effectiveness of methadone as HIV prevention.[30,31] These papers provide a broader analysis of social and health costs than this chapter. They do not consider the range of behavioral and programmatic variables considered here. Though the particulars of their modeling approach differ from this chapter—using cost-utility analysis rather than cost per averted infection—both analyses suggest that methadone maintenance treatment (MMT) is highly cost-effective when compared with other interventions that policy makers value to extend life and improve health.

HOMOGENEOUS MODEL
WITHOUT TREATMENT

Before analyzing the impact of methadone treatment, it is helpful to present a basic susceptible-infected model of HIV transmission in the absence of treatment intervention. The basic model will be familiar to infectious disease epidemiologists.[32] In addition to highlighting basic features of the model, this discussion provides an opportunity to identify major underlying assumptions with their likely implications.

This chapter considers a self-contained population of IDUs. The population recruits new members at a constant rate of θ per day. Entrants are assumed to be HIV-negative though this is not essential. θ determines overall population size but does not influence the qualitative features of the model. It is potentially subject to policy manipulation through deterrence, public education, or social service programs for likely users.

Active users exit the population at random with a constant exit rate of δ/person/unit time. This implies that an individual's drug use "career" is an exponentially distributed random variable with mean duration $(1/\delta)$. In simulations, we assume that $(1/\delta) = 4000$ days (or about 11 years), the approximate mean duration of drug-use behavior. This exit rate is assumed to be independent of HIV status and independent of an IDUs previous experience as a drug user. Drug careers are therefore assumed to be short compared with the natural history of HIV disease.

A more elaborate model would incorporate the cumulative effect of past treatment episodes, and would consider a heterogeneous distribution of drug-using behavior. HIV-positive individuals might also exit the population due to death, treatment, or illness at higher rates than other IDUs.

To simplify a complex pattern of drug-using behavior, we assume that some fixed fraction Ω of IDUs engage in unsafe needle-sharing, while the remaining fraction (1-Ω) practice safer injecting and face no HIV risk. This is a useful model to identify key features of HIV incidence and prevalence. A more realistic model would include varied behaviors from extremely low-risk to extremely high-risk behavior. Many individuals do not attend shooting galleries or share needles with strangers. Yet they may share needles with lovers or close friends, or share cookers, have sex partners who are also IDUs, and engage in other behaviors that bring HIV risk.[33]

Equally important, we assume that sharing occurs in shooting galleries where individuals mix with other injectors. This pattern promotes rapid disease spread as susceptible IDUs encounter many needle partners capable of transmitting the disease. Although heterogeneity is not modeled, shooting galleries are especially dangerous because they create greater opportunity for a minority of high-risk, frequent injectors to encounter other individuals who might otherwise face small individual risks.[33,34]

In this framework, shooting gallery participants are assumed to frequent these locations with a constant arrival rate of λ per unit time. Following Kaplan,[35] IDUs are assumed to frequent galleries once per week. HIV transmission can occur when an uninfected person shares a needle with someone carrying the virus. Because the analysis presumes a homogeneous group of active sharers, a reasonable approximation is the average λ among those injecting at any specific time. Since frequent injectors spend a higher proportion of their time in shooting galleries, the appropriate approximation for λ will exceed the population average.

Given such a discordant pair, we assume a constant infectivity κ, the probability that the virus is actually transmitted. A more complete model would allow κ to vary with infection duration. Jacquez and colleagues[27] argue that HIV-infected individuals are especially infectious during the first two months of infection. For simplicity and due to lack of specific models, we model a constant infectivity here, setting $\kappa = 0.01$. This matches previous work.[36,37]

At any given time t, there are a total of $N(t)$ active IDUs. Of these, $I(t)$ are assumed to be HIV-positive. $I(0)$ is the initial number of infected individuals in the population. It is also useful to write the population HIV prevalence as $\pi(t) = I(t)/N(t)$. We initialize the model assuming that $\pi(0) = 0.3\Omega$. So 30% of active sharers are seropositive at the beginning of the simulation. This appears to be a reasonable estimate of conditions prior to determined policy intervention.[26]

Any positive value of $\pi(0)$ yields the same steady-state value. The population of IDUs is at equilibrium when the number of new entrants balances the num-

Table 6.1. Model Parameters and Baseline Values

Parameter	Definition	Baseline Value
$N(t)$	IDU population	(see text)
$I(t)$	Number of infecteds	(see text)
$\pi(t)$	HIV prevalence	(see text)
Ω	Proportion of shooting gallery participants	0.30
θ	Arrival rate into IDU population	0.5/day
λ	Arrival rates into shooting galleries	1/(7 days)
κ	Infectivity	0.01
δ	Exit rate from active IDU population	1/(4000 days)
Treatment Parameters		
M	Number of treatment slots	(see text)
C	Treatment cost/day	$11.00
β	Reduction in injection rate during treatment	75%
γ	Permanent cure rate of treatment	0.2
μ	Exit rate from treatment	1/(400 days)
Steady-State Values		
N^*	Total IDU population absent treatment	(see text)
π^*	HIV prevalence absent treatment	(see text)
N^+	Total IDU population in the presence of treatment	(see text)
π^+	HIV prevalence given treatment	(see text)

ber of exits. Similarly, the steady-state prevalence π^* is the proportion infected such that the rate of new infections exactly balances the number of infected individuals who exit the population.

Such a random mixing model is most appropriate for drug cultures in which such sharing widely occurs. One large study[33] details HIV risk behaviors among drug users admitted to methadone programs in eight cities during the late 1980s and early 1990s. Attendance at shooting galleries declined in all of these cities. Yet by 1990, more than 20% of respondents in Philadelphia, Baltimore, San Antonio, and New York reported such behavior. Out-of-treatment drug users report higher rates of risky behavior. Methadone clients may also underreport undesired behaviors. These prevalence estimates therefore represent lower bounds on the prevalence of such practices.

This random mixing model can be extended to include overlapping subgroups in which an individual routinely shares needles within her subgroup, with only occasional contact with others. More elaborate contact patterns and social networks can also be modeled using graph-theoretic approaches.[34,37]

The presence of highly segregated subgroups tends to depress HIV incidence by reducing the number of HIV-discordant pairs. Table 6.1 summarizes the relevant parameters and simulation values.

FORMAL MODEL

Expressing these relationships more formally, population size $N(t)$ is governed by the differential equation

$$\frac{dN}{dt} = \theta - \delta N, \qquad N(0) = N_0. \qquad (1)$$

In other words, the rate of population increase is the number of entrances per unit time (θ) minus the per-participant exit rate (δ) time population size ($N(t)$). The system reaches equilibrium when $dN/dt = 0$, or

$$N^* = \frac{\theta}{\delta} \qquad (2)$$

N^* simply scales the problem in this formulation.

The number of infected persons $I(t)$ follows a more complex relationship described in (3):

$$\frac{dI}{dt} = -\delta I(t) + \kappa\lambda[\Omega N(t) - I(t)]\frac{I(t)}{\Omega N(t)}, \qquad I(0) = 0.3\Omega N_0 \qquad (3)$$

The first right-hand term reflects the normal exit process of IDUs from the population, and the fact that all new entrants are uninfected.

The second term deserves more careful consideration. At time t, there are $\Omega N(t)$ active sharers, of whom $[\Omega N(t) - I(t)]$ remain uninfected and therefore susceptible to the disease. Given the arrival rate λ into shooting galleries, $\lambda[\Omega N(t) - I(t)]$ uninfected sharers attend a shooting gallery per unit time.

In similar fashion, $\lambda I(t)$ infected sharers frequent shooting galleries during the same period. (Since shooting galleries are the only source of HIV risk in the model, all infected sharers come from the subgroup that frequents these places.) Thus, a total of $\lambda\Omega N(t)$ people are present in a shooting gallery per unit time.

Each uninfected sharer is randomly paired with another gallery participant. Given random sharing, the odds of *one's partner* being infected is the proportion of infected individuals, or $\lambda I(t)/\lambda\Omega N(t) = \pi(t)/\Omega$. Since shooting galleries contain the individuals at greatest risk, HIV prevalence in these places is far higher than the overall prevalence among all IDUs.

Thus, the number of discordant partnerships is $\lambda[\Omega N(t) - I(t)]*[I(t)/\Omega N(t)]$. Since some fraction κ of these pairs result in new infection, one produces equation (3). Such equations can be analytically solved in many cases.[32]

Setting dI/dt to zero, one can also solve for the steady-state prevalence.

$$\pi^* = \max\left\{0, \Omega(1 - \frac{\delta}{\kappa\lambda})\right\} \qquad (4)$$

Notice that an infected sharer has, on average, $\lambda^*(1/\delta)$ sharing experiences, and she will infect some fraction κ of her uninfected sharing partners. If the gallery prevalence is π^*/Ω, she will, on average, infect precisely one other person before leaving the population. If δ exceeds $\kappa\lambda$, the epidemic will eventually die out because the number of new infections cannot match the number of infected IDUs leaving the population.

Over time, policy interventions that shorten drug careers (raise δ), reduce the frequency of needle-sharing (reduce λ), or reduce the infectivity of needle-sharing contacts (reduce κ) can have a large impact on the course of the epidemic. Reducing Ω—the proportion of individuals who frequent shooting galleries—will reduce steady-state prevalence, but will not eliminate the disease since the steady-state gallery prevalence is always $[1 - \delta/\kappa\lambda]$. Eliminating the disease in these settings requires measures such as the provision of bleach that reduce risk among remaining participants.

Finally, note that the relevant policy goal is to *minimize the number of new infections over time*. Consistent resource allocation requires calculation of present discounted values (*PDV*) to reflect the timing of costs and benefits. If one uses a discount rate of r per unit time,

$$PDV[Incidence] = \int_0^\infty \exp[-rt]\kappa\lambda[\Omega N(t) - I(t)]\frac{I(t)}{\Omega N(t)} dt \qquad (5)$$

In keeping with common practice, we employ an annual discount rate of 3%.

INCLUDING METHADONE IN THE MODEL

This section develops a simple model that incorporates methadone treatment. As discussed above, treatment programs greatly vary in content, quality, and client population. Moreover, published evaluations have used many yardsticks to report program performance and cost. Drug treatment influences drug behavior in many ways. IDUs who relapse often display lower rates of drug use, and may exit more quickly from the drug-using population. Methadone treatment may also link clients with important social and medical services that influence HIV risk, drug use, and general well-being.[14]

Methadone treatment also reduces HIV risk in many ways. Many treatment programs follow harm-reduction principles in teaching clients about the dangers of needle-sharing and providing instruction in the proper cleaning of injection equipment.[18] Treatment may also encourage condom use, though programs report mixed success in influencing sexual risks.

This analysis abstracts from a complex reality by presuming that methadone treatment reduces drug use for a (random) period of T days. T is assumed exponentially distributed with mean $(1/\mu)$. The initial analysis presumes perfect adherence during the treatment period. This assumption is relaxed in the next section.

At the completion of the treatment interval, some fraction γ of IDUs recover and leave the population. All others relapse and resume their pretreatment drug use and HIV risk. Treatment outcomes are assumed independent of HIV status or previous history for the same individual.

The analysis also ignores the complex matching process that links individuals with drug treatment. It is assumed that M treatment slots are provided, and that injection users are randomly assigned to available slots whenever these slots are available. No self-selection or program-initiated sorting policies are modeled in this analysis. M is assumed to be large enough that HIV prevalence among treatment participants closely matches population prevalence. Within the analytic model, M treatment slots are assumed to be added (at time $t = 0$) to a population that was previously in equilibrium absent treatment.

Each treatment slot costs $\$c$ per day in pharmaceutical costs, labor, and other expenses. The analysis presumes that there are no fixed costs of treatment participation. In practice, outreach and standard intake services create significant costs that might be considered in a more elaborate model.

Treatment duration is assumed to be short compared with changes in HIV incidence and prevalence within the IDU population. It is assumed that treatment slots are always used when there are remaining active drug users. The assumption of excess demand matches conditions in many U.S. cities that experience long waiting lists at treatment sites. A more careful model of treatment dynamics and user heterogeneity is the subject of future work.

Baseline estimates for c, γ, and μ are calculated based upon the results of Kraft and collaborators.[8] Using a more pessimistic figure than these authors', it is assumed that 80% of treatment clients eventually return to drug use (so $\gamma = 0.2$). Treatment duration is assumed to have mean duration $(1/\mu)$ of 400 days.

Sensitivity analysis is also performed to determine the impact of these (and other) parameters. Treatment cost is assumed to be $11 per day, matching the cost of methadone treatment with moderate support services.

Treatment services are then embedded in the epidemiological model developed in the previous section, leading to equations (6) and (7) below. Although the model is grossly simplified, it captures important qualitative features of HIV spread. It also allows approximate calculation of the cost-effectiveness of drug services, linking a plausible simplified treatment model with the underlying epidemiology of HIV.

Including the prospect of treatment, population size is governed by the modified population equation.

$$\frac{dN}{dt} = \theta - [N - M]\delta - M\mu\gamma, \qquad N(0) = N^*. \qquad (6)$$

The last term, $M\mu\gamma$, reflects the net exit rate from drug treatment. Note that $M\mu(1 - \gamma)$ treatment clients flow into the population due to relapse. As long as $N(t)$ exceeds the treatment capacity we have

$$\frac{dI}{dt} = [1 - \frac{M}{N(t)}](-\delta I(t) + \kappa\lambda[\Omega N(t) - I(t)]\frac{I(t)}{\Omega N(t)}) - M\mu\gamma\pi, \quad I(0) = 0.3\Omega N^* \qquad (7)$$

Setting dI/dt and dN/dt equal to zero, we find the steady-state values

$$N^+ = N^* - M\left(\frac{\gamma\mu - \delta}{\delta}\right), \qquad \pi^+ = \pi^* - \frac{\Omega M\mu\gamma\delta}{\kappa\lambda(\theta - M\mu\gamma)} \qquad (8)$$

Here N^+ is assumed to be the steady-state IDU population in the presence of treatment, and π^+ is the corresponding steady-state prevalence. (Here N^* and π^* are the steady-state values in the absence of treatment defined in the previous section.) Equation (8) presumes that $N^+ > M$. Otherwise, there are no active injectors and the HIV epidemic dies out.

Equation (8) also implies that a sufficient number of treatment slots will drive steady-state prevalence to zero. A model with imperfect adherence may not satisfy this relationship.

The present discounted cost of M permanent treatment slots is simply $$Mc/r$. At any time t, some fraction $[1 - M/N(t)]$ of IDUs are active users. So the PDV of averted infections is

$$PDV[Incidence] = \int_0^\infty \exp[-rt]\kappa\lambda[\Omega N(t) - I(t)]\frac{I(t)}{\Omega N(t)}[1 - \frac{M}{N(t)}]dt \qquad (9)$$

Discounting becomes important when steady-state prevalence is far from the initial value. If initial prevalence is very low, implementing treatment is less cost-effective than steady-state comparisons imply. One pays for M treatment slots starting from time zero; yet most of the associated benefit is greatly discounted since averted infections occur in later years. These equations are cumbersome to analyze, but their numerical and analytic properties are investigated using the Mathematica package for personal computers.

Figure 6.1 below illustrates qualitative results of this model using baseline parameters for HIV epidemiology, an 80% post-treatment relapse rate. The figure assumes an IDU population of 2000 users. The X-axis represents the number of treatment slots introduced in this population. This model assumes 100% compliance. As discussed in the next section, this is unrealistic. Results for the baseline case of 75% compliance are quite similar.

Given sufficient capacity, treatment reduces HIV incidence and prevalence at an average cost of between $100,000 and $150,000 per averted infection. When drug treatment is very scarce, methadone helps individual clients, but it has a small impact on population prevalence. A more extensive intervention prevents more infections and is more cost-effective. At very low levels of treatment, methadone appears far less cost-effective than it does when applied to a large proportion of active injectors. Based on *average costs,* treatment on demand to all IDUs appears to be an efficient public health intervention.

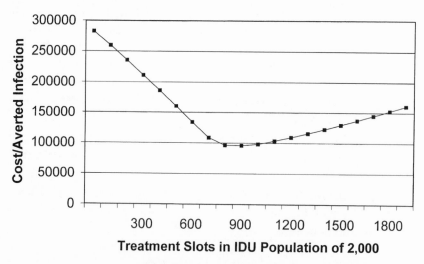

Figure 6.1. Cost-effectiveness of methadone treatment given perfect adherence.

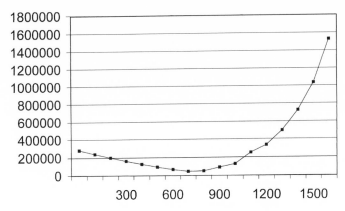

Figure 6.2. Marginal cost-effectiveness of methadone treatment (assuming baseline epidemiological parameters and 100% compliance during treatment).

At the margin, however, treatment on demand appears far less efficient. As shown in Figure 6.2, marginal costs per averted infection rise rapidly. If alternative HIV prevention strategies are available at a cost of $250,000 per averted infection, optimal resource allocation dictates that methadone be implemented until the marginal cost per averted infection reaches this threshold.

With baseline parameters, marginal costs per averted infection exceed $1 million once 80% of IDUs have access to treatment. These scale diseconomies do not reflect declining program effectiveness (though scale diseconomies would aggravate this effect). Declining cost-effectiveness reflects the underlying epidemiology in which treatment has declining marginal impact once steady-state prevalence is driven close to zero.

SENSITIVITY ANALYSIS

The results discussed thus far are predicated on many assumptions and parameter values. In many cases, parameter values are poorly known. Sensitivity analysis is therefore required to identify critical assumptions in the analysis.

Extensive simulations (not reported here) indicate that cost-effectiveness is relatively insensitive to the frequency of needle-sharing, initial prevalence, and treatment duration across the range of empirically plausible values. These parameters alter the optimal allocation of treatment resources but not the resulting cost-effectiveness when resources are optimally deployed.

In contrast, relapse rates and adherence have a more significant impact. These are explored in greater detail below.

RELAPSE RATES AND IMPERFECT ADHERENCE

An actual treatment program elicits imperfect adherence from clients in active treatment. The extent of nonadherence depends on specific programs and specific client groups. Some programs expel clients who are detected with one or more positive urine tests. Other programs adopt more lenient approaches.

The type of nonadherence also varies. One model is that a fixed proportion of treatment clients exhibit no behavioral change as a result of the intervention while the remainder of treatment clients abstain from needle-sharing during active treatment. This model is easily analyzed with minor modification of the above equations, though results are not reported here.

A related, more pessimistic model posits that all treatment clients reduce the frequency of needle-sharing from λ encounters per week to $(1 - \beta)\lambda$. In this case, one can derive the expression

$$\frac{dI}{dt} = [1 - \frac{\beta M}{N(t)}](-\delta I(t) + \kappa \lambda [\Omega N(t) - I(t)]\frac{I(t)}{\Omega N(t)}) - M\mu\gamma\pi \qquad (10)$$

Table 6.2 below illustrates the qualitative features of the resulting model. Each entry represents the average cost per averted infection for a common scenario in which a stable IDU population of 2000 members is provided 1200 new treatment slots. The proportion of sharers, relapse rates, and treatment adherence vary as shown. Baseline values are used for all other parameters.

As shown, methadone is quite cost-effective when large proportions of IDUs engage in this behavior. Because treatment is not targeted to likely sharers in this model, it is far less cost-effective when needle-sharing is rarely practiced in the relevant population. Because needle-sharing among strangers was more prevalent during the mid-1980s than it is today, untargeted treatment is less cost-effective today than it was a decade ago.

Within a given population, such results also highlight the importance of targeting subpopulations of likely sharers in treatment interventions. Treatment entry criteria that identify likely sharers can dramatically increase the cost-effectiveness of subsequent interventions.

Also shown is the surprisingly weak link between in-treatment adherence and cost-effectiveness. Nonadherence of 50% yields similar costs per averted infection as perfect adherence in this model. Treatment regimes that produce eventual exit from the IDU population have a substantial epidemiological impact even when individual adherence to treatment appears poor at any specific point.

Table 6.2. Average Cost Per Averted Infection, 1200 Treatment Slots, Varying Needle-Sharing and Treatment Adherence Rates (Other Parameters Set to Baseline Values)

30% Active Needle Sharing	50% Treatment Compliance	75% Treatment Compliance	Full Treatment Compliance
90% Relapse	$321,304	$278,720	$240,166
80% Relapse	140,655	113,083	103,634
70% Relapse	114,072	104,695	99,540
60% Relapse	107,140	101,912	98,419
20% Active Needle Sharing	**50% Treatment Compliance**	**75% Treatment Compliance**	**Full Treatment Compliance**
90% Relapse	$481,932	$418,062	$360,236
80% Relapse	210,983	169,625	155,458
70% Relapse	171,108	157,042	149,306
60% Relapse	160,710	152,868	147,630
10% Active Needle Sharing	**50% Treatment Compliance**	**75% Treatment Compliance**	**Full Treatment Compliance**
90% Relapse	$963,556	$836,151	$720,491
80% Relapse	421,966	339,249	310,917
70% Relapse	342,217	314,085	298,613
60% Relapse	321,421	305,736	295,260

Post-treatment relapse rates play a much stronger role. An intervention with 90% relapse rates is roughly half as cost-effective as one with an 80% relapse rate. Programs with 60% relapse rates or lower appear highly cost-effective across the range of plausible parameters.

Perhaps surprising, the optimal *number* of treatment slots is generally higher given high relapse rates than it would be in an otherwise comparable, perfectly adherent one. If methadone remains cost-effective with high relapse rates, the optimal policy is to provide a very large number of available slots.

The accompanying figures explain these apparently paradoxical results. Figure 6.3 shows the average cost curves for two interventions, one with an 80% relapse rate, and one with a 90% relapse rate. Average costs per averted infection prove surprisingly similar. However, the high relapse rate requires a much higher treatment capacity to reduce new infections.

Figure 6.4 below shows similar information by computing the *marginal cost* per averted infection for the two interventions. If, for example, alternative HIV

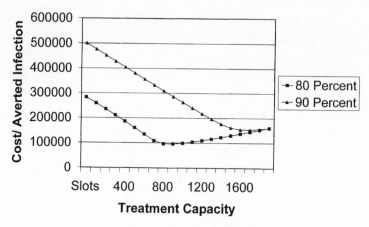

Figure 6.3. The impact of relapse on cost-effectiveness.

prevention interventions are available for $300,000 per averted infection, the optimal number of treatment slots is almost 50% higher for a treatment that brings high relapse rates as for one that greatly reduces post-treatment drug use.

DISCUSSION

This chapter examines a simplified but empirically reasonable model of methadone treatment. Evaluated solely as an HIV prevention measure, widespread availability of treatment is shown to significantly reduce disease prevalence. Baseline assumptions result in costs per averted infection below $200,000

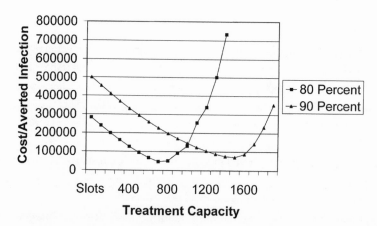

Figure 6.4. Marginal costs and relapse rates.

given the optimal deployment of treatment resources. This is a prudent social investment when compared to other interventions Americans value to prolong and to extend human life.

As in the case of needle exchange, methadone has the greatest epidemiological impact when it is widely available to the population at greatest risk. These analytic results mirror the empirical findings of Des Jarlais and other authors who have studied cross-national HIV prevention strategies. These authors find that Amsterdam and other cities have maintained low HIV prevalence through the provision of extensive and varied services to IDUs.[38]

The stylized model presented includes many simplifications. The remainder of the discussion steps outside of the formal model to consider several important issues.

Including Behavioral Heterogeneity

A more realistic model would include variation in risk-behavior among needle-sharers. For example, an individual may share needles with only her spouse or a close friend. Yet her sharing partner may practice riskier behavior.

Simulation analysis (not reported here) expands the model to accommodate high-risk frequent injectors and low-risk types. A companion paper in progress explores these issues in greater depth. Due to the lack of reliable data, only the qualitative implications of this modeling are summarized here.

If high-risk and low-risk groups are equally responsive to treatment, it is generally optimal to give high-risk individuals top priority in available treatment. High-risk individuals are more likely to be HIV-positive. Because they share more frequently, they create more opportunities for disease spread.

If epidemiological conditions are severe, steady-state prevalence can approach 100% in the high-risk group and can become very high within low-risk groups as well. In such extreme cases, treatment provision has little impact on steady-state prevalence in either group. A cream-skimming strategy may then be optimal. Because low-risk individuals are less likely to be infected, some can be protected by placing them into treatment before they seroconvert.

In many cases, however, high-risk individuals perform poorly in methadone treatment. HIV risk is associated with more frequent needle-sharing, psychiatric disorders, poly-drug use, and other factors that are correlated with poor entry and retention. Many high-risk individuals who enter treatment are expelled due to positive urine tests and other nonadherence with prescribed treatment.

If the objective is to allocate resources to minimize relapse or to maximize the number of drug-free days, it is prudent to allocate scarce treatment to the most promising eligible clients. From the viewpoint of HIV epidemiology, the proper objective is to minimize the number of needle-sharing encounters between infected and susceptible individuals. Small behavior changes among frequent injectors can therefore produce important population effects. Targeting high-risk groups treatment may be optimal even when frequent injectors exhibit lower compliance and have higher relapse rates than other treatment candidates.

Should HIV-Infected Individuals Be Targeted for Drug Treatment?

Some jurisdictions give priority to HIV-positive individuals in allocating treatment slots, though this appears to be unusual.[7] There are many nonepidemiological reasons to enroll HIV-positive individuals since reduced drug use is important for overall well-being. Like pregnant women, HIV-infected individuals have costly, specialized, and complex medical needs that may create obstacles for many treatment programs.

From an epidemiological perspective, targeting treatment based on HIV status has some important advantages. Serostatus is a verifiable condition less vulnerable to ambiguity or deceptive self-reports. Allocating services based on HIV status may also increase incentives for early counseling and testing.

From an epidemiological perspective, targeting individuals based upon current risk behavior is more difficult to implement but has more powerful results. Frequent needle-sharers—even those who are HIV-negative—are more likely to spread infection than HIV-positive individuals who take minimal behavioral risks. If infectivity peaks early in the natural history of HIV disease, there is even more reason to target uninfected risk-takers as the highest priority group.

Are Supplemental Services Cost-Effective in Preventing HIV?

Psychiatric services, job counseling, and other ancillary services are correlated with improved outcomes.[6,39] However, these services increase unit costs and complexity of methadone treatment services. Supplemental services may therefore not represent a cost-effective use of scarce treatment resources.

No uniform answer to this question can be offered, but optimization principles suggest two relevant concerns. Supplemental services are cost-effective only when they are properly targeted. Psychiatric services are not cost-effective when provided to low-risk individuals who are unlikely to contract or spread the disease. Socially advantaged drug users generally face the lowest HIV risks.

Yet the same group has access to the most extensive bundle of treatment services. This is not a cost-effective allocation of social resources.

Cost-effectiveness also depends upon the true alternative uses of resources used to implement supplemental services. If the binding constraint is the overall budget, provision of supplemental services will reduce the available supply of treatment services. If, however, the major constraint is the scarcity of clinical and managerial skill, the optimal policy may be to finance extensive services implemented by the best available treatment organizations.

What is the Role of Corrections in Reducing HIV Spread?

Injection drug use is an illegal and expensive behavior that disrupts users' ability to fulfill legitimate social roles. Most IDUs therefore encounter the correctional system in the course of their drug use.

As documented by Altice and colleagues,[40] corrections offers an important opportunity to locate and to treat individuals who might otherwise avoid or lack access to standard drug treatment services. Extensive criminal behavior is a risk factor for HIV infection and for unsafe and frequent injection. Correction-based intervention therefore provides an opportunity to reach important core groups in HIV spread.

Parole and probation systems offer an especially important opportunity for correctional-based intervention. Demonstration projects and prior research are not definitive, but evidence suggests that close supervision and frequent drug-testing reduce the likelihood and frequency of drug use.[7] Pollack and collaborators provide a recent analysis of these issues, focusing on discharge planning, entitlement security, and case management as essential elements of appropriate health care and preventive services to the growing population of supervised offenders.[41]

Penalties for Nonadherent Methadone Maintenance Treatment Clients

Treatment programs have varying philosophies regarding the proper response to patient nonadherence.[6] Many programs expel clients who appear with "dirty urines" or whose illegal drug use is otherwise detected. Philosophies differ regarding the proper balance between deterrence and support. Most recently, Jonathan Caulkins and Sally Satel argue for stringent policies to deter cocaine use and to improve the overall environment of substance abuse treatment.[42] As these authors argue, "[Expelling clients who repeatedly test positive for cocaine] might substantially reduce cocaine abuse among current methadone patients. Some would fail to control their cocaine use, but expelling them would free up their slots for other, more compliant patients while reinforcing the clinic's commitment to the behavioral standards it sets."

Given long waiting lists for treatment in many areas, these authors are correct that more stringent policies may improve access for more adherent patients, while improving the overall environment of substance abuse treatment. Although these are important benefits, it is noteworthy that treatment providers resist such policies. As Caulkins and Satel themselves report, providers fear that expelled cocaine users will face especially high HIV risk. From an epidemiological perspective, providers have a strong case if permissive policies toward current treatment clients create greater opportunities for eventual cessation of injection drug use.

Is Treatment "On Demand" Cost-Effective?

At the margin, providing treatment to all IDUs becomes cost-ineffective once the supply of available treatment is sufficient to drive steady-state prevalence close to zero. In this sense, treatment on demand is inefficient if all active injectors seek treatment. In practice, however, the current analysis confirms the value of widespread treatment for eligible IDUs. Given the strong scale economies to emerge from the analytic and numerical simulations, providing treatment to the entire IDU population proved far more cost-effective than the treatment environment in many U.S. cities that can only accommodate a small minority of eligible IDUs.

How Does Methadone Treatment Compare with Less Intense Interventions?

Viewed solely as an HIV prevention measure, methadone appears slightly less cost-effective than needle exchange and other low-intensity prevention efforts. In contrast to many harm-reduction interventions, such treatment brings documented reductions in drug use, criminal activity, and other important areas of social performance. Methadone thereby addresses a broader social agenda strongly valued in communities affected by injection drug use.

Linking Prevention to Treatment

In populations that incur significant HIV incidence through needle-sharing, well-implemented methadone treatment appears essential to a balanced HIV prevention strategy. Drug treatment and less-intensive prevention interventions are likely to be most effective as part of a coordinated package of needed care. This is difficult to accomplish given the many institutional practices and incentives to separate these functions.

In recent years, some treatment programs and HIV community prevention planners have attempted to reduce these barriers. Under current law, CDC-provided HIV prevention funds cannot be used to reimburse treatment services. However, several jurisdictions have deployed these funds to support HIV "prevention case managers" who recruit high-risk IDUs and to appropriately place these individuals into treatment. Enhanced needle-exchange programs include outreach and other components designed to link IDUs with drug treatment, psychiatric counseling, and other social services. This more expansive mission brings greater political legitimacy to needle-exchange efforts. It also identifies men and women at the core of the epidemic who in the absence of treatment are most likely to spread new infections.

Can Methadone Treatment Prevent Hepatitis C?

Perhaps the most unsettling questions concern the ability of methadone treatment to prevent other blood-borne diseases. Most important, can it slow the spread of Hepatitis C (HCV), which has already infected the great majority of IDUs?[43] Although HCV and HIV are spread through the same social processes and behavioral risks, HCV is far more efficiently transmitted and is therefore far more difficult to contain through either treatment or harm-reduction interventions.

Preliminary estimates suggest that neither methadone nor needle exchange, acting in isolation, can effectively slow HCV spread.[44] Acting in combination, however, both types of interventions have the potential to slow disease spread.[45] Finding the right combination of feasible low-intensity and intensive interventions remains a central challenge for policy makers. Epidemiologically grounded analytic models are one essential component of this effort.

REFERENCES

1. Kaplan, E. H. Economic analysis of needle exchange. *AIDS* 1995; 9(10):1113–1119.
2. Kahn, J. G. The cost-effectiveness of HIV prevention targeting: How much more bang for the buck. *American Journal of Public Health* 1996; 86(12):1709–1712.
3. Holtgrave, D. R. and J. A. Kelly. Preventing HIV/AIDS among high-risk urban women: The cost-effectiveness of a behavioral group intervention. *American Journal of Public Health* 1996; 86(10):1442–1445.

4. Currie, J. and J. Gruber. Saving babies. *Journal of Political Economy* 1996; 104(6): 1263–1296.
5. Tengs, T. O., M. Adams, et al. Five-hundred life-saving interventions and their cost-effectiveness. *Risk Analysis* 1995; 15:369–390.
6. Ball, J. C. and A. Ross. *The Effectiveness of Methadone Maintenance Treatment: Patients, Programs, Services, and Outcome.* New York: Springer-Verlag, 1991.
7. Kleiman, M. *Against Excess: Drug Policy for Results.* New York: Basic Books, 1993.
8. Kraft, M. K., A. B. Rothbard, et al. Are supplementary services provided during methadone maintenance really cost-effective? *American Journal of Psychiatry* 1997; 154(9):1214–1219.
9. Boyum, D. and M. Kleiman. Alcohol and other drugs. *Crime.* J. Q. Wilson and J. Petersilia. San Francisco: Institute for Contemporary Studies, 1995.
10. Hser, Y.-I., Anglin M. D., et al. A survival analysis of gender and ethnic differences in responsiveness to methadone maintenance treatment. *International Journal of the Addictions* 1990–1991; 25(11A):1295–1315.
11. Kosten, T. R., B. J. Rounsaville, et al. "A 2.5 year follow-up of depression, life crises, and treatment effects on abstinence among opioid addicts." *Archives of General Psychiatry* 1986; 3(3):733–738.
12. Magura, S., P. C. Nwakeze, et al. Pre- and in-treatment predictors of retention in methadone treatment using survival analysis. *Addiction* 1998; 93(1):51–60.
13. Gerstein, D. R. and H. J. Harwood. *Treating Drug Problems.* Washington, DC: National Academy Press, Institute of Medicine, 1990.
14. Egertson, J. A., D. M. Fox, et al., Eds. *Treating Drug Abusers Effectively.* Malden, MA: Blackwell, 1997.
15. Hubbard, R. L. *Drug Abuse Treatment: A National Study of Effectiveness.* Chapel Hill, NC: University of North Carolina Press, 1989.
16. McGlothlin, W. H. and M. D. Anglin. Shutting off methadone: Costs and benefits. *Archives of General Psychiatry* 1981; 38(8):885–892.
17. Caulkins, J. P., C. P. Rydell, et al. *Mandatory Minimum Drug Sentences: Throwing Away the Key or the Taxpayers' Money?* Santa Monica, CA: RAND Drug Policy Research Center, 1997.
18. D'Aunno, T. and T. Vaughn. Variations in methadone treatment practices: Results from a national study. *Journal of the American Medical Association* 1992; 267(2):253–258.
19. Brown, B. and R. Needle. Modifying the process of treatment to meet the threat of AIDS. *International Journal of the Addictions* 1994; 29(13):1739–1752.
20. Ball, J., W. Lange, et al. Reducing the risk of AIDS through methadone maintenance treatment. *Journal of Health and Social Behavior* 1988; 214–226.
21. Metzger, D., G. Woody, et al. Human immunodeficiency virus seroconversion among intravenous drug users in- and out-of-treatment: An 18-month prospective follow-up. *Journal of Acquired Immune Deficiency Syndromes and Human Retrovirology* 1993; 6(9): 1049–1056.
22. Metzger, D., G. Woody, et al. Risk factors for needle sharing among methadone-treated patients. *American Journal of Psychiatry* 1991; 148(5):636–640.

23. Kaplan, E. Probability models of needle exchange. *Operations Research* 1995; 43(4):558–569.

24. Barnett, P. The cost-effectiveness of methadone maintenance as a health care intervention. *Addiction* 1999; 94(4):479–488.

25. Kaplan, E. and D. Soloschatz. How many drug injectors are there in New Haven? Answers from AIDS data. *Mathematical and Computer Modelling* 1993; 17(2):109–115.

26. Holmberg, S. D. The estimated prevalence and incidence of HIV in 96 large U.S. metropolitan areas. *American Journal of Public Health* 1996; 86:642–654.

27. Jacquez, J., J. Koopman, et al. Role of the primary infection in epidemics of HIV infection in gay cohorts. *Journal of Acquired Immune Deficiency Syndromes and Human Retrovirology* 1994; 7:1169–1184.

28. Rydell, C., J. Caulkins, et al. Enforcement or treatment? Modeling the relative efficacy of alternatives for controlling cocaine. *Operations Research* 1996; 44(5):687–695.

29. Hagan, H., D. Des Jarlais, et al. Reduced risk of Hepatitis B and Hepatitis C among injection drug users in the Tacoma Syringe Exchange Program. *American Journal of Public Health* 1996; 85:1531–1537.

30. Zaric, G. S., M. L. Brandeau, and P. G. Barnett. Methadone maintenance and HIV prevention: A cost-effectiveness analysis. *Management Science* 2000; 46:1013–1031.

31. Zaric, G. S., P. G. Barnett, and M. L. Brandeau. HIV transmission and the cost-effectiveness of methadone maintenance. *Am J Public Health* 2000; 90:1100–1111.

32. Anderson, R. M. and R. M. May. *Infectious Diseases of Humans.* Oxford: Oxford University Press, 1991.

33. Battjes, R., R. Pickens, et al. HIV infection and AIDS risk behaviors among injection drug users entering methadone treatment: An update. *Journal of Acquired Immune Deficiency Syndromes and Human Retrovirology* 1995; 10:90–96.

34. Des Jarlais, D. and S. Friedman. Shooting galleries and AIDS: Infection probabilities and 'tough' policies. *American Journal of Public Health* 1990; 80(2):142–144.

35. Kaplan, E. H. Needles that kill: Modeling human immunodeficiency virus transmission via shared needle injection equipment in shooting galleries. *Reviews of Infectious Diseases* 1989; 11(2):289–298.

36. Kaplan, E. and R. Heimer. A model-based estimate of HIV infectivity via needle sharing. *Journal of Acquired Immune Deficiency Syndromes and Human Retrovirology* 1992; 5:1116–1118.

37. Kretzschmar, M. and L. Wiessing. Modelling the spread of HIV in social networks of injecting drug users. *AIDS* 1998; 12(7):801–811.

38. Des Jarlais, D. C. The 1993 Okey Memorial Lecture: Cross-national studies of AIDS among injecting drug users. *Addiction* 1994; 89(4):383–392.

39. McLellan, A. T., I. O. Arndt, et al. The effects of psychosocial services in substance abuse treatment. *Journal of the American Medical Association* 1993; 269(15):1953–1959.

40. Altice, F., F. Mostashari, et al. Predictors of HIV infection among newly sentenced male prisoners. *Journal of Acquired Immune Deficiency Syndromes and Human Retrovirology* 1998; 18(5):444–453.

41. Pollack, H., K. Khoshnood, et al. Health care delivery strategies for criminal offenders. *Journal of Health Care Finance* 1999; 26(1):63–78.
42. Caulkins, J., and S. Satel. Methadone patients should not be allowed to persist in cocaine use. *FAS Drug Policy Analysis Bulletin* 1999; 7.
43. Coutinho, R. HIV and Hepatitis C among injecting drug users: Success in preventing HIV has not been mirrored for Hepatitis C. *British Medical Journal* 1998; 317:424–425.
44. Pollack, H. A. *Cost-effectiveness of methadone as HIV prevention*. National HIV Prevention Conference, Centers for Disease Control and Prevention, CDC, 1999.
45. Pollack, H. Can we protect drug users from Hepatitis C? *Journal of Policy Analysis and Management* 2001; 20(2):358–364.

Chapter 7 Costs and Benefits of Imperfect HIV Vaccines: Implications for Vaccine Development and Use

Douglas K. Owens, Donna M. Edwards, and Ross D. Shachter

HIV VACCINES: RATIONALE
AND CHALLENGES

In less than 20 years, 47 million people have been infected with the human immunodeficiency virus (HIV).[1] New HIV infections now occur at a rate of about 16,000 per day worldwide.[1] Approximately 14 million people have died from HIV infection—2.5 million died in 1998 alone.[1] The HIV pandemic now ranks as one of the worst epidemics in history, taking its place alongside bubonic plague and influenza which caused devastating losses of human life. The introduction of highly active antiretroviral therapy has prolonged survival with HIV infection,[2] but the high cost of these drugs puts them out of reach of the developing world, where over 95% of the people who have HIV live.[1] For the developing world, the options for preventing further spread of HIV are interventions to reduce behaviors that transmit HIV, or the development of an affordable HIV vaccine.

Development of an HIV vaccine is difficult for many reasons, as recently summarized by Letvin.[3] Investigators do not understand which elements of the immune response provide protection from infection.

A primary question is whether an antibody response is sufficient to control or prevent infection, or whether a vaccine must also induce a cellular immune response by inducing HIV-1 specific cytotoxic T-lymphocytes (CTLs)—white-blood cells that are important in the control of many infections.[3] After infection with HIV, viral replication occurs rapidly, with the development of many mutations that may escape recognition by the immune system.[3] In addition, HIV viral RNA is reverse transcribed into DNA that integrates into the infected person's genetic material; this proviral DNA can exist indefinitely, and can begin viral replication at any time.[3] Thus, HIV genetic information is hidden from the immune system. Furthermore, specific mucosal immunity may be essential in preventing HIV infection through sexual activity.[3] Finally, HIV-1 can be classified into clades—strains of viruses that are similar based on nucleotide sequencing.[4] Most infections in North America are caused by clade B viruses, whereas clade A and D viruses cause most infections in Africa. Whether a vaccine that provided immunity to virus from one clade would also protect against viruses from other clades is not known.

Although development of an HIV vaccine has proved challenging,[3,5,6] over 34 candidate vaccines have undergone phase I trials that test safety and antigenicity, and three have undergone phase II trials.[7-12] For example, investigators recently announced the start of the first phase I trial, performed in Africa, to test a vaccine that uses the avian canarypox virus as a vector to introduce HIV genes into cells of the vaccine recipient. Currently, a preventive vaccine, AIDS-VAX, that uses as an immunogen recombinant gp 120, an HIV envelope protein, is in phase III efficacy trials.[7] In late spring of 2000, the U.S. National Institutes of Health (NIH) announced that a phase III efficacy trial of a therapeutic vaccine would begin. The trial will test a vaccine made from an inactivated virus in patients who are taking antiretroviral medication.

As noted, both preventive and therapeutic vaccines are under development. A *preventive vaccine* is given to an uninfected person with the aim of preventing infection, or at least preventing development of disease. A *therapeutic vaccine* is administered to a person who is already infected with HIV, with the aim of slowing or stopping the progression of disease. A therapeutic vaccine would presumably slow disease progression by reducing viral replication, in turn reducing levels of virus in body fluids, and thus might reduce infectivity.[13] However, a therapeutic vaccine also prolongs the life of the vaccine recipient, and thus could perversely lead to increased transmission of HIV. Complicating this picture, some vaccines may both reduce the probability of infection and, in people who do become infected, slow the development of disease. Whether a vaccine is preventive or therapeutic is important because it determines who gets vaccinated and who bears the risks and benefits associated with the vaccine.

Given the challenges inherent in its development, an HIV vaccine may not provide perfect protection against infection. The trials of the AIDSVAX vaccine, now under way in the United States and Thailand, have been controversial because of concerns that the vaccine will not elicit a CTL response and therefore will not provide protection against infection. The NIH initially refused to support the trials because of this concern. The controversy has highlighted a difficult question: how promising should a candidate vaccine be for it to be used in human trials of efficacy?

We summarize here our analyses of the costs and benefits of potential preventive and therapeutic HIV vaccines. We used a mathematical model to evaluate the costs and benefits of vaccines in early-stage epidemics, in which prevalence is low but rising, and in late-stage epidemics, in which prevalence is high but dropping. We assessed the use of a vaccine in a hypothetical group of homosexual men that we designed to reflect the population and conditions in San Francisco, California. We evaluated the effect of vaccine programs on the prevalence of HIV, on the number of new cases of HIV, on quality-adjusted life years (QALYs) in the vaccinated population, and on costs. The cost-effectiveness analyses that we present here showed that vaccines of even modest efficacy can provide enormous health and economic benefits. We shall argue that trials of such vaccines are justifiable, because even such imperfect vaccines would be highly beneficial if used in an appropriate population.

METHODS

We developed a mathematical model that simulated the course of the HIV epidemic in a cohort of vaccinated and unvaccinated homosexual men. The model predicted health outcomes and economic outcomes for each cohort. Detailed descriptions of our model and input data have been published elsewhere.[14-16] In estimating cost-effectiveness, we used a societal perspective and discounted costs and benefits at 5%.

Model Structure

Our dynamic, compartmental epidemic model[17-20] simulated the course of the epidemic in representative of the population of homosexual men in San Francisco.[14-16] The model evaluated the health and economic outcomes for an unvaccinated group, a group vaccinated with a preventive vaccine (Figure

Unvaccinated Cohort　　　Vaccinated Cohort

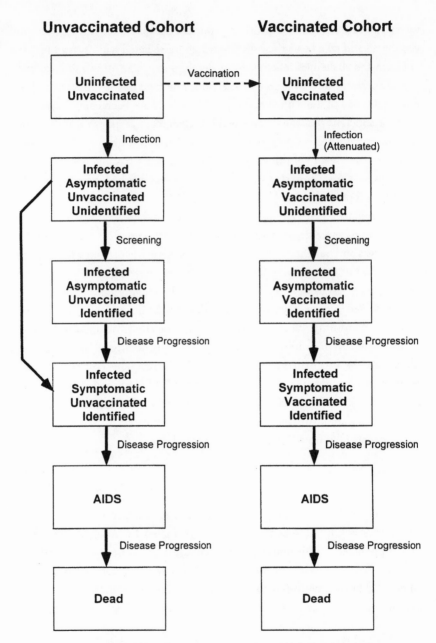

Figure 7.1. Schematic diagram of the preventive vaccine model. Each box represents a homogenous group (or compartment) in the population. Transitions among compartments were governed by the equations shown in the Appendix. Dashed arrow indicates vaccination. Thin arrow represents decreased rate of new HIV infections as a result of vaccination.

7.1), and a group vaccinated with a therapeutic vaccine (Figure 7.2). In such models—which are a standard approach for simulating the course of infectious disease epidemics—mathematical equations characterize the rate at which people move from one compartment to another (see Appendix). Each compartment represents a population subgroup, as shown in Figures 7.1 and 7.2. For example, the top-left box in Figure 7.1 represents the uninfected, unvaccinated portion of the population. The arrows between the boxes represent the mechanisms for moving from one population group to another. For example, people moved from the uninfected, unvaccinated compartment to the infected, asymptomatic, unidentified, unvaccinated compartment by becoming infected with HIV. Thus, the rate of movement between these boxes depends on the rate of incident HIV infection for the population. In each figure, the dotted arrow indicates vaccination. The thin arrow in each figure shows the mechanism by which the vaccine works. A preventive vaccine program reduced incident HIV infections and thus slowed the rate of transition from the uninfected to the infected compartment. For our model, we assumed that a therapeutic vaccine would prolong life during the asymptomatic period. Therefore, the thin arrow in Figure 7.2 indicates slowed transition from the infected, asymptomatic state to the infected, symptomatic state. For both preventive and therapeutic vaccines, we determined the net effect of the vaccine programs by evaluating the change in outcomes between the unvaccinated and the vaccinated cohort after a given period. We assumed that there was preferential selection of sexual partners: in the model, both uninfected and asymptomatic unidentified people select sexual partners preferentially, but not exclusively, from other members of the population who do not have AIDS.[21,22] We implemented the model both in Stella II[23] and in MATLAB. [24]

Vaccine Characteristics

Because the characteristics of an HIV vaccine are not yet known, we analyzed vaccines that had a variety of characteristics, borrowing heavily from the analytic framework developed by Blower and McLean.[19,20] We evaluated vaccines with differing efficacy, duration, and effects on infectivity. For a preventive vaccine, the efficacy is the proportion of partnerships protected from infection. The duration of the vaccine is the length of time that a vaccine recipient is protected from infection. For a therapeutic vaccine, the efficacy is the increase in length of life provided by the vaccine. Our base-case analyses assumed, for simplicity, that the increased duration of life, as well as any associated decrease in infectivity, occurred during the asymptomatic period. The take of a vaccine is

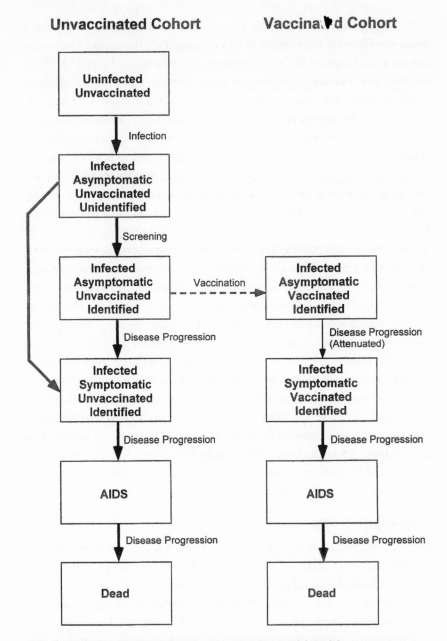

Figure 7.2. Schematic diagram of the therapeutic vaccine model. Each box represents a homogenous group (or compartment) in the population. Transitions among compartments were governed by the equations shown in the Appendix. Dashed arrow indicates vaccination. Thin arrow represents decreased rate of transition to symptomatic HIV disease, as a result of vaccination.

the proportion of people in whom the vaccine has any effect. For the analyses shown here, we assumed vaccine take of 100%. To evaluate the importance of changes in infectivity caused by a therapeutic vaccine, we defined infectivity as the probability of transmission per partnership. Say that we denote a person's infectivity during the asymptomatic period as $b_{1,0}$; we reduced a therapeutic vaccine recipient's infectivity by a factor b_n, so this person's infectivity was equal to $(b_{1,0})(b_n)$.

Health Outcomes

The results of our evaluation of vaccine programs depended substantially on the type of health outcome that we assessed and the time horizon over which we assessed each outcome.[14–16] To provide a comprehensive assessment of vaccine programs, we chose to assess the number of HIV cases averted, the prevalence of HIV in the vaccinated and unvaccinated populations, and the life years saved by the vaccine program. A preventive vaccine results in additional years of life saved in the uninfected healthy population; a therapeutic vaccine results in additional years of life saved in people who are infected with HIV and whose quality of life may vary. To measure on a single scale these outcomes that differ in quality of life, we converted life years saved to QALYs saved (or gained).[25–29] Use of QALYs as an outcome measure enables analysts and policy makers to assess health interventions for different conditions with a common metric; recent guidelines for the conduct of cost-effectiveness analyses recommend the use of QALYs as the preferred approach for valuing health outcomes.[30] We calculated the QALYs gained by a vaccine program by multiplying the length of time that each individual spends in a health state by the quality of life of that health state, assessed on a 0-to-1 scale, where 0 is equivalent to death and 1 is equivalent to perfect health.[25–29] We calculated the total discounted QALYs for the program by summing over all health states that each person experiences during the period of assessment, and then summing over all individuals.

The choice of a time horizon for assessing outcomes also has an important influence on the assessment of a vaccine program.[14–16] We evaluated the effects of a vaccination program that lasted 20 years (that is, vaccine was administered over a period of 20 years). Although the 20-year results are of substantial interest, an analysis that is limited to the 20-year time horizon will underestimate the health benefit of a preventive vaccine program, because the benefit from the program continues beyond the 20-year horizon, even if the vaccine program stops after 20 years. A 20-year time horizon can underestimate or overestimate the health benefits of a therapeutic vaccine program, depending on whether the therapeutic vaccine results in a net increase or decrease in transmission of HIV.[16,31] Paltiel and Kaplan note the hazard of using a short planning horizon for evaluation of interventions.[32] Therefore, we also evaluated the long-term effects (up to 150 years) of a 20-year vaccine program as well.

Economic Outcomes and Costs

We included all incremental costs associated with the implementation of vaccine programs, and treatment costs of any people identified as being infected as a consequence of the vaccine program who would not have been identified without that program. In our base-case analyses, we assumed that an HIV vaccine cost $1000, and we evaluated a wide range of vaccine costs in sensitivity analyses. Our treatment costs were based on the AIDS Cost and Services Utilization Study (ACSUS)[33,34] and from our prior estimates of the cost of treatment.[27] We calculated the marginal cost-effectiveness of vaccine programs by dividing the incremental costs of the program by the incremental health benefit, measured in QALYs.

Input Data

We used published and unpublished data[27,35–41] to estimate the value of input variables for the model (Table 7.1). We used population demographics and estimates of sexual transmission[35,36] to reflect the population of homosexual men in San Francisco. Because risk behaviors may vary across different demographic groups of homosexual men, we evaluated vaccine programs in two types of epidemics. We modeled a late-stage epidemic, in which prevalence was high (49%, consistent with estimates in homosexual men in 1990), risk behavior was attenuated (2 sexual partnerships annually), and prevalence was therefore decreasing; such an epidemic may characterize older homosexual men. We also modeled an early-stage epidemic in which prevalence was low (10%), risk behavior was more common (average 4 partnerships per year), and prevalence was increasing. This level of risk behavior may reflect more closely that of younger homosexual men.[42,43] The initial population size was 55,800; the average age of its members was 30 years.

We evaluated the effects of vaccine programs for a wide range of vaccine characteristics. For our base-case analysis, we evaluated a preventive vaccine with efficacy of 75% and duration of 10 years (Table 7.1). In the base case, we evaluated a therapeutic vaccine that extended the life of all vaccinated people by 5 years and did not change infectivity.

An important consideration about a vaccine program is the effect of the pro-

Table 7.1. Parameter Values and Sources

Name	Base Case	Range
Vaccine Parameters		
Vaccine take (as proportion of those vaccinated), ψ	1	0.1–1
Preventive Vaccines		
Proportion of HIV-susceptible people vaccinated annually, $v_p(t)$	0.75	0.25–0.9
Vaccine efficacy (proportion who are protected from infection), ε	0.75	0.1–0.9
Change in condom use after preventive vaccine, Δ_p	0.75	0.75–1.25
Vaccine duration (years), $1/\omega$	10	5–50
Therapeutic Vaccines		
Proportion of asymptomatic, infected people vaccinated each year, $v_t(t)$	0.75	0.25–0.9
Increase in asymptomatic period due to vaccine (years), $1/\mu_v$	5	1–10
Change in condom use after therapeutic vaccine, Δ_t	0.75	0.75–1.25
Infectivity multiplier for $\beta_{1,0}$, change in infectivity due to vaccine, β_v	1	0.10–1
Transmission Parameters		
Infectivity, asymptomatic period (per-partner probability of transmission of HIV), $\beta_{1,0}{}^a$	0.066	0.044–0.081
Infectivity, symptomatic period (per-partner probability of transmission of HIV), $\beta_{3,0}{}^b$	0.147	0.98–0.179
Annual contact rate, sexual partners, all disease stages except AIDS, late-stage epidemic, p_i^c	2	1.59–5.93
Annual contact rate, sexual partners, all disease stages except AIDS, early-stage epidemic, p_i^c	4	1.59–5.93
HIV Disease Parameters		
Quality of life, uninfected, q_0	1.0	
Quality of life, asymptomatic HIV infection, unidentified, q_1	1.0	
Quality of life, asymptomatic HIV infection, identified $q_2{}^d$	0.83	0.66–1.00
Quality of life, symptomatic HIV infection, $q_3{}^d$	0.42	0.34–0.50
Quality of life, AIDS, $q_4{}^d$	0.17	0.14–0.20

(continued)

Table 7.1. Continued

Name	Base Case	Range
Duration of Disease		
Asymptomatic HIV infection, identified $1/\mu_{1,0}{}^{e}$	8.7	7.1–9.6
Symptomatic HIV infection, $1/\mu_{3,0}{}^{e}$	2.7	2.2–3.2
AIDS, $1/\mu_{4,0}{}^{e}$	2.1	1.7–2.5
Population Parameters		
Population	Homosexual men	—
Initial population size	55,800	—
HIV prevalence, late-stage epidemic	49.3%	10%–50%
HIV prevalence, early-stage epidemic	10%	10%–50%
Average age, years	30	—

Reprinted by permissiom from D. K. Owens, D. M. Edwards, K. D. Schachter, Population effects of preventive and therapeutic vaccines in early- and late-stage epidemics, *AIDS*, 1998; 12(9): 1057–1066. Adapted with permission from D. M. Edwards, R. D. Shachter, D. K. Owens, A dynamic HIV-transmission model for evaluating the costs and benefits of vaccine programs, *Interfaces*, 28: 3 May–June 1998, pp. 144–166. Copyright 1998, the Institute for Operations Research and the Management Sciences, Linthicum, Maryland, USA.

[a]Estimated as 0.45 $\beta_{3,0}$ as in M. L. Brandeau, D. K. Owens, C. H. Sox, R. M. Wachter, Screening women of childbearing age for human immunodeficiency virus: A model-based policy analysis, *Management Science* 1993; 39: 72–92.

[b]Calculated from M. C. Samuel, M. S. Mohr, T. P. Speed, W. Winkelstein, Infectivity of HIV by anal and oral intercourse among homosexual men: Estimates from a prospective study in San Francisco. In E. H. Kaplan and M. L. Brandeau, eds., *Modeling the AIDS Epidemic: Planning, Policy and Prediction,* New York: Raven Press, 1994: 423–438.

[c]Derived from M. C. Samuel, M. S. Mohr, T. P. Speed, W. Winkelstein, Infectivity of HIV by anal and oral intercourse among homosexual men: Estimates from a prospective study in San Francisco. In E. H. Kaplan and M. L. Brandeau, eds., *Modeling the AIDS Epidemic: Planning, Policy and Prediction,* New York: Raven Press, 1994: 423–438, and Communication Technologies in association with the San Francisco AIDS Foundation, HIV-related knowledge, attitudes, and behaviors among San Francisco gay and bisexual men: Results from the fifth population-based survey, San Francisco Department of Public Health, 1990. We assumed that the number of sexual contacts for people with AIDS was one-third the rate noted in the table.

[d]Derived from D. K. Owens, A. B. Cardinalli, R. F. Nease, Jr. Physicians' assessments of the utility of health states associated with human immunodeficiency virus (HIV) and hepatitis B virus (HBV) infection, *Quality of Life Research* 1997; 6: 77–86.

[e]Estimated as in D. K. Owens, R. A. Harris, P. M. Scott, R. F. Nease, Jr. Screening surgeons for HIV infection: A cost-effectivenes analysis, *Ann Intern Med* 1995; 122:641–652.

gram on the vaccine recipients' risk behavior.[19,20] One concern is that a vaccine program might induce a perception of reduced risk and therefore inadvertently increase risk behavior. To account for this concern, we estimated the effect of vaccine programs both with no change in behavior and with a 25% reduction in condom use among vaccine recipients.

Model Validation

To assess the performance of the model, we compared the model output under the assumption of no vaccine program to data on prevalence and incidence of HIV infection estimated or observed in San Francisco from 1990 to 1994. For 1992, the model estimated a prevalence of HIV infection of 41%; estimates from the Department of Public Health indicated a prevalence of 43%. The predicted incidence of AIDS agreed with reported cases to within 15% except for 1992, in which a large number of cases was observed. We performed sensitivity analyses on all model variables.

RESULTS

Preventive-Vaccine Program

A preventive vaccine program in which no change in behavior occurred averted infections and reduced HIV prevalence (Figure 7.3). With the more conservative assumption that vaccine recipients reduced condom use by 25%, a preventive vaccine program nonetheless prevented 2520 infections, accrued 8010 incremental QALYs, and reduced expenditures by $9.4 million in a late-stage epidemic (Table 7.2). Thus, our base-case vaccine, with an efficacy of 75%, provided substantial health benefit and reduced expenditures. As the vaccine efficacy increased, or as duration of protection increased, the health benefits and monetary savings also increased (Figure 7.4A). Especially notable in Figure 7.4A, even vaccines with exceedingly modest efficacy (25%) provide substantial health benefits and are cost-effective by current standards in the United States. For example, a vaccine that has an efficacy of 25% costs less than $50,000 per QALY gained—a commonly used, although arbitrary, benchmark in the United States.[44] A vaccine that provided lifelong protection would reduce costs even if it had an efficacy of only 50% (Figure 7.4A). These results occurred despite the pessimistic assumption that condom use would decrease by 25% in vaccine recipients.

A

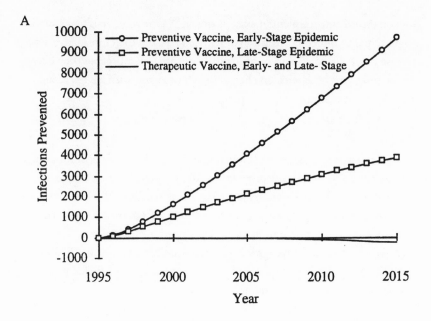

B

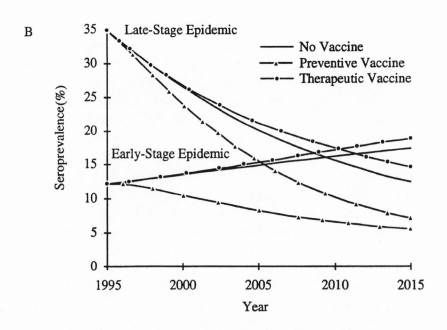

Therapeutic Vaccine Program

A therapeutic vaccine program that engendered no change in risk behavior slightly increased HIV prevalence and the number of HIV infections (Figure 7.3). With the more conservative assumption that vaccine recipients reduced condom use by 25%, the therapeutic vaccine increased total HIV infections by 1040 over a 20-year period (Table 7.2), but nonetheless resulted in an additional 2410 QALYs in the population (Table 7.2). The vaccine program increased expenditures by $9.2 million, and cost $3810 for each QALY gained (Table 7.2). Figure 7.4B shows how changes in the degree to which the vaccine extended life and reduced infectivity affected the costs and benefits of the vaccine program. Of note, therapeutic vaccines that reduced infectivity by 8% or more caused a net decrease in the number of HIV cases and in the HIV prevalence, if there were no reductions in condom use (data not shown); a therapeutic vaccine that reduced infectivity by 50% or more, and added 5 years to the asymptomatic period, reduced net expenditures (Figure 7.4B).

Time Horizon

The time horizon of the analysis had a substantial influence on the estimated costs and benefits of a vaccine program (Figure 7.5). Figure 7.5 illustrates the accrual of costs and benefits of a vaccine program at 1-year intervals. The costs of a preventive vaccine program accumulated quickly, but benefits continued to accrue over time (Figure 7.5A). Thus, a preventive vaccine program appeared less cost-effective when evaluated over shorter time periods. In contrast, a therapeutic vaccine that did not reduce infectivity was less cost-effective over time (Figure 7.5B). In fact, after about 15 years, the net benefit (in QALYs) of the therapeutic vaccine decreased. The decrease occurred because the benefit from increased length of life for vaccine recipients was outweighed by the increased transmission of HIV. For this analysis, we assumed no change in risk behavior, and therefore the net benefit of a therapeutic vaccine program (in

Figure 7.3. Population effects of preventive and therapeutic vaccine programs. Analyses assumed no change in risk behavior due to the vaccine program. (A) Preventive vaccines averted more infections in early-stage than in late-stage epidemics. Therapeutic vaccines slightly increased the number of infections in both early- and late-stage epidemics. (B) The prevalence of HIV is shown for early-stage and late-stage epidemics with no vaccination program and with preventive or therapeutic vaccination programs. Reprinted by permission from D. K. Owens, D. M. Edwards, R. D. Shachter, Population effects of preventive and therapeutic vaccines in early- and late-stage epidemics, *AIDS*, 1998; 12(9):1057–1066.

Table 7.2. Health and Economic Outcomes of Preventive and Therapeutic Vaccines in a Late-Stage Epidemic

	No Vaccine Program		Preventive Vaccine		Therapeutic Vaccine	
	20-Year Outcomes	150-Year Outcomes	20-Year Outcomes	150-Year Outcomes	20-Year Outcomes	150-Year Outcomes
Total Outcomes						
Infections	37,680	38,750	35,160	35,800	38,720	40,230
QALYs	838,670	1,123,790	846,680	1,149,660	841,080	1,118,500
Costs ($M)	6037.1	7195.7	6027.7	7176.8	6046.3	7241.5
Incremental Outcomes						
Infections Averted	—	—	2520	2950	−1040	−1480
QALYs gained	—	—	8010	25,870	2410	−5290
Cost ($M)	—	—	−9.4	−18.8	9.2	45.8
Marginal Cost Effectiveness ($/QALY)	—	—	Dominant[a]	Dominant[a]	3810[b]	Dominated[c]

[a]Dominant indicates that the vaccine program increased QALYs and reduced costs, relative to no vaccine progam.

[b]The marginal cost-effectiveness ratio indicates that a therapeutic vaccine program results in expenditures of $3810 for each additional QALY gained relative to no vaccine.

[c]Dominated indicates that the vaccine program reduced QALYs and increased costs, relative to no vaccine program. This finding does not hold for most therapeutic vaccines that reduce infectivity or for many therapeutic vaccines that are not accompanied by reductions in condom use (see text). Analyses for this table assumed a 25% reduction in condom use in vaccine recipients, a preventive vaccine with 75% efficacy and duration of 10 years, and a therapeutic vaccine that increased the asymptomatic period by 5 years and did not reduce infectivity.

Source: Adapted with permission from D. M. Edwards, R. D. Shachter, D. K. Owens, A dynamic HIV-trasmision model for evaluating the costs and benefits of vaccine programs, Interfaces, 28: 3 May–June 1998, pp. 144–166. Copyright 1998, the Institute for Operations Research and the Management Sciences, Linthicum, Maryland, USA.

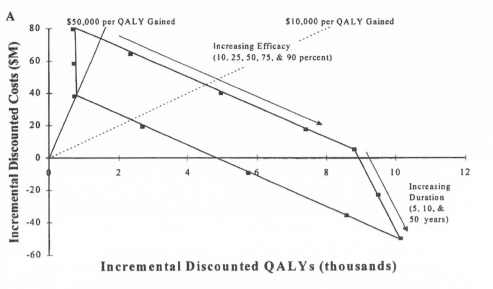

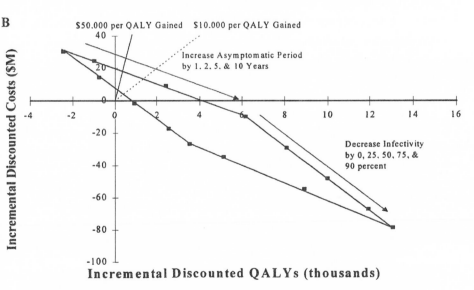

Figure 7.4. Costs and benefits of preventive and therapeutic vaccines. The figure indicates health and economic outcomes for a 20-year period, with a 25% reduction in condom use by vaccine recipients, consistent with Table 7.2. Each polygon indicates the costs and benefits of vaccine with varying characteristics. Points on the polygon that fall below the horizontal axis indicate vaccines that reduce costs; points on the polygon to the right of the vertical axis indicate vaccines that increase quality-adjusted life years (QALYs). The slope of a line from the origin represents the cost-effectiveness ratio in $/QALY. The solid and dotted lines from the origin show the cost-effectiveness ratios of $50,000 per QALY gained and

QALYs) remained positive over long time horizons, in contrast to the more conservative result in Table 7.2.

Epidemic Stage

The relative advantages of preventive and therapeutic vaccines differed in late-stage and early-stage epidemics. Figure 7.6 shows the long-term outcomes for vaccine programs, based on the assumption that no change in behavior occurred. The maximum benefit of the vaccine programs was greater than in our base-case analysis, because of both the longer time frame and the assumption of no behavior change. In a late-stage epidemic, a therapeutic vaccine of intermediate efficacy reduced expenditures more than did a preventive vaccine of intermediate efficacy (Figure 7.6A). The maximum health benefit obtainable (QALYs gained) was similar for preventive and therapeutic vaccines in a late-stage epidemic. In contrast, in an early-stage epidemic, the health gains obtained with a highly efficacious preventive vaccine far exceeded those obtained with a therapeutic vaccine (Figure 7.6B). These results reflected the larger number of infections that were potentially avertable in an early-stage epidemic relative to a late-stage epidemic. Results for a 20-year time horizon showed similar patterns.

Vaccine Costs

Our base-case analysis assumed a vaccine cost of $1000. Such a price would make the vaccine prohibitively expensive for most people at risk for HIV in the developing world. If a therapeutic vaccine cost $100, virtually all preventive and therapeutic vaccines would be cost-saving (Figure 7.7). If a therapeutic

---

Figure 7.4. *continued*

$10,000 per QALY gained, respectively. Thus, a point on the polygon to the right of the solid line indicates a vaccine that costs less than $50,000 per QALY gained. (A) Preventive vaccine. Each solid square on the polygon indicates a vaccine with characteristics shown in parentheses. For example, the squares on the top line of the polygon indicate vaccines that have a duration of 5 years, and efficacy of 10%, 25%, 50%, 75%, and 90%. The solid squares on the bottom line of the polygon indicate cost and benefits for vaccines with 50-year duration and varying efficacy. Points inside the polygon can be inferred by connecting the squares with straight lines. (B) Therapeutic vaccine. The polygon indicates the costs and benefits of vaccines with varying increases in the length of the asymptomatic period and reductions in infectivity. Reprinted by permission from D. M. Edwards, R. D. Shachter, D. K. Owens, A dynamic HIV-transmission model for evaluating the costs and benefits of vaccine programs, *Interfaces*, 28:3 May–June 1998, pp. 144–166. Copyright 1998, the Institute for Operations Research and the Management Sciences, Linthicum, Maryland, USA.

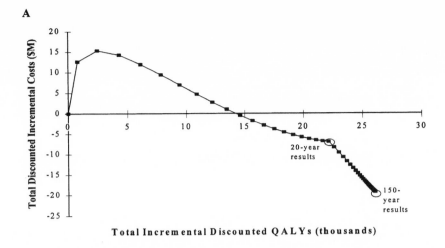

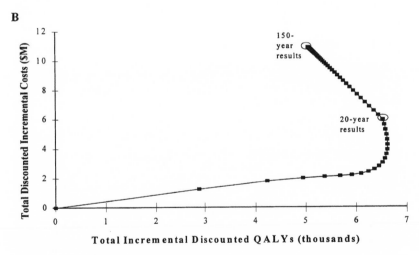

Figure 7.5. Time dependence of costs and benefits of HIV vaccines. The figure indicates the net present value of costs and benefits that accrued to members of the population until time t and assumed no change in risk behavior; therefore, these results differ from our base-case analysis. (A) Preventive vaccine with 75% efficacy and duration of 10 years. The vaccine program becomes cost-saving approximately 15 years after inception. (B) Therapeutic vaccine. The net benefit, measured in quality-adjusted life years (QALYs), of the vaccine diminishes after about 15 years, as noted in the text. If the vaccine reduced infectivity by more than 8%, such a decrease in benefit did not occur.

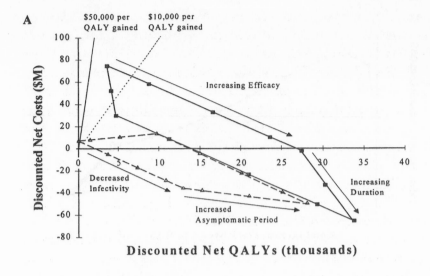

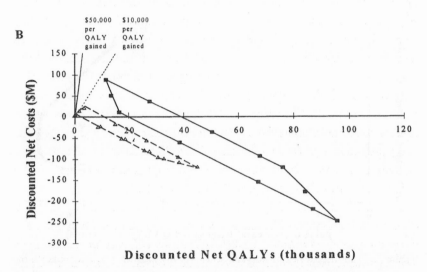

Figure 7.6. Costs and benefits of vaccines in late-stage and early-stage epidemics. Long-term results (150 years) of vaccine programs that do not change risk behavior. See Figure 7.4. for explanation of polygons. (A) In a late-stage epidemic, therapeutic vaccines (dashed polygon) of moderate efficacy reduce costs more than do preventive vaccines (solid polygon) of moderate efficacy. (B) In an early stage epidemic, preventive vaccines have greater maximum benefit, as measured in quality-adjusted life years (QALYs).

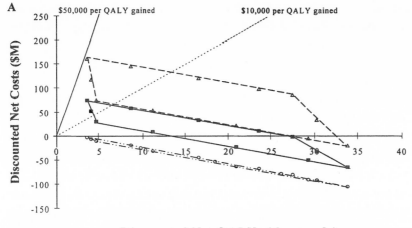

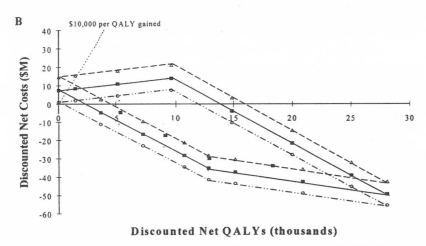

Figure 7.7. Effect of vaccine cost on costs and benefits of a therapeutic vaccine program. Long-term results (150 years) of vaccine programs that do not change risk behavior. See Figure 7.4 for explanation of polygons. The polygons drawn with a dashed, solid, and broken line indicate vaccines that cost $2000, $1000, and $100, respectively. Vaccine benefit was measured in quality-adjusted life years (QALYs). (A) Preventive vaccine. (B) Therapeutic vaccine.

vaccine cost $2000, it would still cost less than $10,000 per QALY gained for most combinations of vaccine characteristics (Figure 7.7B).

DISCUSSION

We used a transmission model to evaluate the costs and benefits of preventive and therapeutic vaccines in a population of homosexual men. We highlight three major findings of our analysis. First, vaccines of extremely modest efficacy provide substantial health benefits; vaccines of only moderate efficacy reduce expenditures. Second, use of different health outcomes and time horizons results in substantially different assessments of vaccine programs; some health outcomes provide incomplete and potentially misleading assessments of vaccine programs. Finally, if both therapeutic and preventive vaccines become available, the strategy for using these vaccines should depend on the characteristics of the epidemic in the population that will undergo vaccination.

Our most important finding is that vaccines of moderate efficacy nonetheless provide enormous health benefits and can reduce net spending. A preventive vaccine that provided protection for 10 years and reduced the probability of infection by 75% would avert infections, reduce prevalence, and reduce net expenditures even if it cost $1000 and was associated with reduced use of condoms. A vaccine that provided lifelong protection would be cost-saving even if it had an efficacy of only 50%. Even when we made the pessimistic assumption that condom use would decrease by 25% in vaccine recipients (Table 7.2 and Figure 7.4), vaccine programs were beneficial under a wide range of assumptions. Modestly effective vaccines provide substantial benefit owing to the complete or near-complete fatality of HIV and because HIV affects young adults, who lose many years of life from premature death. Similarly, therapeutic vaccines that increased length of life by 5 years or more cost less than $10,000 per QALY gained; if they also reduced infectivity, they reduced expenditures. Although most of the vaccines that we evaluated are cost-effective by U.S. standards, a vaccine that cost $1000 would be far too expensive for most parts of the world. We chose $1000 as the vaccine cost to illustrate a pessimistic scenario; clearly, a less expensive vaccine is needed.

As we mentioned, there has been substantial debate about when candidate vaccines should proceed to efficacy trials in humans. To date, the focal point of this debate has been the AIDSVAX vaccine, which the U.S. National Institutes of Health refused to fund for trials. In part, this debate is philosophical. Some investigators believe that efficacy trials should await both an understanding of the immune response that is protective and a candidate vaccine that appears to provide such an immune response. Underlying this position is the notion that without such an understanding, vaccines are unlikely to be effective. The alternative viewpoint is that trials should not wait for such an understanding, which may be years away. On this side, proponents can point to previous successful vaccines, such as those for poliomyelitis, that were widely used long before researchers understood how they worked.

Does our analysis shed any light on this debate? We suggest that vaccines that would provide significant health benefit when used in a population should be evaluated in clinical trials. Our analysis strongly indicates that HIV vaccines do not need to be perfect or nearly perfect to provide substantial health and economic benefit. Thus, we believe that candidate vaccines that are likely to be of modest efficacy should be tested in trials of efficacy, absent better candidate vaccines. If trials are postponed until a candidate is found that has a high probability of near-perfect efficacy, the cost of the delay may be substantial. A useful extension of our work would be to evaluate the cost of delay formally; for now, we do know that, with 16,000 new HIV infections occurring daily, the cost of even short delays will be a staggering loss of life.

Our analysis also demonstrates how the choices of an outcome measure and of the time horizon can influence the assessment of a vaccine program. Although preventive vaccine programs appeared beneficial regardless of the health outcome assessed, therapeutic vaccine programs appeared harmful if we assessed them by only their effect on prevalence or cases averted. When assessed by a more comprehensive outcome—QALYs—therapeutic vaccine programs displayed evident merit. Use of QALYs imposes an additional burden on the analyst, who must translate changes in the number of cases of HIV infection into changes in life-years, and then further make the appropriate quality adjustments. Although each of these steps can introduce additional uncertainty, use of simpler measures underestimated the benefit of therapeutic vaccine programs. In addition, use of QALYs to express the benefit of a vaccine program facilitates comparisons with other health interventions, for HIV and for other diseases.

The choice of time horizon was important because costs and benefits of vaccine programs accrued at different rates. Our finding that costs of a preventive vaccine accrued more quickly than did the benefits is not unexpected, but highlights a drawback of using short time frames for program evaluation. In addition, for therapeutic vaccines, evaluation at periods longer than about 15 years indicated that the cumulative health benefit stopped increasing and eventually decreased (for vaccines that do not decrease infectivity). Thus, an evaluation over short time periods could underestimate the benefit of a preventive vaccine program and overestimate the benefit of a therapeutic vaccine program. In evaluating a 20-year vaccine program, we computed QALYs and the costs for the population at the end of 20 years by projecting the effects of the program over an extended period (150 years). These analyses indicate that, absent other changes, a 20-year vaccine program affected health and economic outcomes into the future, even though we discounted health and economic outcomes at 5%. We did not attempt to account for potential changes in HIV therapy, which are occurring rapidly.

Our analysis indicated that preventive vaccines had greater maximum benefit in early-stage epidemics than did therapeutic vaccines—a result that fits well with our intuition. In a late-stage epidemic, a therapeutic vaccine of moderate efficacy reduced expenditures more than did a preventive vaccine of moderate efficacy. Should both therapeutic and preventive vaccine become available, the characteristics of the epidemic in the population will be relevant if resources are insufficient to administer both vaccines throughout the appropriate populations.

Our analysis required assumptions about sexual behavior and estimates of transmission probabilities that are inherently difficult to verify. In much of the world, heterosexual transmission of HIV is the usual mechanism of infection; our transmission parameters were based on a population of homosexual men. In addition, our cost estimates were developed prior to the advent of highly active antiretroviral therapy; they probably underestimate costs associated with early disease and may overestimate costs associated with advanced disease. Furthermore, our cost estimates assume the cost of vaccine development is included in the per-person cost of the vaccine; the evaluation of vaccines that are candidates for clinical trials could consider vaccine development costs explicitly. Given these limitations, our quantitative results should be interpreted with caution and do not apply directly to populations with other modes of transmission. In addition, our results depend on estimates of parameters—for example, vaccine cost—that are unknown. Once these data are available, our analyses should be updated. We believe that the qualitative insights for our analysis are robust, however, and that our main conclusions are not likely to be affected by these uncertainties.

Over the next decade, the HIV pandemic will claim the lives of most of the 33 million people now infected. Given this devastating forecast, a vaccine that produced even small decrements in transmission or small increments in longevity would result in enormous benefit, if it were affordable worldwide.

Our analysis underscores the urgency of the search for an HIV vaccine and reminds us that we should not let the search for a perfect vaccine prevent us from realizing the benefits of a good vaccine.

APPENDIX

Details of our model have been published previously.[14,15] Our analytic framework builds on the work of Blower and colleagues;[19,20] the model notation is defined in Table 7.3. We assumed that homosexual men entered the population at a constant rate. We further assumed that a proportion of asymptomatic men learned of their infection status through screening, and that all men learned of their infection status when they developed symptoms of HIV disease. Infectivity and partnering behavior varied with disease stage.[16] The model accounted for HIV transmission by sexual contact only.

As an example of how we developed equations for the model, consider the equation for the number of people in the uninfected, unvaccinated population (Figure 7.1). Let this number be $Y_{0,0}(t)$, at time t (for $Y_{ij}(t)$, where the subscript $i = 0, j = 0$ indicates a population that is uninfected and unvaccinated, as explained in Table 7.3). $Y_{0,0}(t)$ was calculated as follows. The number of new uninfected, unvaccinated susceptible people who entered the population was $I_{0,0}$. The number of people who were vaccinated, and thus left this compartment, was the product of the number of uninfected unvaccinated people, $Y_{0,0}(t)$, the percentage of the population that participated in the vaccine program, $v_p(t)$, and the vaccine take, ψ, or $v_p(t)\psi Y_{0,0}(t)$. Our model assumed that a proportion of the population died from causes other than HIV (not shown in Figure 7.1); this number was given by the product of the number of uninfected unvaccinated people, $Y_{0,0}(t)$, and the non-AIDS death rate, μ, or $\mu Y_{0,0}(t)$. The number of people who became infected with HIV was the product of the number of susceptible individuals $Y_{0,0}(t)$, the average annual number of sexual partnerships, p_0, and the probability, per partnership, of acquiring HIV, $\lambda(t)$, or $p_0\lambda(t)Y_{0,0}(t)$. We also assumed that as vaccine protection waned in vaccine recipients, these people would reenter the uninfected, unvaccinated population; we calculated the number of these newly susceptible people as the product of the number of uninfected, vaccinated people, $Y_{0,1}(t)$, where $j = 1$ indicates a vaccinated population, and the rate of loss of vaccine protection, ω, or $\omega Y_{0,1}(t)$. Thus, the total number of uninfected, unvaccinated people, $Y_{0,0}(t)$, was given by

$$\frac{dY_{0,0}(t)}{dt} = I_{0,0} - v_p(t)\psi Y_{0,0}(t) - \mu Y_{0,0}(t) - p_0\lambda(t)Y_{0,0}(t) + \omega Y_{0,1}(t). \quad (1)$$

Table 7.3. Definition of Model Variables

Disease Stage (i)

$i = 0$ Uninfected (HIV−)
$i = 1$ Infected (HIV+) asymptomatic (unidentified)
$i = 2$ Identified infected (HIV+) asymptomatic
$i = 3$ Infected (HIV+) symptomatic
$i = 4$ AIDS

Vaccination Status (j)

$j = 0$ Unvaccinated
$j = 1$ Vaccinated

Disease-Stage Specific Variables

$Yi,j(t)$ Number of people in disease stage i with vaccination status j at time t
$\lambda(t)$ Probability of acquiring the infection at time t from any one partner
$\lambda_v(t)$ Probability of acquiring the infection at time t from any one partner, under behavior modifications due to vaccine
$\beta_{i,j}$ Per-partner infectivity (chance of transmitting HIV) of individual in disease stage i with vaccination status j (note that this is per-partner, and not per-contact, infectivity)
p_i Contact rate (number of new partners per year) of individual in disease stage i
$1/\mu_{i,j}$ Mean duration (in years) of disease stage i under vaccination status j
q_i Quality-adjustment for a year of life in disease stage i
$I_{i,j}$ Annual immigration of people in disease stage i with vaccination status j
$n_{00,ij}$ Probability of condom use in a partnership between an uninfected, unvaccinated person and a person with disease and vaccination status i,j
$n_{01,ij}$ Probability of condom use in a partnership between an uninfected, vaccinated person and a person with disease and vaccination status i,j

Outcome Variables

Q Total discounted quality-adjusted life years (QALYS) lived by the members of the population

Population Variables

μ Non-AIDS-related annual death rate
σ Fraction of population that is screened annually for HIV

Other variables

r Annual discount rate
ξ True-positive rate of screening process

Source: Reprinted by permission from D. K. Owens, D. M. Edwards, R. D. Shachter, Population effects of preventive and therapeutic vaccines in early- and late-stage epidemics, *AIDS*, 1998; 12(9): 1057–1066. Adapted with permission from D. M. Edwards, R. D. Shachter, D.K. Owens, A dynamic HIV-transmission model for evaluating the costs and benefits of vaccine programs, *Interfaces,* 28: 3 May–June 1998, pp. 144–166. Copyright 1998, the Institute for Operations Research and the Management Sciences, Linthicum, Maryland, USA.

Table 7.4. Model Equations

State Equations

$$\frac{dY_{0,0}(t)}{dt} = I_{0,0} - v_p(t)Y_{0,0}(t) - \mu Y_{0,0}(t) - p_0\lambda(t)Y_{0,0}(t) + \omega Y_{0,1}(t) \tag{1}$$

$$\frac{dY_{0,1}(t)}{dt} = v_p(t)Y_{0,0}(t) - \mu Y_{0,1}(t) - \omega Y_{0,1}(t) - p_0(1-\varepsilon)\lambda_v(t)Y_{0,1}(t) \tag{2}$$

$$\frac{dY_{1,0}(t)}{dt} = I_{1,0} + p_0\lambda(t)Y_{0,0}(t) - \sigma\xi Y_{1,0}(t) - v_p(t)Y_{1,0}(t) + \omega Y_{1,1}(t) - \mu_{1,0}Y_{1,0}(t) - \mu Y_{1,0}(t) \tag{3}$$

$$\frac{dY_{1,1}(t)}{dt} = p_0(1-\varepsilon)\lambda_v(t)Y_{0,1}(t) + v_p(t)Y_{1,0}(t) - \omega Y_{1,1}(t) - \sigma\xi Y_{1,1}(t) - \mu_{1,1}Y_{1,1}(t) - \mu Y_{1,1}(t) \tag{4}$$

$$\frac{dY_{2,0}(t)}{dt} = I_{2,0} + \sigma\xi\left(Y_{1,0}(t) + Y_{1,1}(t)\right) - v_t(t)Y_{2,0}(t) - \mu_{2,0}Y_{2,0}(t) - \mu Y_{2,0}(t) \tag{5}$$

$$\frac{dY_{2,1}(t)}{dt} = v_t(t)Y_{2,0}(t) - \mu_{2,1}Y_{2,1}(t) - \mu Y_{2,1}(t) \tag{6}$$

$$\frac{dY_{3,0}(t)}{dt} = I_{3,0} + \sum_{i=1}^{i=2}\sum_{j=0}^{j=1}\mu_{i,j}Y_{i,j}(t) - \mu_{3,0}Y_{3,0}(t) - \mu Y_{3,0}(t) \tag{7}$$

$$\frac{dY_{4,0}(t)}{dt} = \mu_{3,0}Y_{3,0}(t) - \mu_{4,0}Y_{4,0}(t) - \mu Y_{4,0}(t) \tag{8}$$

$$\lambda(t) = \frac{\displaystyle\sum_{j=0}^{j=1}\sum_{i=1}^{i=4}p_i\beta_{i,j}n_{00,ij}Y_{i,j}(t)}{\displaystyle\sum_{j=0}^{j=1}\sum_{i=0}^{i=4}p_iY_{i,j}(t)} \tag{9}$$

$$\lambda_v(t) = \frac{\displaystyle\sum_{j=0}^{j=1}\sum_{i=1}^{i=4}p_i\beta_{i,j}n_{01,ij}Y_{i,j}(t)}{\displaystyle\sum_{j=0}^{j=1}\sum_{i=0}^{i=4}p_iY_{i,j}(t)} \tag{10}$$

Outcome Equation

$$Q = \int_0^T\sum_{j=0}^{j=1}\sum_{i=0}^{i=4}q_1Y_{i,j}(t)e^{-rt}\,dt \tag{11}$$

Source: Reprinted by permission from D. K. Owens, D. M. Edwards, R. D. Shachter, Population effects of preventive and therapeutic vaccines in early- and late-stage epidemics, *AIDS*, 1998; 12(9): 1057–1066. Adapted with permission from D. M. Edwards, R. D. Shachter, D. K. Owens, A dynamic HIV-transmission model for evaluating the costs and benefits of vaccine programs, *Interfaces*, 28: 3 May–June 1998, pp. 144–166. Copyright 1998, the Institute for Operations Research and the Management Sciences, Linthicum, Maryland, USA.

The equations that governed transitions between other compartments (equations 1–10) are shown in Table 7.4, along with equation 11, which calculated QALYs. For simplicity, we have omitted the term for vaccine take, ψ, because our base-case analyses assumed a vaccine take of 100%.

We accounted for the effect of vaccines by modifying the rate of transition between the appropriate compartments in the model. For a preventive vaccine, we reduced the rate of HIV infection in susceptible, vaccinated people relative to susceptible, unvaccinated people. The number of new HIV infections in unvaccinated, susceptible individuals was $p_0\lambda(t)Y_{0,0}(t)$. The number of new infections in the vaccinated susceptible group was $p_0(1 - \varepsilon)\lambda_v(t)Y_{0,1}(t)$, where $\lambda_v(t)$ indicated the probability of acquiring HIV from one partnership, given any changes in risk behavior that accompanied vaccination. If no behavior change occurred ($\lambda_v(t) = \lambda(t)$), vaccination reduced the rate of HIV infection of susceptible people by the term $(1 - \varepsilon)$. If the preventive vaccine efficacy was 75% ($\varepsilon = 0.75$), as we assumed in our base case, the rate of HIV infection among vaccine recipients was reduced to 25% of the rate among unvaccinated individuals. For a therapeutic vaccine, we modeled the effect of the vaccine as a reduced rate of transition from the asymptomatic to the symptomatic state, as indicated in Figure 7.2.

ACKNOWLEDGMENTS

We thank Lyn Dupre for comments on the manuscript and Heather Varughese for preparation of the figures. Douglas K. Owens was supported by a VA Health Services Research and Development Career Development Award. Donna M. Edwards was supported by the United States Department of Energy through the Doctoral Studies Program at Sandia National Laboratories. This research was supported in part by a grant to the Societal Institute of the Mathematical Sciences from the National Institute on Drug Abuse, National Institutes of Health (R-01-09531-01A2).

REFERENCES

1. UNAIDS Joint United Nations Programme on HIV/AIDS. AIDS Epidemic Update: December 1998. Available at: *http://www.unaids.org* 1998.
2. Palella FJ, Delaney KM, Moorman AC. Declining morbidity and mortality among patients with advanced human immunodeficiency infection. *N Engl J Med* 1998; 338: 853–860.
3. Letvin N. Progress in the development of an HIV-1 vaccine. *Science* 1998; 280:1875–1880.
4. Hu DJ, Dondero TJ, Rayfield MA, et al. The emerging genetic diversity of HIV: the importance of global surveillance for diagnostics, research and prevention. *JAMA* 1996; 275:210–216.

5. Haynes BF. Scientific and social issues of human immunodeficiency virus vaccine development. *Science* 1993; 260:1279–1286.

6. Haynes, BF, Pantaleo G, Fauci AS. Toward an understanding of the correlates of protective immunity to HIV infection. *Science* 1996; 271:324–328.

7. Heyward WL, MacQueen KM, Goldenthal KL. HIV vaccine development and evaluation: Realistic expectations. *AIDS Res Hum Retroviruses* 1998; 14: Suppl 3:S205–210.

8. Graham BS, Wright PF. Candidate AIDS vaccines. *N Engl J Med* 1995; 333:1331–1339.

9. Dolin R, Graham BS, Greenberg SB, et al. The safety and immunogenicity of a human immunodeficiency virus type 1 (HIV-1) recombinant gp 160 candidate vaccine in humans. *Ann Intern Med* 1991; 114:119–127.

10. Redfield RR, Birx DL, Ketter N, et al. A phase I evaluation of the safety and immunogenicity of vaccination with recombinant gp 160 in patients with early human immunodeficiency virus infection. *N Engl J Med* 1991; 324:1677–1684.

11. Wintsch J, Chaignat C-L, Braun DG, et al. Safety and immunogenicity of a genetically engineered human immunodeficiency virus vaccine. *J Infect Dis* 1991; 163:219–225.

12. World Health Organization. Scientific and public health rationale for HIV vaccine efficacy trials. *AIDS* 1995; 9:WHO1–WHO4.

13. Sperling RS, Shapiro DE, Coombs RW, et al. Maternal viral load, zidovudine treatment, and the risk of transmission of human immunodeficiency virus type 1 from mother to infant. *N Engl J Med* 1996; 335:1621–1629.

14. Edwards DM, Shachter RD, Owens DK. A dynamic HIV-transmission model for evaluating the costs and benefits of vaccine programs. *Interfaces* 1998; 28:144–166.

15. Owens DK, Edwards DM, Shachter RD. Population effects of preventive and therapeutic HIV vaccines in early- and late-stage epidemics. *AIDS* 1998; 12:1057–1066.

16. Edwards DM. A cost-effectiveness analysis of potential preventive and therapeutic HIV vaccines. Stanford, CA: Stanford University, 1995.

17. Anderson RM, Gupta S, May RM. Potential of community-wide chemotherapy or immunotherapy to control the spread of HIV-1. *Nature* 1991; 350:356–359.

18. Nowak MA, McLean A R. A mathematical model of vaccination against HIV to prevent the development of AIDS. *Proc R Soc Lond* [Biol] 1991; 246:141–146.

19. McLean AR, Blower SM. Imperfect vaccines and herd immunity to HIV. *Proc R Soc Lond* [Biol] 1993; 253:9–13.

20. Blower SM, McLean AR. Prophylactic vaccines, risk behavior change, and the probability of eradicating HIV in San Francisco. *Science* 1994; 265:1451–1454.

21. Service SK, Blower SM. HIV transmission in sexual networks: An empirical analysis. *Proc R Soc Lond* [Biol] 1995; 260:237–244.

22. Philipson T, Dow WH. Infectious disease transmission and infection-dependent matching. Department of Economics, University of Chicago, 1995.

23. Newcomb M, Liu W, Officer C, et al. Stella II. Hanover, NH: High Performance Systems, Inc., 1996.

24. The MathWorks Inc. The student edition of MATLAB. Englewood Cliffs, NJ: Prentice-Hall, Inc., 1992.

25. Torrance GW. Social preferences for health states. An empirical evaluation of three measurement techniques. *Socio-Econ Planning* 1976; 10:129–136.

26. Owens DK, Sox HC, Jr. Medical decision making: Probabilistic medical reasoning. In: Shortliffe EH, Perreault LE, Fagan LM, Wiederhold G, eds. *Medical Informatics: Computer Applications in Health Care.* Reading, MA: Addison-Wesley, 1990:70–116.

27. Owens DK, Harris RA, Scott PM, Nease RF, Jr. Screening surgeons for HIV infection: A cost-effectiveness analysis. *Ann Intern Med* 1995; 122:641–652.

28. Owens DK, Cardinalli AB, Nease RF, Jr. Physicians' assessments of the utility of health states associated with human immunodeficiency virus (HIV) and hepatitis B virus (HBV) infection. *Quality of Life Research* 1997; 6:77–86.

29. Tsevat J, Solzan JG, Kuntz KM, et al. Health values of patients infected with human immunodeficiency virus. *Med Care* 1996; 34:44–57.

30. Gold MR, Siegel JE, Russell LB, Weinstein MC. *Cost-Effectiveness in Health and Medicine.* New York: Oxford University Press, 1996.

31. Edwards DM, Shachter RD, Owens DK. Comparison of methods for valuing health and economic effects of interventions with delayed outcomes: Application to HIV vaccine programs. *Med Decis Making* 1995; 15:420.

32. Paltiel AD, Kaplan EH. The epidemiological and economic consequences of AIDS clinical trials. *J Acquir Immune Defic Syndr* 1993; 6:179–190.

33. Hellinger FJ. Forecasts of the costs of medical care for persons with HIV: 1992–1995. *Inquiry* 1992; 29:356–365.

34. Hellinger FJ. The lifetime cost of treating a person with HIV. *JAMA* 1993; 270:474–478.

35. Brandeau ML, Owens DK, Sox CH, Wachter RM. Screening women of childbearing age for human immunodeficiency virus: A model-based policy analysis. *Management Science* 1993; 39:72–92.

36. Samuel MC, Mohr MS, Speed TP, Winkelstein W. Infectivity of HIV by anal and oral intercourse among homosexual men: Estimates from a prospective study in San Francisco. In: Kaplan EH, Brandeau ML, eds. *Modeling the AIDS Epidemic: Planning, Policy and Prediction.* New York: Raven Press, 1994:423–438.

37. Communication Technologies in association with the San Francisco AIDS Foundation. HIV-related knowledge, attitudes, and behaviors among San Francisco gay and bisexual men: Results from the fifth population-based survey: San Francisco Department of Public Health, 1990.

38. Ward JW, Bush TJ, Perkins HA, et al. The natural history of transfusion-associated infection with human immunodeficiency virus: Factors influencing the rate of progression to disease. *N Engl J Med* 1989; 321:947–952.

39. Muñoz A, Wang M-C, Bass S, et al. Acquired immunodeficiency syndrome (AIDS)-free time after human immunodeficiency virus type 1 (HIV-1) seroconversion in homosexual men. *Am J Epidemiol* 1989; 130:530–539.

40. Muñoz A, Kirby AJ, He YD, et al. Long-term survivors with HIV-1 infection: Incubation period and longitudinal patterns of CD4+ lymphocytes. *J AIDS Hum Retrovir* 1995; 8:496–505.

41. Winkelstein WJ, Wiley JA, Padian NS, et al. The San Francisco Men's Health Study: Continued decline in HIV seroconversion rates among homosexual/bisexual men. *Am J Pub Health* 1988; 78:1472–1474.

42. Lemp GF, Hirozawa AM, Givertz D, et al. Seroprevalence of HIV and risk behaviors

among young homosexual and bisexual men: The San Francisco/Berkeley Young Men's Survey. *JAMA* 1994; 272:449–454.

43. Elkstrand ML, Coates TJ. Maintenance of safer sexual behavior and predictors of risky sex: The San Francisco Men's Health Study. *Am J Public Health* 1990; 80:973–977.

44. Owens DK. Interpretation of cost-effectiveness analyses [Editorial]. *Journal of General Internal Medicine* 1998; 13:716–717.

Part Three **Case Studies**

Chapter 8 Harm Reduction in Rome: A Model-Based Evaluation of Its Impact on the HIV-1 Epidemic

Massimo Arcà, Teresa Spadea, Giulia Cesaroni,

Marina Davoli, Annette D. Verster, and Carlo A. Perucci

In August 1994, the Lazio Region Health Authority in Italy started a two-year pilot harm reduction program (HRP) aimed at contacting drug users currently not in treatment and reducing the health risks related to injecting drugs. The integrated program, implemented in the city of Rome, involved street outreach, needle exchange programs, distribution of condoms, information and counseling, first aid (for overdose), drop-in centers for day and night care, and referral to methadone maintenance treatment.

In two years of activity, three outreach units made 148,000 contacts, 87% of which were with 5047 different drug users. About 200,000 sterile syringes and more than 60,000 condoms were distributed, and 526 drug users were referred for methadone treatment. The emergency unit and the street outreach teams together intervened in 519 events of overdose. Overall, the Lazio Region Health Authority spent 9 billion lire (at that time, about $5.2 million) to fund the HRP. We have reported a more detailed outline of the program and a descriptive analysis of the full range of activities elsewhere.[1,2]

One objective of the HRP was to reduce the incidence of HIV-1 infections among both drug users and their noninjecting sexual partners. A prospective follow-up of the people contacted through the program, to measure HIV-1 incidence and estimate possible changes attributable to the HRP, was rejected as practically unfeasible. Consequently, mathematical modeling seemed to be the only way to assess the HRP's prevention effectiveness.

In this analysis we used a compartmental mathematical model of the transmission dynamics of HIV-1 infection with the threefold aim to:

- estimate the effect of the HRP in terms of reduction of HIV-1 incidence and prevalence;
- study the influence of the HRP implementation time on its estimated impact;
- assess and discuss advantages and limitations of mathematical models as tools for evaluating prevention programs.

METHODS

Model Structure and Baseline Parameters

In previous works[3,4] we thoroughly discussed the development of a model for the transmission dynamics of HIV-1 in Italy, and the estimation of the key parameter values based on the available observational evidence. Here, we briefly describe the main characteristics of the model, including some changes made in the structure to address the objectives of this analysis.

The model involves the population aged 15 to 44 years, stratified in four groups with respect to sex (male/female) and intravenous drug use (yes/no). HIV-1 can be transmitted either through needle sharing among drug injectors or through heterosexual contact; we have chosen to disregard homosexual transmission, due to the epidemiological situation in Italy, where data document a limited number of AIDS cases among men who have sex with men[5] and a growing trend for new HIV-1 infections attributable to heterosexual transmission.[6] Consequently, in the evaluation we disregarded the cases of HIV-1 prevented through the HRP among same-sex partners of drug users.

Ten subgroups are created by further stratifying the four groups with respect to behaviors related to HIV-1 transmission: sharing needles among injecting drug users (IDUs) of both sexes, having sex for money, drugs, or other goods among female IDUs, and rate of sexual partner change among non-drug-user heterosexuals (NDUHs).

The total NDUH population amounts to 1.2 million males and 1.2 million females, with stable dynamics, thus mirroring the demography of Lazio, the region that includes Rome. We used data from vital statistics to calculate rates of entry (due to age and immigration) and exit (due to age, deaths, and emigration). We derived the parameters concerning the rates of partner change for NDUHs from a cross-sectional study on a probabilistic sample of the Italian population aged 18 to 30 years.[7]

The number of IDUs was initially set at 18,200, with a male-to-female ratio of 4.8. We have specified a 10-fold increase in mortality among male IDUs and a 20-fold increase among female IDUs, in agreement with the results of an earlier cohort study.[10] The model allows for 3% of IDUs to enter the NDUH group every year, which is more than balanced by new entries that increase the IDU population at an annual rate of 2%.[11] In the absence of data on IDU behavior during the early years of the HIV-1 epidemic (late 1970s), we estimated the model parameters from three surveys of drug injectors carried out in Rome in 1990, 1992, and 1995.[8,9] We adjusted the values to account for increasing knowledge and consciousness about behavior related to HIV-1 transmission, concurrently trying to reproduce HIV-1 incidence trends consistent with those observed in the first decade of the epidemic.

The interaction between and within the subgroups is ruled by probability matrices that define the mixing pattern, that is, the degree at which individuals in a subgroup mix with individuals from other subgroups.[3] In our model, we assume proportional mixing (i.e., the proportion of partnerships that group A reserves from group B is proportional to the total number of partnerships offered by group B) with respect to needle sharing, while sexual partnerships follow a more assortative pattern. This means that partnerships between IDUs are more likely than they would be under proportional mixing and that low-sex-activity NDUHs establish relationships only with other NDUHs, and preferably with individuals with similar characteristics.

We used evidence from observational studies to estimate the parameters describing the distribution of the incubation period (the time elapsed from the infection with HIV-1 to the diagnosis of AIDS) and the probability of transmitting HIV-1. The first is a generalized Gamma, obtained by partitioning the "infected" compartment in three subcompartments and assuming constant rates of transition out of each. Transition rates are computed to reproduce the median incubation times reported by the Italian Seroconverter Study.[12] The longer incubation period assumed among NDUH males than among other groups reflects observational data[13] and depends on their older age at seroconversion[6] and on the negative association between this variable and AIDS-free survival.[13]

We put the probability of becoming infected from a used needle at 0.007, as estimated by Kaplan.[14] The probability of transmitting HIV-1 in a sexual partnership involving an infected individual and a susceptible one is modeled by a discrete Weibull distribution, as suggested by Jewell and Shiboski,[15] with a factor allowing for non-Bernoulli compounding (over the number of contacts) of the probability of transmission per single intercourse. Moreover, the model allows for variable infectiousness during the incubation period, and posits that the male-to-female transmission probability exceeds the female-to-male by a factor of three. The prevalence of condom use (in the absence of the HRP) increases during the incubation period from 20% to 65%, and its preventive effectiveness is set at 98.6%. The values for the main parameters described above are reported in Table 8.1.

Neither spontaneous changes over time in behavior (apart from those induced by the HRP) nor changes in the incubation period distribution are allowed. The simulated epidemic is started (at time $t = 0$) by seeding the population with four infected IDUs (three males and one female) and run for 30 years. The simulated trends in HIV-1 incidence resulting from this model were used as baseline values in evaluating potential reductions owing to the HRP.

Modeling the Impact of the HRP

Among the operational data collected within the two-year HRP, we chose the activity measures that could have most directly affected the transmission dynamics of HIV-1, as schematically represented by our model. These are the numbers of syringes and condoms distributed and the number of drug users referred to methadone maintenance treatment. We assumed that all 199,590 syringes were used by IDUs, in addition to (and not substituting) those already circulating. As for condoms, we hypothesized that IDUs used only 85% of the total amount distributed, corresponding to 51,500 condoms. The last measure used in the simulations was based on the 526 IDUs referred to methadone treatment, about half of whom were assumed to have stopped injecting drugs during the two years (132 per year).

The following steps adapted the selected outcome measures to the model structure, in order to obtain values appropriate for the parameters of the model. First, we reallocated the total number of syringes distributed to the six IDU subgroups. In this regard, we had two options: the first was to suppose that syringes had been given to all subgroups, proportionally to group size, while

Table 8.1. Baseline Parameters of the Model

Incubation Period (duration in months)	IDU	NDUH-M	NDUH-F
I stage	36	37.5	37
II stage	94	62.5	94
III stage	26	26	26

Transmission Probability			
Per used needle	0.007		
Per sexual intercourse		M → F	F → M
I stage		0.05	0.05/3
II stage		0.04	0.04/3
III stage		0.07	0.07/3
Nonconstancy factor		0.21	

	IDU-M	IDU-F	NDUH-M		NDUH-F	
Sexual behavior			LS	HS	LS	HS
			(75%)	(25%)	(90%)	(10%)
Rate of sexual partner change (per year, excluding prostitution)	1.5	2.0	0.28	1.6	0.32	3.2

Proportion of NDUHs among	IDU-M	IDU-F
sexual partners of IDUS	0.8	0.3

Frequency of condom use	All groups
I stage	0.20
II stage	0.45
III stage	0.65

Needle Sharing	IDU-M	IDU-F
Proportion of needle sharers	0.40	0.55
Rate of change of sharing partner (average number of partners to borrow needles from, per year)	6.6	8.7
Average number of borrowed needles, per year	85.6	156

Prostitution	IDU-F
Proportion of IDU females who have sex for money, drugs, or other goods	0.31
Average number of clients, per year	500
Frequency of condom use with clients	0.99

the second postulated that they had been given only to needle sharers. This second alternative gives us an upper limit for the impact of the needle exchange, which we will refer to as the "maximum effect" hypothesis, as opposed to the first, "basic effect," option. The strategy of a proportional distribution across all the IDU subgroups was adopted for condoms as well.

Table 8.2. Parameter Changes Representing the Different Services Offered by the HRP

		Baseline	Basic Effect Hypothesis	Maximum Effect Hypothesis
Syringes				
Average number of borrowed	M	85.6	81.6	75.2
needles, per year	F	156	152	145.6
Condoms				
Increase in protected	M		+5%	
sexual partners	F		+2%	
Methadone		Baseline	HRP	
Annual rate of IDU moving to NDUH		3%	3.5%	
Annual IDU population growth		2%	1.5%	

The number of syringes given to each group was then parameterized in terms of reduction in the average frequency of borrowing used needles for reuse: therefore, in the "basic effect" option, the syringes given to nonsharers had no preventive effect. Analogously, we parameterized the number of condoms distributed to IDUs as an increase in the proportion of protected sexual partnerships; the resulting increase was higher in males than in females owing to the different baseline frequencies of sexual intercourse. Finally, considering that the estimated 2% annual growth in the IDU population accounts for around 24,000 subjects at the beginning of the 1990s,[11] we had to assume a yearly exit rate of 0.5% to simulate 132 IDUs quitting drugs due to the HRP. Thus, we increased by such a value the yearly rate of IDUs moving to NDUHs and reduced concurrently the annual growth by the same amount, to simulate the exit of IDUs not balanced by new entries. Changes in the parameter values are summarized in Table 8.2.

The HRP started in August 1994, which in the model corresponds to $t = 19.75$, and the modified parameter values were kept constant from that time onward. To assess the influence of the HRP's starting time on its estimated effect, and in particular to see whether an earlier implementation would have had a greater impact on the epidemic, we simulated starting a program with the same outcome measures at two time points: June 1987 ($t = 12.5$, corresponding to time of the observed peak of HIV-1 incidence among IDUs,[6] and June 1989 ($t = 14.5$, soon after this peak).

Last, we tried to estimate the independent effect of each component of the integrated HRP on the HIV-1 incidence time trends.

RESULTS

All the results are reported in terms of number of incident HIV-1 cases per quarter. Figure 8.1 shows the temporal changes in this quantity with respect to sex and drug use, as predicted by the baseline model. Initially, the virus spreads primarily and very rapidly among IDUs, reaching a peak of 440 new cases per quarter (323 males and 117 females) during the twelfth year from the start of the epidemic. At the same time, while the high-risk groups become saturated with infection, a significant though slow rise in HIV-1 among NDUHs takes place, affecting females more than males. The model predicts that the counts for IDU and NDUH females will cross after 14 years, at about 80 new HIV-1 infections per quarter. These predictions fit reasonably well with the estimates for Lazio region derived by surveillance data,[6] when the initial time is set at January 1975, although the observed decline in the number of newly diagnosed HIV-1 infections among IDUs was sharper than was predicted by this model. It must be recalled, however, that the model includes none of the changes in drug-related behaviors observed in the early 1990s and documented by the surveys.[8]

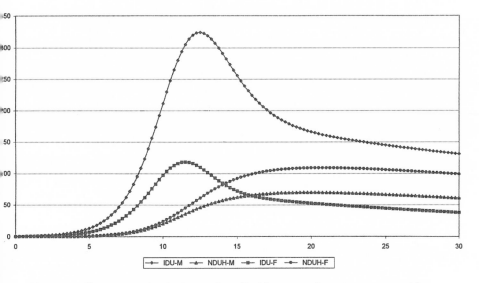

Figure 8.1. Changes over time in the number of incident cases of HIV-1 per quarter with respect to sex and intravenous drug use. Baseline model.

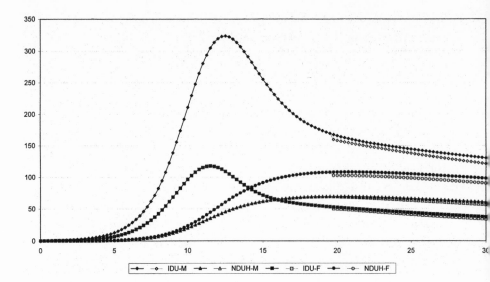

Figure 8.2. Changes over time in the number of incident cases of HIV-1 per quarter with respect to sex and intravenous drug use. Estimated impact of the 1994 HRP (basic effect option).

Figure 8.2 shows the estimated effect of the HRP. Soon after the program starts, we observe a decrease of 16 new infections per quarter; of these, 10 cases (8 M and 2 F) are prevented among IDUs, and 6 cases (1 M and 5 F) among NDUHs. This reduction remains constant up to the thirtieth year, indicating that although the simulated program is effective in preventing several new infections during its course, it has no impact on the shape of the epidemic curves.

The implications of the two hypotheses about syringe distribution (basic effect, in which needles are given to all IDUs, and maximum effect, in which they are given only to sharers) are compared in Figure 8.3, where we reduced the time axis scale in order to focus on the period after the HRP implementation. As expected, IDUs get the greatest benefit from the HRP when new syringes are given only to sharers, with an extra 66 infections averted in two years. As a consequence, over the two years, 5 more cases are prevented among NDUH females who have sex with male IDUs. In the long term, the basic effect and the maximum effect curves overlap for all subgroups.

Figure 8.4 shows the influence of the HRP implementation time on its over-

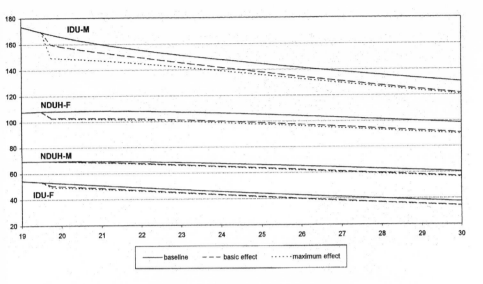

Figure 8.3. Changes over time in the number of incident cases of HIV-1 per quarter with respect to sex and intravenous drug use. Maximum versus basic effect estimate of the 1994 HRP impact.

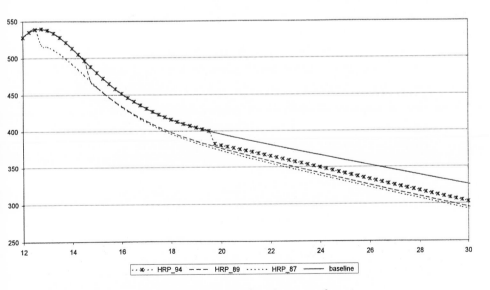

Figure 8.4. Changes over time in the number of incident cases of HIV-1 per quarter. Influence of the HRP implementation time on its estimated impact.

Table 8.3. Estimated Number of New HIV-1 Infections Prevented Through a Two-Year HRP and Cost-Effectiveness Ratio: Comparisons Among Different Implementation Hypotheses

	Basic Effect Hypothesis			Maximum Effect Hypothesis		
	1987	1989	1994	1987	1989	1994
IDU-M	105	78	54	243	171	114
IDU-F	25	21	18	42	30	24
NDUH-M	6	6	5	9	8	7
NDUH-F	36	43	44	47	50	49
Total	172	148	121	341	259	194
Cost-effectiveness (thousand USD per averted infection)	30	35	43	15	20	27

all impact. An HRP which had started in 1987, and had produced the same operational data as those observed in 1994, would have prevented 51 more infections in its first two years than the actual HRP did (+42%). Maintaining the early implemented HRP would have resulted, over the long period, in about 32 prevented infections per quarter, 10 more than it is estimated for the actual HRP. The gain would have been less marked had the program started in 1989. In neither case does the earlier implementation modify substantially the epidemic trend over the long period.

A summary of the results achieved through the simulated HRP under the different scenarios depicted above is reported in Table 8.3, in terms of cumulative number of new HIV-1 infections averted in the first two years. Rough estimates of the cost-effectiveness ratio (cost per averted infection)[16] have also been calculated, using the total HRP funding ($5.2 million) as the overall program cost.

Finally, in Figure 8.5 we assess the independent effect of each of the three services offered within the HRP and incorporated in the model simulation. The sudden decrease in incidence results from the cumulated effects of distributing condoms, which affect mainly the incidence among NDUH females, and sterile syringes, which reduce the transmission through needle sharing among IDUs. Although the impact of an increased condom use remains constant during the conduct of the program, increasing the number of circulating needles tends to become less important as time goes by. In contrast, the referral of IDUs to methadone maintenance treatment produces an effect only in the long term, overcoming the prevention effectiveness of condom distribution after seven years of a prolonged HRP.

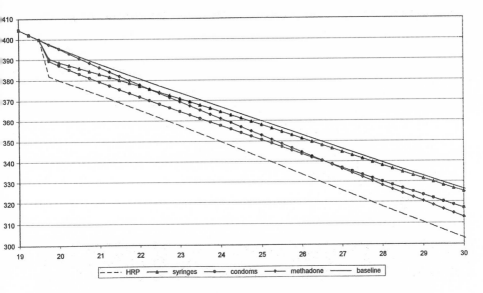

Figure 8.5. Changes over time in the number of incident cases of HIV-1 per quarter with respect to sex and intravenous drug use. Relative contributions of the services offered within the 1994 HRP on the program impact (basic effect option).

DISCUSSION

Before discussing the results of the HRP evaluation with respect to the main program outcome—the reduction in HIV-1 incidence—we wish to comment on some of the program process and output measures. The two-year pilot harm reduction program carried out in Rome from 1994 to 1996 succeeded in contacting about 5000 IDUs, which is more than 20% of the estimated number of users who were injecting drugs at the program start. Many of these IDUs (37%) did not attend the general drug services. When compared to those who regularly used drug services, they were younger and reported more frequent use of noninjectable drugs.[2] About 10% of those contacted by the program were referred to treatment centers, mainly for methadone maintenance therapy.

In two years the HRP emergency unit took care of more than 500 overdose episodes. We cannot say how many of these episodes would have been assisted by the ordinary emergency system and how many saved lives can be credited to the program in this respect.

As for the operational data we used in the model, we should have increased the value of about 200,000 sterile syringes distributed by the street units by the number of syringes IDUs got from exchange machines. Because this second number was not known it was not included in the simulations.

We do not know how many HRP syringes replaced needles that would have been borrowed from other IDUs, thus potentially preventing HIV-1 transmission, and how many HRP syringes replaced needles that would have been bought, with no effect on the transmission dynamics. However, even in the maximum effect hypothesis (all the sterile syringes were given to IDUs who share and were used instead of borrowed needles), the reduction in the average number of borrowings per time unit is slight (Table 8.2). Indeed, although this reduction results in preventing several new HIV-1 infections, it does not get R_0, the basic reproduction number, below 1 for IDUs, and leaves epidemic trends substantially unchanged.

The baseline rates of needle sharing used in our model are higher than those reported by IDUs in Rome in 1990. This is consistent with a lowering of HIV-1 risk behaviors after the AIDS epidemic emerged (1985) and results in an early epidemic trend similar to that observed in the Lazio region, once the infectivity of an infected needle is set at 0.007. If we used much higher values for this probability of transmission, as recent analysis of data on Thai IDUs seems to suggest (Satten, personal communication), we would need proportionally lower rates of sharing to get the same baseline solutions. In that case, the number of syringes distributed through the HRP would represent a higher proportion of those already circulating, and a stronger preventive effect could be estimated.

The harm reduction strategy was first, and unsuccessfully, proposed in Lazio in 1988; a more timely implementation of the HRP would have had a greater impact on HIV-1 incidence, although it would not have modified the epidemic trend over the long period. We cannot know, however, whether an earlier HRP would have produced the same operational data as the real one.

The three components of the HRP modify the HIV-1 transmission dynamics in different ways. The impact of the distribution of condoms is especially evident among NDUH females, and it remains constant over time. As for the other two results of the integrated program, the decrease in needle sharing and the increase in the number of IDUs who quit injecting, the first has a sudden effect that vanishes after a few years, while the second manifests only in the long term.

The estimated cost of each HIV-1 infection averted through the prevention program ranges from $15,000 to $43,000, according to the assumed scenario. The lifetime cost of medical care associated with HIV and AIDS in the United States has increased from $56,000 in 1992 dollars and a 5% discount rate[17] to

$157,000 in 1996,[18] while the number of quality-adjusted life years saved per one HIV infection averted has decreased from 9.26 to 7.10. Using these figures, which are not far from cost estimates produced in Italy,[19] we obtain negative cost-utility ratios (cost per quality-adjusted life year), indicating that the program actually saved resources and can be judged as cost-saving.

Although Table 8.3 refers to the number of new HIV-1 infections averted in the two years of program activity, in most simulations we extended the effects of the HRP to several years after its conclusion. In fact, at the end of the pilot phase, the emergency unit and the drop-in center continued to operate using other funds, while the street unit activities were substantially reduced due to lack of financing.

In 1998, as the National Conference on Drugs acknowledged the cost-effectiveness of the Lazio pilot program and indicated harm reduction as part of an integrated strategy to fight drug abuse, the Lazio Regional Authority decided to reserve one-third of its Drug Fund (about $1.7 million) for financing HRPs. Consequently, Rome street units have now fully resumed operations (though a greater coordination among them would be desirable). In the meantime, general drug services have increased their use of methadone maintenance treatments (in Italy, methadone consumption increased from 133 kilos in 1993 to 513 kilos in 1997).

In this respect, we conclude that the impact of the Rome HRP, although limited in extent, was not limited in time, as it induced long-term changes in both IDUS' behavior and the health and social care systems' attitudes toward drug abuse.

REFERENCES

1. Verster AD, Davoli M, Perucci CA et al. Harm reduction in Rome. *Int J Drug Policy* 1996; 7:73–79.
2. Davoli M, Patruno F, Pasqualini F et al. Programma integrato di riduzione del danno nei tossicodipendenti a Roma. *Progetto Salute* 1997; 36.
3. Arcà M, Perucci CA, Spadea T. The epidemic dynamics of HIV-1 in Italy: Modeling the interaction between intravenous drug users and heterosexual population. *Stat Med* 1992; 11:1657–1684.
4. Perucci CA, Abeni D, Arcà M, Davoli M, Pugliese A. Modeling the HIV-1 and AIDS epidemic among drug injectors. In: Stimson G, Des Jarlais DC, Ball A (Eds.) *Drug Injecting and HIV Infection.* London: UCL Press, 1998:115–129.
5. Centro Operativo AIDS (COA) dell'Istituto Superiore di Sanità. Aggiornamento dei casi di AIDS notificati in Italia al 30 giugno 1998. Notiziario ISS, vol. 11, no. 9 (suppl. 1).

6. Brancato G, Perucci CA, Abeni DDC et al. The changing distribution of HIV infection: HIV surveillance in Lazio, Italy, 1985 through 1994. *Am J Public Health* 1997; 87: 1654–1658.

7. D'Arcangelo E, Marasca G, Vitiello C. I comportamenti sessuali della popolazione giovanile italiana in riferimento alla problematica AIDS: Primi risultati di un'indagine nazionale. *Dip Stat Prob e Stat Appl, Univ Roma "La Sapienza." Serie A-Ricerche* 1990; 22.

8. Davoli M, Perucci CA, Abeni DDC et al. HIV risk-related behaviors among injection drug users in Rome: Differences between 1990 and 1992. *Am J Public Health* 1995; 85: 829–832.

9. Verster AD, Davoli M, Montiroli PM, Abeni DDC, Perucci CA. Risk behaviour among injecting drug users in Rome, 1990–1995. *7th Int Conference on the Reduction of Drug-Related Harm.* Hobart, Australia, 1996:108.

10. Perucci CA, Davoli M, Rapiti E, Abeni D, Forastiere F. Mortality of intravenous drug users in Rome: A cohort study. *Am J Public Health* 1991; 81:1307–1310.

11. Perucci CA, Davoli M, Papini P, Bargagli AM, Arcà M. Evidence of increasing numbers of intravenous drug users (IVDUS) in Lazio, Italy, 1988–1992. *Proc 5th Int Conference on the Reduction of Drug-Related Harm.* Toronto, Canada, 1994:63.

12. Pezzotti P, Galai N, Vlahov D, Rezza G, Lyles CM, Astemborski J. Direct comparison of time to AIDS and infectious disease death between HIV seroconverter injection drug users in Italy and the United States: Results from the ALIVE and ISS studies. *J Acquir Immune Defic Syndr Hum Retrovirol* 1999; 20:275–282.

13. Mariotto A, Mariotti S, Pezzotti P et al. Estimation of the AIDS incubation period in intravenous drug users: A comparison with male homosexuals. *Am J Epidemiol* 1992; 135: 428–437.

14. Jewell NP, Shiboski SC. Statistical analysis of HIV infectivity based on partner studies. *Biometrics* 1990; 46:1133–1150.

15. Kaplan EH, Heimer R. A model-based estimate of HIV infectivity via needle sharing. *J Acquir Immune Defic Syndr* 1992; 5:1116–1118.

16. Pinkerton SD, Holtgrave DR, DiFranceisco WJ, Stevenson LY, Kelly JA. Cost-effectiveness of a community-level HIV risk reduction intervention. *Am J Public Health* 1998;88:1239–1242.

17. Guinan ME, Farnham PG, Holtgrave DR. Estimating the value of preventing a Human Immunodeficiency Virus infection. *Am J Prev Med* 1994; 10:1–4.

18. Holtgrave DR, Pinkerton SD. Updates of cost of illness and quality of life estimates for use in economic evaluations of HIV prevention programs. *J Acquir Immune Defic Syndr Hum Retrovirol* 1997; 16:54–62.

19. Visco Comandini V. Analisi economica dell'AIDS: Strumenti per la programmazione regionale. *Quaderni per la ricerca. Serie studi/36.* Roma: ISR-CNR, 1995.

Chapter 9 Evaluating Israel's Ethiopian Blood Ban

Edward H. Kaplan

In January 1996, the Israeli daily *Ma'ariv* reported that donations to Israel's national blood supply from Ethiopian immigrants were routinely discarded without informing the donors. Blood bank physicians adopted this policy in response to the factor-of-fifty higher prevalence of HIV among Ethiopian immigrants relative to the rest of the Israeli population. Revelation of this exclusion policy resulted in a violent protest by 10,000 Ethiopian immigrants, accounting for one-sixth of the 60,000 Ethiopians living in Israel at that time, in which 70 persons were injured.[1,2,3] Subsequently, a committee chaired by former Israeli President Yitzhak Navon was formed to conduct an official investigation into Israel's Ethiopian blood ban.[4]

The director of the Magen David Adom (the Israeli equivalent of the Red Cross) defended the exclusion policy by stating: "Everyone can judge for themselves that if the opposite had occurred (someone had been infected by Ethiopian blood), then there also would have been an upheaval."[5] An expert in medical ethics stated, "Clearly, from a medical standpoint, there is no question the policy was correct."[3,6] And an editorial in the *Jerusalem Post* argued: "In fact, there is nothing wrong in the decision to disqualify blood from immigrants who come from AIDS-afflicted countries. . . . Had even one such donation caused the death of its recipient, the country would have been up in arms against the health authorities for being criminally lax."[7]

In contrast, Novel Prize–winner Elie Wiesel stated, "An entire community has been thus humiliated,"[8] while Jewish Agency Chairman Avraham Burg declared, "Every member of Israeli society is my brother—I would give my blood to them all and receive blood from them all."[9] Israel's Minister of Health, Ephraim Sneh, accused the Magen David Adom of behavior that was "irregular, unethical and unfair. . . . Ethiopian immigrants were laid down, a needle was pushed into their veins and a pint of blood was taken, but they were misled. . . . This is a good example of how the path to hell may be paved by the best of intentions."[10]

This chapter presents the details underlying previously reported evaluations of Israel's blood exclusion decision.[11,12] I begin with a brief review of recent HIV incidence estimates in both Ethiopian and non-Ethiopian Israelis, and use these studies to create estimates of HIV incidence among potential blood donors. I then report a simple model of the probability that a donation testing negative for HIV antibody is contaminated with HIV, and estimate this infectious donation risk for both Ethiopian and other Israelis. I employ this model to estimate the impact of exclusion on the annual number of infectious donations, and use this result in an implicit cost-effectiveness analysis. I then determine thresholds for the monetary benefits of healthy donations and social costs of blood exclusion that enable deciding when, on the basis of cost-benefit analysis, the exclusion option is defensible (or not). Throughout the analysis, I adopt a series of assumptions that favor the exclusion decision. In spite of this deliberate bias, the analysis reveals that the public health basis for the exclusion decision is weak.

ESTIMATED HIV INCIDENCE IN ISRAEL

From 1981 through March 1997, Israel's Ministry of Health reported a total of 440 AIDS cases, 93 of whom continued to reside in Israel.[13] In addition, 1436 HIV-infected persons who had not progressed to AIDS were reported alive in Israel as of March 1997.[13]

Aggregate HIV incidence rates among adult non-Ethiopian Israelis were estimated previously from reporting delay-corrected AIDS case reports via the method of back-calculation.[14] The estimated annual rates of infection were as follows (± standard deviation in parentheses): 75 (±6) for the years 1980–82; 68 (±6) for 1983–85; 62 (±9) for 1986–89; and 61 (±12) for 1990–93.

The remaining infections in Israel are among Ethiopian Jewish immigrants. This immigration was punctuated by two large waves: approximately 17,000 arrived between 1982 and 1985, while an additional 25,000 have arrived since 1991.[15] Coupled with immigration in intervening years, roughly 50,000 Ethiopian Jews arrived in Israel.[4,15,16] Net births in this community within Israel have further increased the population to its current size of 60,000.[4]

While nearly 40% of known HIV infections in Israel occurred among Ethiopian immigrants, virtually all of these occurred among adult Ethiopians who immigrated to Israel since 1991.[4,15] The HIV incidence rate among these recent immigrants aged 15 or above was estimated statistically as 7 (±2) infections per 1000 uninfected persons annually as of May 1995 via the use of a snapshot estimator.[17,18]

To estimate the probability that a contaminated blood donation occurs, we will require HIV incidence rates for potential blood donors. To create comparable rates, we assume that in both the non-Ethiopian and the Ethiopian Israeli populations, the rate of new infections among persons below age 15 is negligible, and the incidence rates among potential donors equal the incidence rates in the population aged 15 or greater. Doing so leads to overestimates of the HIV incidence rates among potential donors. First, the incidence rate among potential donors is probably lower than in the population at large due to self-selection; those recognizing that they are at risk for infection might simply choose not to donate, for example, or alternatively the voluntary nature of blood donation could simply correlate with lower rates of HIV risk behaviors. Second, donors at greater risk for HIV infection might be excluded for reasons other than the HIV antibody test (as has been explained for the case of the United States).[19] Donors could be excluded for testing positive for some other disease (e.g., hepatitis) or for revealing a greater risk of exposure to HIV (e.g., via injection drug use).

Nonetheless we will adopt these assumptions, for as will be shown below, they overstate the preventive impact of the exclusion policy. Noting that virtually all infections among Ethiopian immigrants occurred among those who immigrated since 1991, while 70% of the Ethiopian population in Israel is of age 15 or above,[20] we arrive at an HIV incidence rate of 3 infections per 1000 uninfected persons per year. Similarly, noting that the overall number of non-Ethiopian Israelis aged 15 or above equals 3.9 million[21] and that the prevalence of HIV in this population equals 0.0002, extrapolating the most recent back-calculation results yields an incidence of 1 in 64,000 or 1.6 per 100,000 uninfected persons per year.

MODELING THE PROBABILITY
OF INFECTIOUS DONATION

What is the risk of an infectious donation? In Israel, all donated blood and organs have been screened for HIV antibody since 1986.[22] Consequently, the only infected blood donations capable of entering the blood supply are those producing false negative antibody tests. Such false negative results can occur if the blood donation occurs in the window period between the time of infection and the development of HIV antibodies.[19,23] The conditional probability $p(t)$ that an antibody-negative donation at time t is infected is thus given by

$$p(t) = \frac{\text{Pr\{Donor is infected and donation tests antibody negative\}}}{\text{Pr\{Donation tests antibody negative\}}}.$$

The probability that a donation tests antibody negative at time t is the sum of two terms: the probability that the donor is uninfected at time t (where we ignore the negligible false positive test rate), and the probability that the donor is infected but in the window. Let $\iota(x)$ denote the HIV incidence rate among potential donors at time x, and define the cumulative incidence between two dates a and b as

$$I(a,b) = \int_a^b \iota(x)dx.$$

With this notation, we see that

$$\text{Pr\{Donor is uninfected at time } t\} = e^{-I(-\infty,t)}.$$

Now let W denote the duration of the window period, and $f(w)$ be the associated probability density. For an antibody-negative donation at time t to be infected, the donor must have been infected somewhere between time $t - W$ and time t. The probability of this event equals $E[e^{-I(-\infty,t-W)} - e^{-I(-\infty,t)}]$. We thus conclude that

$$\text{Pr\{Donor is infected and donation tests antibody negative\}}$$

$$= E[e^{-I(-\infty,t-w)} - e^{-I(-\infty,t)}]$$

$$= \int_0^\infty (e^{-I(-\infty,t-w)} - e^{-I(-\infty,t)}) f(w)dw$$

$$= e^{-I(-\infty,t)} \int_0^\infty (e^{I(t-w,t)} - 1) f(w)dw.$$

Combining the results above, we find that

$$p(t) = \frac{e^{-I(-\infty,t)} \int_0^\infty (e^{I(t-w,t)} - 1) f(w) dw}{e^{-I(-\infty,t)} \int_0^\infty (e^{I(t-w,t)} - 1) f(w) dw + e^{-I(-\infty,t)}}$$

Now, the average duration of the window period ($\overline{w}$) has been reported to equal 25 days with a 95% confidence interval ranging from 9 to 41 days.[19,23] This fact combined with the low incidence rates observed in Israel enables the excellent approximation

$$e^{I(t-w,t)} \approx 1 + I(t - w,t).$$

The brevity of the window period also precludes rapid changes in the HIV incidence rate over the time period of interest prior to donation, which implies that the simplification $I(t - w,t) \approx \iota(t)w$ will be very accurate. Substituting these two approximations into our model for $p(t)$ yields the result

$$p(t) = \frac{\iota(t)\overline{w}}{1 + \iota(t)\overline{w}} \approx \iota(t)\overline{w}$$

with the final approximation following from the very small value of $\iota(t)\overline{w}$ for the problem at hand.

We can now estimate the probability that an antibody-negative donation is infected for potential non-Ethiopian and Ethiopian Israeli donors via the incidence rates reported above. Given a mean window period of 25 days = 0.07 years, we obtain probabilities of 1.1 in one million for non-Ethiopian Israelis, and 2.1 in 10,000 for Ethiopian immigrants to Israel. Note that the relative risk of a potentially infectious donation from an Ethiopian relative to a non-Ethiopian Israeli donor depends only on the ratio of the *incidence* rates, as opposed to the prevalence. As the incidence rate among potential Ethiopian donors exceeds that of non-Ethiopian Israelis by a factor of 190, one might argue that the officials actually underestimated the additional risks posed by potential Ethiopian donors to the blood supply (as the prevalence ratio discussed earlier implied a factor of 50 elevation in risk).

However, as the above calculations make clear, the absolute risks involved are very small. By way of comparison, in the United States, it has been estimated that the probability an antibody-negative donation is in the window equals 1 in 430,000,[23] about twice the risk for non-Ethiopian Israelis. It is probably true that the risks estimated above are too high given the inflated donor HIV incidence rates employed. Nonetheless we will use the estimates above, for they will lead to an upper bound on the preventive impact of the exclusion policy.

IMPLICIT COST-EFFECTIVENESS ANALYSIS

To establish the impact of excluding Ethiopian donors on the number of infectious donations to the Israeli blood supply, we need to consider the mix of donations that would have occurred had Ethiopian donors not been excluded.[11] This information is available, for as stated previously, the policy as implemented was to draw blood from Ethiopian donors and then discard it. From mid-1990 through mid-1995, there were 942,517 donors of whom 2,055 were Ethiopian immigrants.[4] This annualizes to a rate of 188,000 and 411 donors for non-Ethiopian and Ethiopian Israelis, respectively. However, in 1995 it was reported that there were 225,000 *donations* from 190,000 *donors,* or 1.18 donations per donor.[4] For purposes of analysis we will assume that this ratio applies to both groups of donors. Doing so probably overestimates the numbers of donations that could be expected from Ethiopians, for reportedly most of the Ethiopian donations resulted from organized drives of army units.[24] However, overestimating Ethiopian participation in the blood supply will also overestimate the public health effectiveness of excluding Ethiopian donors. Application of the multiplier to the annual number of donors suggests that 222,000 and 485 donations could be expected among non-Ethiopian and Ethiopian Israelis annually.

A good measure of the risk associated with including or excluding Ethiopian donors is the annual number of potentially infectious donations resulting from either policy. Letting π equal the fraction of blood donations that test antibody positive, d equal the number of annual donations, and p equal the probability that an antibody-negative donation is in fact HIV-infected, the expected number of potentially infectious donations n is given by

$$n = d \times (1 - \pi) \times p.$$

Applying this formula to non-Ethiopian Israeli donors ($d = 222,000$, $\pi = 0.0002$, $p = 1.1 \times 10^{-6}$) yields an annual expected number of 0.24 infectious donations. For Ethiopian Israeli donors ($d = 485$, $\pi = 0.015$, $p = 2.1 \times 10^{-4}$), one would expect a total of 0.1 infectious donations annually.

With respect to HIV, then, the total public health effectiveness of excluding Ethiopian donors can be viewed as a reduction in the total annual number of infectious donations from 0.34 to 0.24, a *relative* reduction of 29%. Note that this relative reduction in the number of infectious donations admitted to the blood supply sounds much more modest than the "factor of 50" argument based on comparative HIV prevalence rates. But more important, the *absolute* reduction in infectious donations equals only *0.1 per year* across the *entire* blood supply. Since the effectiveness of exclusion depends solely on the number of infected donations that would have been given by Ethiopian Israeli donors, all of our assumptions taken together *overestimate* this quantity. If incidence rates among potential Ethiopian donors were lower than estimated among adult Ethiopian immigrants, or if the number of donations per donor was less for Ethiopian than for non-Ethiopian Israeli donors, then the effectiveness of exclusion would be even less than the estimated annual rate of 0.10 infectious donations.

An implicit cost-effectiveness argument can now be stated: excluding Ethiopian immigrants from donating blood is defensible only if the incremental costs associated with such a policy are worth less to society than an annual increase of 0.10 infectious donations to the blood supply. Viewed simply from this perspective, it is not clear that excluding Ethiopian donors is justified on the grounds of maximizing public health effectiveness. To consider some of the social costs of this policy, recall that 70 persons were injured in the demonstration protesting the blood exclusion decision. The costs of treating these injuries alone might compete with the expected medical cost increase resulting from an additional 0.1 infected donations annually for a few years, especially when one realizes that HIV disease and AIDS do not develop in all recipients of infected blood. In the United States, for example, 25% to 50% of transfusion recipients die within one year from transfusion from their underlying medical problems.[19] The impact of this policy on the Ethiopian community in Israel also should not be understated. According to anthropologist Shalva Weill of the Hebrew University, "Blood is symbolic. An insult to their blood is an insult to the community's identity. It goes beyond AIDS. It's their physical identity which is being violated."[2] Also threatened was the adequacy of the blood supply in Israel, for following the disclosure of the exclusion policy, there was a significant drop in blood donations to the Magen David Adom.[25] And of course, commentators cited earlier implicitly argued that there is a cost to deception itself. One might argue that most of these costs accrued only because the policy was exposed; absent the knowledge that the blood was being discarded, there would have been no riot, for example. However, one can also argue that a priori, there existed a high likelihood that the policy would become exposed at some point in the future, and thus considering social costs of the sort described above is not inappropriate.

The Navon Commission's official inquiry regarding this affair concluded that the officials who adopted the blood exclusion policy were not evil, and that in fact they did worry about stigmatizing the community.[4,26] Though the panel found that it was wrong to lie to Ethiopian donors, they also noted that the decision was taken for public health purposes. Given our analysis above, perhaps the best explanation of what happened is that Israeli health officials vastly overestimated the additional risk to the blood supply posed by Ethiopian donors.

IMPLICIT COST-BENEFIT ANALYSIS

One criticism of our cost-effectiveness analysis is that by focusing only on averted infected donations, we ignore other important sources of costs and benefits. For example, we have ignored the benefits derived from the donation of healthy units of blood to the national supply, and we have not related the magnitude of these benefits to the costs associated with infectious donations.

To proceed, we need to introduce three new parameters.[12] Let b denote the benefit in dollars associated with each uninfected blood donation, c the cost in dollars for each infected donation, and s the annual social cost in dollars associated with implementing the exclusion decision. We could also incorporate the wasted expense of HIV testing for blood discarded irrespective of the test result, but the effect of doing so is negligible.[12] As before, let d denote the number of donations, π denote HIV antibody prevalence, and p denote the probability that an antibody-negative donation is in fact infected.

Omitting social costs, the expected annual net benefits associated with accepting blood are given by

$$d \times (1 - \pi) \times (b \times (1 - p) - c \times p).$$

To obtain the overall annual net benefits in the absence of exclusion, we add the net benefits for non-Ethiopian and Ethiopian Israeli donors. To obtain the overall net benefits of the exclusion policy, we take the annual net benefits for non-Ethiopian Israeli donors and then subtract the social cost of exclusion. The exclusion policy is justified on the basis of cost-benefit analysis only if it produces larger annual net benefits. This situation will prevail when the annual social costs of exclusion are smaller than the annual net costs associated with Ethiopian Israeli donors, that is, exclusion is justified on cost-benefit grounds when

$$s < d \times (1 - \pi) \times (c \times p - b \times (1 - p))$$

where all of the parameters on the right-hand side pertain to Ethiopian Israeli donors.

The inequality above can be used to establish thresholds for determining when exclusion is justifiable on cost-benefit grounds. First, suppose that the social costs s are equated to zero. Exclusion is justified in this instance if the marginal cost of including Ethiopian blood (given by $c \times p$) exceeds the marginal benefit of inclusion (given by $b \times (1 - p)$). Otherwise it does not make sense to exclude Ethiopian donors. Second, and perhaps more interestingly, the analysis also suggests social cost thresholds where exclusion is indefensible for any presumed benefit per healthy donation. Setting $b = 0$, excluding Ethiopian Israeli donors remains defensible only if $s < d \times (1 - \pi) \times c \times p$.

We have previously estimated that $d = 485$, $\pi = 0.015$, and $p = 2.1 \times 10^{-4}$ for Ethiopian donors. We can establish a point estimate for c by assuming that each infectious donation leads, over all time, to m infections, each of which carries a cost to society. We can estimate an upper bound on this multiplier m by assuming that HIV incidence in the population is proportional to HIV prevalence. Doing so enables the bound[27]

$$m \leq \frac{1}{1 - r\overline{D}}$$

where r is the ratio of incidence to prevalence, and $\overline{D}$ is the mean duration of infection. This formula is applicable only if the quantity $r\overline{D}$ (the reproductive rate of infection) is less than 1, and represents the expected total number of infections generated over all time from an initial infected person in an infinite population of susceptibles (including the index case).[27] Since almost all recipients of donated blood are non-Ethiopian Israelis, we use the previously estimated incidence and prevalence rates for this population and obtain $r \approx 0.07$. Taking $\overline{D}$ to equal ten years (the mean incubation period from HIV infection to the development of AIDS), we estimate that $m = 3.33$.

For each of these infections, we consider the sum of the lifetime direct medical costs required to treat a new HIV infection, and the indirect costs accruing from lost productivity, among other factors. Others have estimated the lifetime medical costs per HIV infection as being near \$200,000.[28] Discounted future earnings lost are often used as a proxy for indirect costs in health research. While no estimates are available for the magnitude of such a loss for newly infected Israelis, U.S. figures suggest these costs are on the order of \$500,000.[29]

Though it would take many years for future infections to accrue, we will proceed as if each infectious donation leads to 3.33 infections immediately, which again biases the argument to favor the exclusion policy. Incorporating direct medical costs, indirect costs, and the infection multiplier suggests that the societal cost per infectious donation c should be on the order of ($\$200,000$ + $\$500,000$) $\times$ 3.33 = $\$2.33$ million.

Rather than attempting to estimate the benefits of healthy donations b and the social costs of exclusion s, we will instead consider decision thresholds implied by the estimated values of the other parameters. At $c = \$2.33$ million, the exclusion decision is not defensible on cost-benefit grounds if the benefits from healthy blood donations exceed $\$490$ per donation. It is not at all clear that a healthy unit of blood is in fact worth $\$490$ at the margin; thus it is important to consider social costs in evaluating the exclusion decision. Doing so leads to the conclusion that the exclusion decision is not defensible if the social costs of exclusion s exceed $\$234,000$ annually. With a population of 60,000 Ethiopian immigrants in Israel, a useful question to ask is whether the annual negative social consequences of the exclusion decision amount to more than $\$234,000/60,000 = \$3.90$ per Ethiopian immigrant. If one believes this to be the case, then the exclusion decision cannot be defended on cost-benefit grounds.

While better estimates of all the parameters employed in this model could lead to different numerical thresholds, the general point transcends the particulars of the numerical example offered: the exclusion decision can be justified only if the social costs of the policy are very small. However, many if not most observers would agree that the social costs to Israel of excluding Ethiopian donors are not small, again calling into question the decision to exclude Ethiopian Israelis from donating blood.

CONCLUSION

In reviewing Israel's policy of excluding Ethiopian donors, the Navon Commission found that deceiving blood donors was wrong, but concluded that those responsible for the decision acted in the interests of public health, and not out of bigotry or racism.[4,26] The analysis in this chapter suggests that the public health benefits of the exclusion policy were overestimated. On average, excluding Ethiopian donors prevents at most one HIV infectious donation every ten years, a benefit that is outweighed by the social costs of exclusion if the latter exceed $\$234,000$ per year in total, or $\$3.90$ per Ethiopian immigrant per year.

In closing, although the analysis reported here was conducted after the fact, a similar study could have been performed prospectively. Even lacking the statistical estimate of HIV incidence among Ethiopian immigrants required to model the probability of undetected infectious donations (for this too was determined only recently), the framework used in this chapter could have served as an organizing principle for the systematic exploration of alternative assumptions regarding HIV incidence among Ethiopian Israeli donors, the safety of the blood supply, and the rationale for exclusion. Blood supplies around the world continue to face threats from HIV and other infectious diseases, and excluding those donors believed to pose high risks remains a viable option in such circumstances. Whether donor exclusion is justified in any given scenario of course depends on the particulars. The models illustrated in this chapter, I believe, comprise a defensible approach to evaluating such specifics.

ACKNOWLEDGMENTS

This research was supported in part by the Societal Institute of the Mathematical Sciences via grant DA-09531 from the National Institute on Drug Abuse, the Center for Interdisciplinary Research on AIDS at Yale University via grant MH/DA-56826 from the National Institutes on Mental Health and Drug Abuse, and the Lady Davis Fellowship Trust, Jerusalem.

REFERENCES

1. Schmemann S. Ethiopians in Israel riot over dumping of donated blood. *New York Times* 1996, January 29:1.
2. Tsur B. The insult was too much to bear. *Jerusalem Post* 1996, January 29:1.
3. Vikhanski L. Israel's blood policy causes furor. *Nature Medicine* 1996, 2:260.
4. Navon Y, Winograd E, Hillel N, Nagan L, Rachmilevich E, Zakai Y. *Summoning to Clarify the Blood Donation Affair of Ethiopian Immigrants* (in Hebrew). Jerusalem: Government of Israel, 1996.
5. United Press International. Israel medical head defends destroyed blood. UPI wire service 1996, January 30 (accessed via NEXIS).
6. Siegel J. Policy on Ethiopian blood donors is correct. *Jerusalem Post* 1996, January 28:12.
7. *Jerusalem Post* Editorial Staff. Ethiopian protest (editorial). *Jerusalem Post* 1996, January 29:6.
8. Reuters. Elie Wiesel blasts Israel on Ethiopian blood donations. Reuters wire service 1996, January 29 (accessed via NEXIS).
9. *Jerusalem Post* staff. Burg slams Navon Committee findings. *Jerusalem Post* 1996, July 31:3.

10. Siegel J. Sneh: Lying about Ethiopian blood was "unethical." *Jerusalem Post* 1996, March 18:12.

11. Kaplan EH. Israel's ban on use of Ethiopian's blood: How many infectious donations were prevented? *Lancet* 1998, 351:1127–1128.

12. Kaplan EH. Implicit valuation of a blood exclusion decision. *Medical Decision Making* 1999, 19:207–213.

13. National Tuberculosis and AIDS Unit. *HIV/AIDS Quarterly Report.* Jerusalem: Israel Ministry of Health, 1997, no. 1.

14. Kaplan E, Slater P, Soskolne V. How many HIV infections are there in Israel? Reconstructing HIV incidence from AIDS case reporting. *Public Health Reviews* 1995, 23:215–235.

15. Pollack S, Israel AIDS Study Group. Epidemiological and immunological study of HIV-seropositive Ethiopian immigrants in Israel. *Israel Journal of Medical Sciences* 1993, 29 (suppl):19–23.

16. Central Bureau of Statistics. Table 5.4: Immigrants and potential immigrants by period of immigration, country of birth and last country of residence. In: *Statistical Abstract of Israel.* Jerusalem: Government of Israel, 1995 (retrieved via *www.cbs.gov.il/shnaton/st05-04.gif*).

17. Kaplan EH, Kedem E, Pollack S. HIV incidence among Ethiopian immigrants to Israel. *J Acquir Immune Defic Syndr* 1998, 17:465–469.

18. Kaplan EH, Brookmeyer R. Snapshot estimators of recent HIV incidence rates. *Operations Research* 1999; 47:29–37.

19. Lackritz EM, Satten GA, Aberle-Grasse J, Dodd RY, Raimondi VP, Janssen RS, Lewis WF, Notari EP IV, Peterson LR. Estimated risk of transmission of the human immunodeficiency virus by screened blood in the United States. *N Engl J Med* 1995; 333:1721–1725.

20. Central Bureau of Statistics. Table 2.23: Jews, by country of origin, place of birth and age. In: *Statistical Abstract of Israel.* Jerusalem: Government of Israel, 1995 (retrieved via *www.cbs.gov.il/shnaton/st02-23.gif*).

21. Central Bureau of Statistics. Table 2.10: Population, by age, sex, religion, district, sub-district and area. In: *Statistical Abstract of Israel.* Jerusalem: Government of Israel, 1995 (retrieved via *www.cbs.gov.il/shnaton/st02-10.gif*).

22. Slater PE, Costin C. The epidemiology of adult AIDS and HIV infection in Israel. *Israel Journal of Medical Sciences* 1993, 29 (suppl):2–6.

23. Satten GA. Steady-state calculation of the risk of HIV infection from transfusion of screened blood from repeat donors. *Mathematical Biosciences* 1997, 141:101–113.

24. Siegel J. "Ma'ariv" report will stigmatize Ethiopian immigrants. *Jerusalem Post* 1996, January 26:3.

25. Siegel J. Blood donations drop significantly. *Jerusalem Post* 1996, February 6:12.

26. Siegel J. Navon panel finds fault with MDA, falls short of calling for dismissals. *Jerusalem Post* 1996, July 29:1.

27. Kaplan EH, Cramton PC, Paltiel AD. Nonrandom mixing models of HIV transmission. In: *Mathematical and Statistical Approaches to AIDS Epidemiology.* Edited by C. Castillo-Chavez. *Lecture Notes in Biomathematics* 1989, 83:218–239.

28. Holtgrave DR and Pinkerton SD. Updates of cost of illness and quality of life estimates for use in economic evaluations of HIV prevention programs. *J Acquir Immune Defic Syndr* 1997, 16:54–62.

29. Brandeau ML, Owens DK, Sox CH, Wachter RM. Screening women of childbearing age for human immunodeficiency virus: A model-based policy analysis. *Management Science* 1993, 39:72–92.

Chapter 10 Feeding Strategies for Children of HIV-Infected Mothers: Modeling the Trade-Off Between HIV Infection and Non-HIV Mortality

James G. Kahn, Elliot Marseille, and Joseph Saba

Each year, approximately half a million infants worldwide acquire the human immunodeficiency virus (HIV) from their mothers, according to the United Nations Combined AIDS Program (UNAIDS). The risk of transmission from mother to child varies up to 50% in breastfeeding populations.[1] Much transmission occurs in utero and intra partum, but risk during breastfeeding itself is about 14% on average, and higher with long duration breastfeeding.[2,3] Mother-to-child HIV transmission risk is largely avoidable through the use of perinatal antiretroviral therapy and formula feeding.[4] These strategies are widely used in the developed world.[5]

In many countries hardest hit by the AIDS epidemic, however, especially in Africa and Asia, there are serious barriers to implementing such interventions. Financial resources for health care are extremely limited, forcing difficult choices among possible programs. Short-course perinatal antiretroviral therapy can be cost-effective compared with other public health interventions, provided that HIV prevalence is moderate and antiretroviral regimens are inexpensive, such as nevirapine single dose.[6,7] Formula feeding interventions also raise financial challenges.

Furthermore, in settings with poor sanitation and high infant mortality, there is a risk that formula feeding will increase mortality from illnesses such as diarrhea and pneumonia by removing the protective benefits of breastfeeding. For decades public health advocates have encouraged breastfeeding as a cheap and effective means to reduce infant mortality and morbidity. This trade-off between reduced HIV transmission and increased non-HIV infant mortality has been examined in several simulation models. These analyses conclude that overall mortality is reduced with formula feeding if non-HIV infant mortality is low.[8-14]

There are several reasons to revisit and extend these analyses. First, there are now much better data on the magnitude and timing of breastfeeding-associated HIV transmission.[3] Thus, the trade-off between HIV and non-HIV risk can be better estimated. Second, the advent of effective short-course antiretroviral therapy to reduce vertical transmission alters the HIV prevention benefits of formula feeding. Finally, as countries develop strategies to reduce mother-to-child transmission, there is a need to understand the magnitude of benefit and cost-effectiveness compared with current treatment and feeding practices. These factors were considered in a recent analysis for South Africa,[15] but have not been incorporated into a more general model.

We constructed a model to formally assess different infant feeding strategies, using the most recent information about the effects of perinatal antiretrovirals and risk of HIV transmission during breastfeeding. We ask two questions: How does formula feeding affect combined HIV and non-HIV mortality in the infants of HIV-infected mothers? And, what is the optimal duration of breastfeeding? We apply our model in eight geographic settings (rural and urban South Africa, Tanzania, Thailand, and Brazil) and for varied assumptions about perinatal antiretroviral therapy.

METHODS

Overview

Our model assesses month-by-month risks of fatal adverse events (death or HIV infection) for five infant feeding strategies. We consider current breastfeeding patterns and four alternatives: long-term (24 month) breastfeeding, breastfeeding for 6 months, breastfeeding for 3 months, and formula feeding from birth.

In each feeding alternative we assume that breastfeeding or formula is the primary food until six months, after which one or the other is continued to 24 months in combination with other foods.

The analysis tracks a cohort of 100 infants born to HIV-infected mothers. A certain proportion of the infants are infected with HIV during pregnancy and delivery. We estimate this proportion both with and without a perinatal antiretroviral (ARV) intervention. The remainder of infants are at risk of both non-HIV death and HIV transmission. The model sums these two risks to determine the number of fatal adverse events in the cohort in each month and over the full 24 months.

In settings or scenarios where formula feeding is not the preferred strategy, we estimate the optimal duration of breastfeeding. Optimal duration is defined as the age of the child when the added risk of non-HIV death due to formula feeding (i.e., the increment in the non-HIV hazard rate) drops to the level of the ongoing risk of HIV transmission with breastfeeding. Expressed in terms of the total hazard of fatal adverse events (non-HIV death plus HIV infection), optimal duration corresponds to the age when the hazard with formula feeding equals the hazard with breastfeeding.

We also describe cost data required to assess cost-effectiveness.

Health Inputs

The model uses the health inputs summarized in Table 10.1 and below. The percent of newborns at risk (HIV-uninfected at birth) is 100% minus the risk of HIV transmission during pregnancy and delivery. This risk has recently been estimated at about 18% in several clinical trials in Africa, with some variation by country.[16-19] Thus 81% to 87% are at risk of HIV infection at birth. Two short-course perinatal ARV regimens have been reported as approximately 50% effective: zidovudine alone[17] and zidovudine in combination with lamivudine.[16] Thus, in the presence of ARV perinatal therapy, we assume that more newborns are susceptible during breastfeeding because only half as many were infected with HIV prior to breastfeeding. There is considerable concern that the rebound in HIV serum viral load seen after the end of the perinatal ARV therapy will lead to higher transmission during breastfeeding,[20,21] but empirical data on this issue are still pending from clinical trials.

Estimates of the risk of HIV transmission during breastfeeding are based on studies comparing breastfeeders with non-breastfeeders. The mean risk associated with any breastfeeding, including short duration, has been estimated at 14%.[2] Most risk is in the first two to three months[22,23] and likely largely in the

Table 10.1. Model Inputs, by Site

	South Africa		Tanzania		Thailand		Brazil	
	Urban	Rural	Urban	Rural	Urban	Rural	Urban	Rural
Newborns at risk (HIV-uninfected at birth)								
No antiretroviral (ARV) program	80.0%	80.0%	82.0%	82.0%	81.4%	81.4%	87.0%	87.0%
ARV pre-partum (50% efficacy)	90	90	91.0	91.0	90.7	90.7	93.5	93.5
HIV transmission during breastfeeding								
Full 24 months, no ARV program	27.0%	24.0%	20.0%	20.0%	20.0%	20.0%	8.6%	8.0%
Full 24 months, ARV pre-partum	27.0	27.0	22.2	22.2	22.3	22.3	8.6	8.6
Late postnatal (3–24 mo) risk	5.9	5.9	5.1	5.1	5.0	5.0	2.2	2.2
Non-HIV mortality								
1 month	0.010	0.025	0.034	0.038	0.012	0.017	0.021	0.026
1 year	0.030	0.070	0.083	0.095	0.020	0.041	0.041	0.065
2 years	0.040	0.093	0.107	0.122	0.023	0.052	0.050	0.083
Relative risk with formula feeding	3	4	3	4	3	4	3	4
Current breastfeeding patterns								
1 month—substantial	60%	69%	77%	77%	36%	72%	73%	84%
any	93	96	99	99	46	93	95	97
3 months—substantial	50%	53%	56%	63%	25%	56%	43%	58%
any	85	92	98	98	44	87	65	75
6 months—substantial	25%	38%	50%	52%	21%	44%	30%	45%
any	65	81	97	97	41	82	50	70

first month (Glenda Gray, unpublished data). Late postnatal risk, from 2.5 to 24 months, has been calculated in one meta-analysis at 7.4% of those uninfected at 2.5 months;[3] depending on risk prior to 2.5 months, this is approximately 5% of all infants born to HIV-positive mothers. For our model, we assume that HIV transmission risk for a full 24 months of breastfeeding is 20 per 100 infants born to HIV-positive mothers. This includes risk to age 3 months of 15 per 100, and for age 3 to 24 months of 5 per 100. Data from South Africa suggest higher overall risk,[19] while data from Brazil suggest lower overall risk.[18] The monthly risk pattern is specified by calibrating a Weibull probability density function to these values.

We selected the Weibull function because it is well suited to portraying risk functions that evolve over time. It can be calibrated to known characteristics of a survival or risk function, such as instantaneous or cumulative risk at specified times, and provides a reasonable basis for interpolation for times lacking empirical data. A previous analysis of this health problem used the Weibull to portray non-HIV mortality risk by age.[13] We extend this technique to other inputs that follow a similar temporal pattern: relative risk of non-HIV mortality, breastfeeding patterns, and HIV risk through breastfeeding.

The Weibull survival function is given by:

$$S(t) = Pr\{T > t\} = \exp(-\alpha t^{\beta}) \tag{1}$$

where T is the random variable denoting survival time, α determines survival at $t = 1$ and β determines the evolution of risk over time (a value >1 yields increasing risk and <1 yields decreasing risk). We use this form of the function to portray cumulative risk of HIV through breastfeeding by age as well as the inputs discussed below. We calibrated curves to available empirical data, the timing of which varies by input (e.g., 3 and 24 months for HIV risk, versus 1, 12, and 60 months for non-HIV mortality).

The instantaneous Weibull hazard is:

$$h(t) = \alpha^{*}\beta^{*}t^{(\beta-1)} \tag{2}$$

indicating risk to those still susceptible to this outcome at time t, e.g., risk of HIV infection to those uninfected. The instantaneous probability density function, which indicates risk using the entire initial cohort as the denominator, is the product of hazard and the proportion surviving. We calculated interval survival probabilities to permit direct calibration to empirical data that report risk for time intervals (usually months) rather than points in time. The calculation is:

$$Pr\{t_n < T \leq t_{n+1}\} = S(t_n) - S(t_{n+1}) \tag{3}$$

Non-HIV mortality rates are estimated where possible based on standardized demographic and health surveys conducted in each country.[24-26] These surveys report mortality at 1 month, 1 year, and 5 years, by region and major city (except Brazil, for which mean countrywide data are reported). For South Africa, we obtained similar but less complete estimates from multiple sources[27] (Glenda Gray, personal communication, March 3, 1998). We estimated mortality at 2 years by interpolating with a Weibull function calibrated to the reported data points.

Multiple studies suggest that formula feeding increases mortality, typically two- to three-fold.[28] We relied on a study conducted with data from Malaysia in 1977,[29] since it provides the most detailed estimates by age. Relative risk was 3.2 over the first year of life, dropping from 10 in days 8–28, to 2.5 in months 2–6, and 1.3 in months 7–12 (derived from Tables 3 and 5 of Habicht).[29] No elevated risk was noted in the second year of life. In our model, we used a relative mortality risk of 3 for urban locations and 4 for rural locations. These both represent high estimates, potentially biasing the analysis in favor of breastfeeding. Risks by month were interpolated using the Weibull function calibrated to these relative risk benchmarks.

Current breastfeeding patterns by month of age are determined from the same demographic and health surveys used to estimate mortality except in South Africa, where additional sources were consulted[30] (Neil Soderlund, personal communication, March 4, 1998) and some extrapolation was required (e.g., from urban South Africa and rural Tanzania to rural South Africa). We estimate two levels of breastfeeding. "Any breastfeeding" is tracked as the basis to calculate risk of HIV transmission. "Substantial breastfeeding" is also estimated (as the mean of exclusive and any breastfeeding) to facilitate extrapolation from current non-HIV infant mortality rates to mortality rates expected with all breastfeeding or all formula feeding (see below). One limitation of these data is their age (e.g., for Thailand from 1987); we were unable to find more recent estimates.

Calculation of Health Outcomes

Empirical data on non-HIV mortality reflect existing feeding patterns, including a mix of feeding practices in each month of life. We estimate month-specific non-HIV mortality with pure breastfeeding and with formula feeding by simple mathematical transformations of that month's observed mortality, prevalence of feeding patterns, and relative risk of mortality with formula feeding.

The basic equation that relates feeding pattern to risk of mortality is:

$$b \cdot m_b + f \cdot m_b \cdot RR = m_o \qquad (4)$$

where each parameter is defined for a particular month: $b =$ the prevalence of breastfeeding, $m_b =$ mortality with breastfeeding, $f =$ the prevalence of formula feeding ($= 1 - b$), $RR =$ the relative risk of mortality with formula feeding, and $m_o =$ observed mortality. For this calculation, breastfeeding prevalence is defined as the total of exclusive and primary breastfeeding, excluding limited breastfeeding. We use this approach because the protection conferred by breastfeeding is proportional to its exclusivity, and the relative risks we use are based on exclusive breastfeeding. Empirical estimates of all variables except m_b are available. Transformed, the mortality with breastfeeding can be calculated as:

$$m_b = m_o / (b + f \cdot RR) \qquad (5)$$

This estimate is imperfect because mortality may be a complex function of feeding practices in previous months, and several inputs are known only imprecisely. However, for our purposes the estimate suffices to adjust observed mortality to mortality with a specified feeding type.

For each month, the total risk of a fatal adverse event is calculated by summing the two independent risks of non-HIV mortality and HIV infection. Double-counting is avoided (i.e., a child who is HIV-infected and dies later of non-HIV causes is counted as only one adverse event). Survival is tracked for 24 months.

Our outcome measure is total fatal adverse events per 100 infants born to HIV-infected mothers. This outcome is calculated by comparing the number of infants born HIV-uninfected in the cohort of 100 to the number alive and HIV-uninfected at 2 years of age.

RESULTS

The optimal feeding strategy in seven settings (all but rural Brazil) is formula feeding (Table 10.2, Figures 10.1A and 10.1B). In these seven settings, short-term breastfeeding strategies are better than current feeding where extended breastfeeding is the norm, but worse where a high proportion of women al-

Table 10.2. Adverse Events (HIV Infections and Non-HIV Deaths), by Site and Antiretroviral Program Status

	South Africa		Tanzania		Thailand		Brazil	
	Urban	Rural	Urban	Rural	Urban	Rural	Urban	Rural
No antiretroviral progam								
Current breastfeeding patterns	22.5	27.2	26.0	27.0	10.3	20.5	10.0	13.2
Breastfeeding 24 months	25.3	27.4	24.8	25.1	20.6	21.9	10.5	12.4
Breastfeeding 6 months	21.5	23.8	21.7	22.2	17.3	18.8	9.1	11.3
Breastfeeding 3 months	19.8	22.6	20.7	21.6	15.8	17.6	8.7	11.3
Formula feeding (no breastfeeding)	3.9	11.6	15.0	18.6	2.4	7.3	7.5	14.9
Difference current vs. best alternative	−18.6	−15.6	−11.0	−8.4	−7.9	−13.2	−2.4	−1.8
ARV perinatal								
Current breastfeeding patterns	25.3	30.6	28.8	29.9	11.5	22.9	10.7	14.1
Breastfeeding 24 months	28.5	30.8	27.6	27.8	22.9	24.4	11.3	13.4
Breastfeeding 6 months	24.2	26.8	24.1	24.6	19.2	20.9	9.8	12.2
Breastfeeding 3 months	22.3	25.5	23.0	23.9	17.6	19.6	9.3	12.2
Formula feeding (no breastfeeding)	4.3	13.0	16.6	20.6	2.7	8.2	8.1	16.0
Difference current vs. best alternative	−20.9	−17.6	−12.2	−9.4	−8.8	−14.7	−2.6	−2.0

A

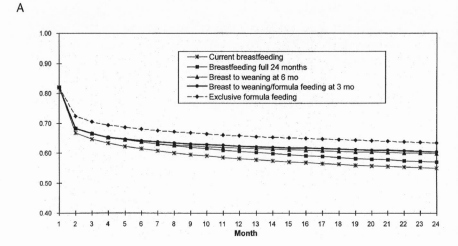

B

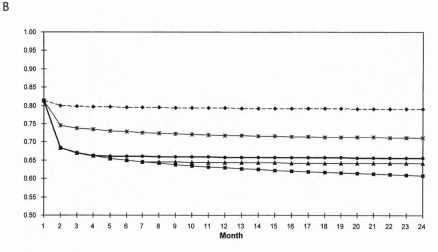

Figure 10.1. (A) Survival without adverse outcome (HIV or death), Tanzania, rural. (B) Survival without adverse outcome (HIV or death) Thailand, urban.

ready formula feed. In general, adverse outcomes decrease as formula feeding increases. Expected risks and gains are slightly higher with perinatal antiretrovirals due to the greater number of infants who are HIV-uninfected initially. The one setting where short-term breastfeeding is preferred is rural Brazil, which combines high non-HIV mortality and low HIV risk in breastfeeding (extrapolated from a study in São Paolo).

In the seven settings where formula feeding appears optimal, the difference between current feeding and formula feeding varies from 2 to 19 fatal adverse events per 100 children. This difference is largest in settings with low non-HIV mortality and high HIV risk through breastfeeding, such as urban South Africa. The difference is lower in settings with high non-HIV mortality, such as rural Tanzania. It is also lower with high current use of formula so that the gains and losses of switching to all formula feeding are muted, such as in urban Thailand. And it is low when HIV risk appears to be low, as in urban Brazil.

We found with our best estimate inputs that in these seven sites none of the breastfeeding strategies could take advantage of differences in timing for HIV transmission and non-HIV mortality. Both are heavily concentrated in the first months of life (Figures 10.2A and 10.2B), with HIV risk higher from the start as well as more enduring. In most scenarios, there appear to be no months in which breastfeeding yields a greater reduction in non-HIV mortality than the increase in HIV transmission. For rural Tanzania (Figure 10.2A), breastfeeding has a lower risk than formula feeding in month 2, but it is impossible to capture this benefit because the advantage for formula feeding is so pronounced in month 1. We assume that strategies to delay onset of breastfeeding are impractical, and in any case may result only in the delay of the high initial breastfeeding risk. In rural Brazil, the risk lines cross at about 6 months (Figure 10.2C), which happens to correspond with a strategy that we defined prospectively.

Sensitivity Analyses

The relative risk of non-HIV mortality with formula feeding may be higher or lower than we assumed; empirical estimates range widely. A lower relative risk strengthens the finding that formula feeding is optimal, since it results in a smaller increase in non-HIV mortality. We attempted to find the relative risk required to make formula feeding equivalent to current feeding in two sites (urban Thailand and rural Tanzania), but could not owing to the two ways in which the model uses relative risk. A high relative risk input has roughly balanced opposing effects. It increases the added mortality risk of formula feeding, which in isolation would favor breastfeeding. However, it also lowers the estimate of infant mortality with pure breastfeeding (per equation 5, above), which has precisely the opposite effect. Thus, it is possible to reduce but not eliminate the benefit of formula feeding by raising relative risk. We believe that this insight from the model, though perhaps counterintuitive at first consideration, is valid for predicting the impact of real programs.

We also examined the possibility that perinatal antiretrovirals affect HIV transmission risk in breastfeeding through mechanisms other than altering the

A

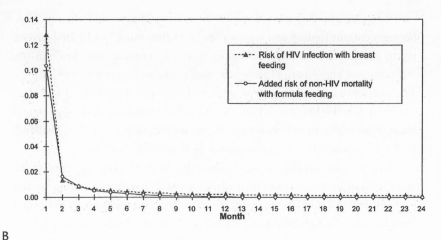

B

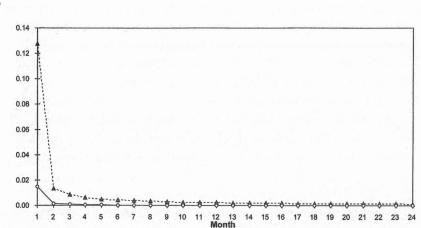

C

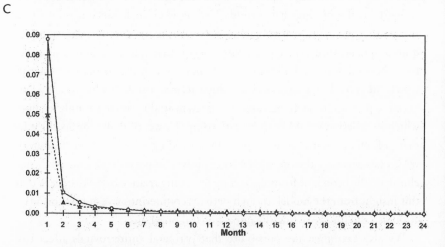

Figure 10.2. (A) Competing risks of HIV infection and non-HIV death, rural Tanzania. (B) Competing risks of HIV infection and non-HIV death, urban Thailand. (C) Competing risks of HIV infection and non-HIV death, rural Brazil.

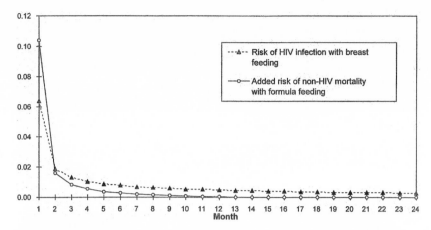

Figure 10.3. Competing risks of HIV infection and non-HIV death, rural Tanzania with perinatal antiretroviral (ARV) therapy and delayed HIV transmission via breastfeeding.

number of susceptibles. These regimens are typically administered to the mother up to one week post-partum and the child for one week. One possibility is that they decrease HIV transmission early in life, by decreasing viral load and transmission both during and for a short period following administration. We examined this scenario in rural Tanzania, lowering the Weibull β to reduce by half the risk of HIV transmission via breastfeeding in the first month of life, leaving total HIV risk the same. In this scenario, formula feeding is no longer preferred. The optimal duration of breastfeeding is about one month (Figure 10.3). It must be emphasized that this delayed benefit is hypothetical; as noted earlier, a rebound in viral load following antiretroviral therapy has been reported and may actually increase HIV risk in the first month of life, which would increase the benefit of formula feeding.

Another important caveat is evident from the analysis presented immediately above. Our model assumes, based on our best reading of very limited empirical data and the way the Weibull function calibrates to match 3-month data, that breastfeeding risk is heavily concentrated in the first month of life: the risk is almost tenfold that in the second month of life. This is consistent with the latest empirical data.[31] Still, future analyses of the timing of breastfeeding-associated HIV transmission may indicate that it is distributed more evenly. If so, then in the absence of other changes in inputs, very short-term (e.g., one month) breastfeeding may be optimal in settings with high infant mortality (e.g., rural Tanzania). The data suggesting that risk is concentrated in the first three months (vs. late postnatal) appear more convincing. Thus it is unlikely that 3-month breastfeeding would be optimal in those settings for which formula feeding currently appears optimal.

The model is flexible, allowing modification of the magnitude and timing of key risks. As better empirical data become available, we will adjust the default inputs. In addition, we have worked with UNAIDS to develop a user-friendly version of this modeling as part of an overall model of preventing mother-to-child HIV transmission. Ministries of health can use the user-friendly model with accompanying instructions to examine different program configurations and epidemiologic inputs in their countries.

Cost-Effectiveness Analysis

Cost inputs required to estimate cost-effectiveness fall into three categories: intervention recruitment, the intervention itself, and changes in medical care costs. Intervention recruitment may include the cost of HIV counseling and testing of pregnant women, if expectant women were not already tested for another reason (e.g., perinatal antiretroviral therapy). The costs of HIV counseling and testing have been estimated previously at $4 per person.[6] Women found to be HIV-infected are then counseled on the options of infant feeding, which includes formula feeding and exclusive breastfeeding, incurring primarily the costs of counselor salary and benefits. The proportion who are HIV-positive and choose formula feeding is a key consideration. It determines the number of intervention recipients across which the costs of HIV testing and intervention counseling must be distributed. Acceptance may be relatively low due to traditional social norms encouraging breastfeeding, as well as fear of censure for HIV infection and other reasons.

The intervention itself includes training sessions (on how to formula feed safely) and monitoring visits (to assess growth and feeding success). The exact numbers and duration are not well established, since emphasis in the past has been on training for breastfeeding. Estimates will need to be refined as programs gain experience. A large cost is the formula itself, which may be available only at market prices, or may be discounted through bulk or subsidized purchases. The quantity required is approximately 20 kg of powdered formula for the first 6 months of life. Formula or cow's milk is needed in comparable quantities for months 7 to 12 and 13 to 24.

Medical care costs for non-HIV disease are expected to be higher with formula feeding, but for HIV disease higher with breastfeeding. Estimates of relative morbidity and use of health services range widely, from 1.1 to 50 depending on the geographic setting and age of subjects.[28] HIV costs have been estimated at $195 per person.[6] Finally, consideration must be given to the cost of contraception, which would be used more often in connection with formula feeding to compensate for greater fertility experienced in the absence of breastfeeding.

In doing a cost-effectiveness analysis, it may also be worthwhile to calculate the cost per disability-adjusted life year (DALY) to facilitate comparison with older health interventions. DALYs are total expected years of life weighted to reflect both health-related quality of life and productivity. In this context, productivity includes monetized earnings of older children and adults as well as the socioeconomic value of managing the household and caring for children and the aged.

The number of DALYs lost due to a fatal adverse event is the difference between expected DALYs for a child with these events and expected DALYs for a child with no such events. For a healthy child, estimated DALYs reflect expected survival in each geographic setting, combined with age-specific productivity adjustments. At a 3% discount rate, expected DALYs are 28 in Tanzania, 31 in South Africa, and 32 in Brazil and Thailand. For a child who dies during the first two years of life from non-HIV causes (i.e., primarily in the first months of life), one could calculate expected DALYs or reasonably assume that all DALYs are lost since the disability-weighted value of the first year of life is only 0.16.

For a child who is HIV-infected, we estimate expected DALYs of 1.0 using methods previously described.[6] We do this by adding disability factors of 0.123 for HIV and 0.505 for AIDS into standard calculations. Our calculation assumes that 25% of infected children progress to AIDS by age 12 months, 80% by 60 months, and 100% at 120 months; children with AIDS are assumed to live for a mean of 12 months. Thus, DALYs lost with HIV infection is DALYs expected at birth minus 1.0.

Precise calculation of DALYs, and of any input distinguishing HIV infection and non-HIV mortality, is complicated in our feeding model by efforts to avoid double counting. A child who becomes HIV infected may die later in infancy of non-HIV causes (thus losing one additional DALY), yet the model is not designed to track such events. However, the error is small: the probability of such events is low because non-HIV mortality risk is low, particularly after the first months of life, and when it occurs only one additional DALY is lost.

DISCUSSION

This analysis suggests that formula feeding is the optimal strategy to reduce mortality in the children of HIV-infected women in most but not all settings.

This conclusion differs from past analyses in the wider range of conditions for which formula feeding appears superior. Confidence in this analysis may also be greater due to recent gains in the understanding of breastfeeding-associated HIV transmission and our use of geographic setting-specific data on HIV, mortality, and breastfeeding patterns. However, uncertainty remains in the distribution of risk within the first three months of life, leaving open the possibility that very short-term breastfeeding (e.g., one month) may be preferred in some settings in which formula feeding currently appears optimal.

The limitations in this method are important. First, the analyses and conclusions are only as good as the input data. We were able to find apparently valid data for many inputs, but remain uncertain about some important subtleties. For example, some data on mortality and breastfeeding may be out of date, and some inputs were lacking entirely for South Africa. The exact temporal pattern of mortality and of the relative risk for higher mortality with formula feeding are generalized from a single study. We did find, however, that uncertainty in the relative risk for non-HIV mortality may not affect major conclusions. Second, our use of the Weibull function to interpolate and extrapolate several inputs, while always tethered to the best empirical data, may misrepresent values of certain inputs in certain months. This is probably of most concern in the predicted values for the first month, where the preferability of formula feeding is irrevocably established.

Feeding programs will often be implemented as part of an overall program to reduce HIV vertical transmission, in concert with perinatal antiretroviral therapy. The overall effectiveness of a combined program is likely to be better than a formula feeding program alone. The cost-effectiveness, in particular, is likely to benefit because of the ability to defray the high cost of HIV testing across two interventions.

There are considerable social, cultural, and public health obstacles to offering formula feeding for HIV-infected women. In a setting where few women formula feed, doing so may signal family members and others that the woman is HIV-infected, which may lead to her being ostracized. Cultural norms favoring breastfeeding may be so strong that formula feeding is interpreted as the mother unacceptably distancing herself from the child. Conversely, it is conceivable that formula feeding can be misunderstood as "modern," leading to HIV-uninfected women adopting the practice when breastfeeding may be preferable for their babies. Care must therefore be taken to encourage formula feeding only among HIV-infected mothers so that the advantages of breastfeeding are sustained in uninfected mothers. These are critical issues which must be effectively addressed prior to implementing a formula feeding program.

ACKNOWLEDGMENTS

This research was supported by UNAIDS and by the National Institute on Drug Abuse via grant DA09531 to the Societal Institute for the Mathematical Sciences.

REFERENCES

1. Dabis F, Msellati P, Dunn D, et al. Estimating the rate of mother-to-child transmission of HIV. Report of a workshop on methodological issues Ghent (Belgium), 17–20 February 1992. *AIDS* 1993; 7:1139–1148.
2. Dunn DT, Newell ML, Ades AE, Peckham CS. Risk of human immunodeficiency virus type 1 transmission through breastfeeding. *Lancet* 1992; 340:585–588.
3. Leroy V, Newell ML, Dabis F, et al. International multicentre pooled analysis of late postnatal mother-to-child transmission of HIV-1 infection. *Lancet* 1998; 352:597–600.
4. UNAIDS/UNICEF/WHO. HIV and infant feeding: A review of HIV transmission through breastfeeding. 1998; WHO/FRH/NUT/CHD/98.3.
5. European Collaborative Study. Therapeutic and other interventions to reduce the risk of mother-to-child transmission of HIV-1 in Europe. *Br J Ob Gyn* 1998; 105: 704–709.
6. Marseille E, Kahn JG, Saba J. Cost-effectiveness of antiviral drug therapy to reduce mother-to-child HIV transmission in sub-Saharan Africa. *AIDS* 1998; 2:939–948.
7. Marseille E, Kahn JG, Mmiro F, Guay L, Musoke P, Fowler MG, and Jackson JB. Cost-effectiveness of single-dose nevirapine regimen for mothers and babies to decrease vertical HIV-1 transmission in sub-Saharan Africa. *Lancet* 1999: 354:803–809.
8. Heymann SJ. Modeling the impact of breast-feeding by HIV-infected women on child survival. *Am J Public Health* 1990; 80:1305–1309.
9. Kennedy KI, Fortney JA, Bonhomme MG, Potts M, Lamptey P, Carswell W. Do the benefits of breastfeeding outweigh the risk of postnatal transmission of HIV via breastmilk? *Trop Doc* 1990; 20:25–29.
10. Hu DJ, Heyward WL, Byers RH, et al. HIV infection and breast-feeding: Policy implications through a decision analysis model. *AIDS* 1992; 6:1505–1513.
11. Lederman S A. Estimating infant mortality from human immunodeficiency virus and other causes in breast-feeding and bottle-feeding populations. *Pediatrics* 1992; 89: 290–296.
12. Del Fante P, Jenniskens F, Lush L, et al. HIV, breast-feeding and under-5 mortality: Modelling the impact of policy decisions for or against breast-feeding. *J Trop Med Hyg* 1993; 96:203–211.

13. Nagelkerke NJ, Moses S, Embree JE, Jenniskens F, Plummer F. The duration of breast-feeding by HIV-1-infected mothers in developing countries: Balancing benefits and risks. *JAIDS* 1995; 8:176–181.

14. Kuhn L, Stein Z. Infant survival, HIV infection, and feeding alternatives in less-developed countries. *Am J Public Health* 1997; 87:926–931.

15. Soderlund N, Zwi K, Kinghorn A, Gray G. Prevention of vertical transmission of HIV: Analysis of cost effectiveness of options available in South Africa. *BMJ* 1999; 318: 1650–1656.

16. Saba J on Behalf of the PETRA Trial Study Team. Interim analysis of early efficacy of various short-term ZDV/3TC combination regimens in preventing mother-to-child transmission of HIV-1: The PETRA Trial. Oral presentation, *6th Conference on Retroviruses and Opportunistic Infections,* Feb 1, 1999.

17. Centers for Disease Control and Prevention. Administration of zidovudine during late pregnancy and delivery to prevent perinatal HIV transmission—Thailand, 1996–1998. *Morb Mortal Wkly Rep* 1998; Mar 6; 47(8):151–154.

18. Tess BH, Rodrigues LC, Newell ML, et al. Infant feeding and risk of mother-to-child transmission of HIV-1 in Sao Paulo State, Brazil. *JAIDS* 1998; 19:189–194.

19. Gray GE, McIntyre JA, Lyons SF. The effect of breastfeeding on vertical transmission of HIV-1 in Soweto, South Africa. *Int Conf AIDS* 1996; Jul 7–12; 11(2):237 (abstract no. Th.C.415).

20. Nicoll A, Newell ML. Preventing perinatal transmission of HIV: The effect of breast-feeding (letter). *JAMA* 1996; 276:1552.

21. Preble E, Piwoz EG. *HIV and Infant Feeding: A Chronology of Research and Policy Advances and Their Implications for Programs.* Washington, DC: The Linkages Project, 1998.

22. Bertollis J, St. Louis ME, Simonds RJ, et al. Estimating the timing of mother-to-child transmission of human immunodeficiency virus in a breast-feeding population in Kinchasa, Zaire. *J Infec Dis* 1996; 174:722–726.

23. Becquart P, Garin B, Sepou A, et al. High incidence of early postnatal transmission of human immunodeficiency virus type 1 in Bangui, Central African Republic. *J Infec Dis* 1998; 177:1770–1771.

24. Chayovan N, Kamnuansilpa P, Knodel J. *Thailand Demographic and Health Survey, 1987.* Institute of Population Studies, Chulalongkorn University, Bangkok, Thailand, and Institute for Resource Development/Westinghouse, 1988.

25. Bureau of Statistics, Planning Commission, Dar es Saalam, Tanzania; Macro International Inc. *Tanzania Demographic and Health Survey.* 1996.

26. Sociedade Civil Bem-Estar Familiar no Brasil, BEMFAM; Programa de Pesquisas de Demografia e Saude (DHS) Macro International Inc. *Brasil Pesquisa Nacional Sobre Demografia e Saude 1996.* 1997.

27. Chimere-Dan O. *Household Survey 1994, Transkei, Eastern Cape Province.* Transkei Department of Welfare and Pensions, Central Statistical Service, Department of Health, and Population Centre Wits University. 1996.

28. Jason JM, Nieburg P, Marks JS. Mortality and infectious disease associated with infant-

feeding practices in developing countries. *Pediatrics* 1984; Supplement "Task Force on Infant-Feeding Practices":702–727.

29. Habicht JP, DaVanzo J, Butz W. Does breastfeeding really save lives, or are apparent benefits due to biases? *Am J Epidemiol* 1986; 123:279–290.

30. Wagstaff L, de Wet T, Anderson A. Infant feeding: Birth to ten, *MRC Urbanisation and Health Newsletter* (Part 2) 1993; 18:9–13.

31. Nduati R, John G, Mbori-Ngacha D, et al. Effect of breastfeeding and formula feeding on transmission of HIV-1: A randomized trial. *JAMA* 2000; 283:1167–1174.

Part Four **New Methods**

for New Problems

Chapter 11 Design of HIV Trials
for Estimating External Effects

Tomas Philipson

This chapter examines the statistical inference problems associated with external effects for the purpose of evaluating and designing HIV-prevention trials. It reports on the application to vaccination trials of some results reported in Philipson,[1] which discusses more generally the topic of external effects in the canonical evaluation framework. In this framework, a set of treatments are randomly assigned, and the impact of these treatments on a defined outcome is studied. In this evaluation problem, the paper defines an external effect to operate when the treatment assignments of other individuals affect the outcome of a given individual. The key aspect of external treatment effects is that the distribution of treatments within a population, and not only the treatment of the investigated person, affects that person's outcomes—others' treatments matter depending on a given treatment assignment.

As an example, I consider the types of HIV prevention trials that are presently conducted on the African continent. The communities involved in these trials often have over one-third of the population infected with HIV, making the continued growth of the virus arguably one of the most important public policy issues in these regions.[2] When the vaccination is used as a treatment, external effects may arise when the infection rate of the control group in a vaccination trial depends on how many are treated—the vaccination rate in the trial. In other words, although the individuals in the control group all receive the same treatment, the assignment of treatments to others affects their outcomes. This chapter discusses the issues raised by such external effects in relation to HIV prevention trials.

The main motivation we offer for the importance of external effects in HIV prevention trials is that they are central to understanding what can be learned from an experimental evaluation about the effect of a larger program implementing the treatment evaluated. This is often a central issue for agencies that fund HIV prevention, such as the World Bank or the United Nations, in deciding whether to support on a large scale a program that has been evaluated to perform on a small-scale basis. If external effects are not dealt with appropriately, evaluations showing small or no effects may turn out to have great effects when implemented, and evaluations showing significant effects may turn out to be insignificant when implemented. In addition I show that costly large-scale experimental evaluations may involve *larger* implementation bias compared to smaller evaluations, even though the aim is to extrapolate implementation of an intervention to a large scale.

The fact that external effects are important for extrapolating from experimentation to implementation suggests that designs of HIV prevention studies should identify them. I argue that a way to identify external treatment effects is randomization of the allocations of treatments across communities (e.g., partners in sexually transmitted disease interventions or villages in vaccination interventions). This is in addition to randomizing the assignment of treatments themselves within these communities. Thus I suggest two stages of randomization: one of allocations of treatments to communities and another of treatments within communities as specified by those allocations. The groups across which the first step of the randomization occurs should be large enough to feasibly "internalize" the externality among themselves. In other words, it should include all those affected externally in their outcomes by other members of the group. For example, if the external treatment effects occur at the level of couples, then couples should be the unit of randomization. In contrast, if external effects occur at the level of the whole community, communities should be randomized. The randomization across individuals within communities identifies the standard private treatment effects, as opposed to the randomization across communities, which identifies the external treatment effects. The external effects are picked up by comparing the outcomes of individuals who received the same treatment but were exposed to different treatment allocations, for example, comparing unvaccinated people across communities with different vaccination rates. The two-step randomization suggests that some criticisms of evaluations with random assignments, such as that they do not take into account contamination, macro, or herd effects, are overcome by redefining the unit of randomization to better incorporate external effects.

Given that a two-step randomization process can identify external and private effects, I discuss design issues when estimating them through finite samples. There is a tension here between the optimal design for estimating the private and external effects. Private effects tend to be best estimated by having the same sized control and treatment groups, but external effects are best estimated by having extreme treatment shares across populations. In a vaccine trial, external effects are most efficiently estimated with very large and small vaccination rates across communities, but this would sacrifice power to detect the private effects of vaccination within those communities.

This chapter relates to many strands of previous work. Although the types of effects discussed here, or related phenomena, certainly have been recognized in a qualitative fashion in previous discussions,[3-10] the attempt here is to put forth a general formal framework in which such effects can be defined explicitly, identified, and assessed in a quantitative fashion. Also, the chapter relates to a large literature on both observational and experimental cluster sampling and randomization.[11] However, the main rationale motivating such cluster sampling is, whether explicitly analyzed or implicitly assumed, to reduce the costs of producing the data. Indeed, without cost differences, cluster sampling is only a disadvantage, as it inflates standard errors beyond random sampling. Here, in contrast, cluster randomization occurs for identification purposes, that is, for statistical as opposed to monetary reasons, and may therefore be advantageous relative to simple random sampling even when ignoring trial production costs. It is worth emphasizing from the start that the chapter deals exclusively with an idealized experimental setting, abstracting from issues such as noncompliance and attrition, as well as other issues of choice or selection that may also make experiments and implementations differ. This is not because they are not important, but because the isolated effects of external effects are more transparently discussed by initially abstracting from such issues.

PRIVATE AND EXTERNAL TREATMENT EFFECTS

I first illustrate and define external treatment effects by considering the simplest case of two treatments and a single population in which the effect operates. I then extend this to multiple treatments and populations. Let treatment assignment be represented by the treatment indicator d; an experimental treatment ($d = 1$) being allocated to a share q of the population and a control treatment ($d = 0$) being allocated to the remaining share $1 - q$. The individual outcome of interest is denoted Y and the distribution of concern is $F(y|d,q)$, which represents the outcomes of those receiving treatment d given that the treated population is q. The issue of external treatment effects is the dependence of this conditional distribution on q—that outcomes of a given treatment group depend not only on their own treatment assignments but also externally on those of others. In other words, treatment consumption of others affects the outcome of a given individual. External treatment effects are thereby defined as outcomes conditional on treatment assignment varying with the allocation of treatments. Denote the mean outcome as a function of the treatment share in the community by $\mu(q) = E[Y|q]$ with $\mu_d(q) = E[Y|d,q]$ being treatment specific means. The mean outcome in the entire population is then the treatment-specific outcomes weighted by the sizes of the two treatment groups.

$$\mu(q) = q\mu_1(q) + (1 - q)\mu_0(q).$$

External effects may reveal themselves through the impact the treated portion has on this overall population mean. Under only private effects, when $d\mu_d/dq = 0$, the relationship is linear with the marginal impact of raising the share of treated by one percent coinciding with the treatment effect: $d\mu/dq = \mu_1 - \mu_0$. It is important to note that this would hold even when the treatment effects were heterogeneous across individuals, as long as the treatment assignments were random, because then the distribution of heterogeneous treatment effects would be the same in the treatment and control groups. However, under external effects, the aggregate outcome as a function of the treatment share may be nonlinear even under random assignment of treatments. It will be convex if the share treated has a reinforcing positive external effect on the private treatment effect, and it will be concave if it has a counteracting negative external effect. More precisely, the effect of raising the share of treated under external effects is

$$\frac{d\mu}{dq} = [\mu_1(q) - \mu_0(q)] + [q\frac{d\mu_1}{dq} + (1 - q)\frac{d\mu_0}{dq}].$$

The first term within the brackets represents the linear effect, as discussed above, when holding the private effect constant as the share of treated increases. However, the terms within the second bracket represent the impact of external effects on outcome means conditional on treatments so that the overall impact is a weighted average of those external effects. If there are no external effects, the second bracket vanishes and the marginal effect of expanding the program decreases to the standard private treatment effect.

Mixing and Aggregation of External Effects

The existence of external effects in smaller subpopulations is related to their existence in larger populations. Understanding the effects of aggregation on the identified external effect seems particularly relevant to HIV prevention trials where mixing among population groups may mask the external effects present. Consider when the communities are made up of couples. Then the share of treated partners takes on only two possible values: $q \in \{0, 1\}$. Now consider the matching within a homogeneous group. The unconditional mean of a given individual equals

$$\mu_d = \sum_{d'} m_{dd'} \mu_d(d')$$

where $\{m_{dd'}\}$ is the matching matrix across treatments for couples. For example, under random matching and random assignment of two treatments with shares $(q, 1 - q)$, the matching matrix is

$$\begin{pmatrix} m_{00} & m_{01} \\ m_{10} & m_{11} \end{pmatrix} = \begin{pmatrix} (1-q)^2 & q(1-q) \\ (1-q)q & q^2 \end{pmatrix}.$$

This implies that the treatment means of the two treatment groups of a given individual are

$$\mu_d = (1 - q)\mu_d(0) + q\mu_d(1).$$

This implies that the populationwide external effects are

$$\frac{d\mu_d}{dq} = \mu_d(1) - \mu_d(0)$$

which says that populationwide external effects are a necessary consequence of an effect within couples. When there are many covariate groups, the external effect is determined by how the treatment-induced matching interacts with the matching of covariate groups. The matching matrix $W = \{w_{gg'}\}$ across the covariate groups and the allocation of treatments across covariate groups induces the matching of treatments $M(W,q)$. Consider an HIV vaccine trial in which there are two covariate groups of males and females; $N = 2$, where $q = (q_M, q_F)$ denotes the vaccination rates of the two sexes. For males the mean outcomes are (μ_{M0}, μ_{M1}), the infection rates among unvaccinated and vaccinated males. For females the analog means are (μ_{F0}, μ_{F1}). The covariate matching matrix W here determines the shares of homosexual and heterosexual matches or sexual contacts. It, together with the vaccination rates of males and females, determines the male means by treatment according to

$$\mu_{M0} = w_{MM}[\mu_{01}q_M + \mu_{00}(1 - q_M)] + w_{MF}[\mu_{01}q_F + \mu_{00}(1 - q_F)],$$
$$\mu_{M1} = w_{MM}[\mu_{11}q_M + \mu_{10}(1 - q_M)] + w_{MF}[\mu_{11}q_F + \mu_{10}(1 - q_F)].$$

Now the external effects are determined by the effect not only of the treatment share in its own covariate group, here males, but also of other covariate groups.

Extrapolation and External Effects

External effects are important for determining the inframarginal effects on population outcomes that arise when going from small experimental evaluations to full-scale program effects. These effects are central to learning about the consequences of implementing a treatment by observing its experimental performance—a central goal of many evaluations. One may distinguish between *experimental* versus *implementation* effects, with the former resulting from the allocation of treatments in the experiment and the latter from the allocation of treatments when implementing the program. External effects are important for this extrapolation because a major difference between experimentation and implementation is the share treated.[12] More precisely, going from the share of treated q in the experiment to a share q' being implemented we have the difference in the population mean

$$\mu(q') - \mu(q) = [q'\mu_1(q') + (1 - q')\mu_0(q')] - [q\mu_1(q) + (1 - q)\mu_0(q)]$$

which may be rewritten as

$$\mu(q') - \mu(q) = -[(q - q')(\mu_1 - \mu_0)] + [q'(\mu_1(q') - \mu_1) + (1 - q')(\mu_0(q') - \mu_0)].$$

These inframarginal implementation effects mimic the marginal effects discussed; the terms within the first bracket represent the difference due to private effects generated by the expansion of treated relative to controls when the program is implemented. Even when there are private effects only, the implemented population outcomes differ from the experimental ones whenever there is a treatment effect: $\mu_1 \neq \mu_0$. The terms within the second bracket represent the impact of external effects weighted by the implementation allocation. It is comprised of the changes through the external effect on the treated and controls as the program moves from experimentation to implementation. The extreme case is when implementation involves all individuals being treated and experimentation involves the (approximate) case of none being treated. In this case, the implementation effect differs from the experimentation effect whenever

$$\mu(1) - \mu(0) \neq \mu_1(0) - \mu_0(0) \Rightarrow \mu_1(1) \neq \mu_1(0)$$

which is illustrated most easily for a linear specification such as

$$\mu_d(q) = \alpha d + \beta q.$$

Here the first term is the private effect and the second term the external effect. The experimental effect is

$$\mu_1(q) - \mu_0(q) = \alpha$$

which differs from its implementation effect

$$\mu_1(1) - \mu_0(0) = \alpha + \beta.$$

The two effects therefore differ by the magnitude of the external effect, β. As illustrated in Figures 11.1A and 11.1B, implementing the program adds not only the private treatment effect to all individuals in the population but also the external effect that the expansion of the program implies.

Figure 11.1A shows the case when there are no external effects so that the full implementation effect is simply the standard private treatment effect: $\mu(1) - \mu(0) = \mu_1(1) - \mu_0(0) = \alpha$. Figure 11.1B shows the case when outcomes fall in the share of treated, as when higher vaccination rates lower infection rates in both vaccinated and unvaccinated groups. As illustrated in Figure 11.1B the implementation effect is larger than the private treatment effect because when a large-scale vaccination program is implemented, infection rates fall among both vaccinated and unvaccinated, which inflates the private treatment effect alone in a small program. Note that even though external effects are the same across the two groups, $d\mu_1/dq = d\mu_0/dq = \beta \leq 0$, implementation effects may differ from experimental effects. In other words, even though there are no interactions between the allocation of treatments and the private treatment effect—the standard private treatment effect is α regardless of what the allocation of treatments are in the population—implementation effects may differ

A

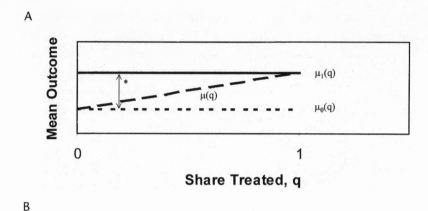

Share Treated, q

B

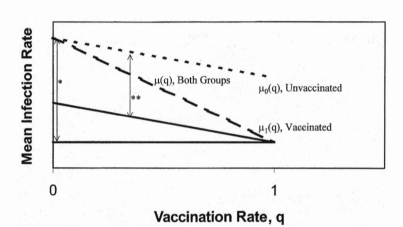

Vaccination Rate, q

Figure 11.1. (A) No external effects. $^*\mu(1) - \mu(0) = \mu_1(q) - \mu_0(q) = \alpha$. (B) External effects for vaccines. *Implementation effect, $\mu_1 - \mu_0$. **Experimental effect, $\mu_1(q) - \mu_2(q)$.

from experimental effects. The issue is not that the private treatment effect cannot be identified through experiments; rather, it is not informative about the implementation effect. For example, for public health programs such as vaccinations, we are ultimately interested in the overall health impact on the population when those programs are implemented as opposed to what happens in small-scale demonstrations.

Inferring the effects of implementation from experimentation is particularly troublesome when external effects are non-monotonic. An example of this would be the case of vaccine trials when there are other methods of avoiding infection. Consider when vaccination is one of several types of protection, as for

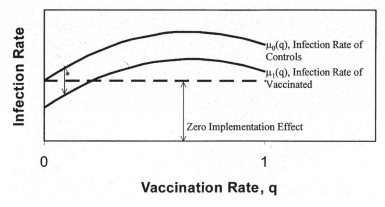

Figure 11.2. Implementation bias when external treatment effect is non-monotonic. *Experimental effect.

example in the case of HIV in the United States where safe sex is another method of protection. However, when there are low vaccination rates everyone protects by other means than vaccination, yielding low infection rates, but when there are high vaccination rates the rate of new infection is low as well, because now people use vaccines instead of other forms of protection. This would suggest that the share of treated may have an inverted U-shaped effect on the rate of infection in both unvaccinated and vaccinated groups. As illustrated in Figure 11.2, such non-monotonicities in external effects are very troublesome for distinguishing implementation effects from experimental effects.

Figure 11.2 shows that although the experimental effect is positive regardless of the vaccination rate, the implementation effect is zero because the rate of new infections when many are vaccinated equals the rate of infection when few are. This occurs because the share of treated lowers the demand for other forms of protection such as safer sexual practices in the case of HIV.

IDENTIFICATION OF EXTERNAL EFFECTS

This section discusses how experiments should be designed to generate the necessary independent variation to identify and separate external and private effects. The important question is how to perform the randomization. Once the randomization has been done, the identification of the two types of effects is usually trivial.

Experimental Identification
of Implementation Effects

Before discussing identification of external effects we first discuss the pitfalls in
the standard practice of using experimental effects to identify implementation
effects after the experiment. A basic question of interest is how well the population effect of implementing a program is mimicked by the experimental effect in an experiment. In other words, if one uses the estimated treatment effect
of an experiment how close does that come to the effect of the larger scale program when implemented? This concern differs from how to identify external
effects by asking when the standard method, not attempting to identify such
effects, is useful or when it is misleading. One concern is whether the *sign* of the
implementation effect can be identified. If this is not possible, a treatment may
be deemed favorable in an experiment although harmful when implemented. A
second issue is whether the magnitude can be identified. In other words, even if
the direction of improvement is identified by the experiment, when does it get
the magnitude right? It turns out that the qualitative characterization of population outcomes provides the key to gain insight into when both the sign and
the magnitude are identified.

   If an experiment involves the share q and the program implementation involves the share q', we define the implementation bias B of the experimental effect by how much it differs from the effect when implementing the program

$$B = [q'\mu(q') - q\mu(q)] - [q'\mu(q) - q\mu(q)].$$

This is the true effect of implementing the program less the experimental treatment effect scaled up to cover the additional part of the population treated under an implementation.

   The experimental effect preserves the sign whenever

$$[q'\mu(q') - q\mu(q)][q'\mu(q) - q\mu(q)] \geq 0$$

where $\mu(q') = (\mu_0(q'), \dots, \mu_K(q'))$ and $\mu(q) = (\mu_0(q), \dots, \mu_K(q))$. For the
sign to be identified by an experiment involving two treatments, it must be that
the contrast $\mu_1(q) - \mu_0(q)$ does not change with the share treated q. If it did,
then the experiment may identify one sign of the contrast, and then when implemented at another treatment share, the sign could be different. Put simply,
it requires that the two functions $\mu_1(q)$ and $\mu_0(q)$ do not cross. This may well
involve that the signs of the slopes of the two functions may be different; the
external effect may operate differently on outcomes of controls and treated.

The uniformity in dominance is exactly captured by the share-independence assumption. Since this assumption says that if controls are worse than treated, then a population with some treated is always better than only having controls. However, when the two curves cross, this is violated.

The difference between implementation and experimental effects is particularly important when external effects *interact* with private effects. In that case, the definition of a treatment effect is in terms of a function as opposed to a number when no such interaction occurs. An important implication of private effects that interact with treatment allocations in general, or the share of treated in particular, is that larger experimental evaluations may involve larger implementation bias than smaller ones. In other words, it is not enough simply to expand the size of the evaluation to better estimate the effect of program implementation. Consider the full-scale implementation bias defined as the difference between the population effect of fully implementing an intervention and the experimental effect extrapolated up to the entire population $B = [\mu(1) - \mu(0)] - [\mu_1(q) - \mu_0(q)]$. This represents how much an intervention that was implemented for the population would affect it, compared to scaling up the experimental effect to the larger size of the population that would receive the intervention if fully implemented. Larger evaluations do not always do better when this bias rises with the share of treated, which occurs whenever the private treatment effect falls with the share of treated, that is, $dB/dq \geq 0$ holds whenever $d[\mu_1 - \mu_0]/dq \leq 0$.

Identification of External Effects Through Two-Stage Randomization

The important function of experimental design to identify external effects is to generate variation in treatment allocations across groups, in addition to the variation in treatments across individuals within groups. We suggest a two-step randomization scheme in which treatment allocations are randomized across groups, and then treatments are randomized within the groups. Although two-stage randomization has been used in practice, as in community-based trials, its role in identifying external effects has not been stressed. In the first step of this process, it is imperative that the unit of analysis (e.g., individual, couple, community) chosen for randomization corresponds to the unit of analysis that is susceptible to external treatment effects. For example, if the external treatment effects occur at the level of couples, then couples should be randomized using the four possible treatment combinations. In contrast, if external effects occur at the level of the whole community, communities should be randomized. The

type of community-based trials that are needed for these identification purposes can be executed within the existing format of many community or mul-
ticenter trials. An example would be the trials used to evaluate the effectiveness
of strategies of reducing HIV infection in African countries which often involve
many communities.

Note that generally, external effects do not impose any restrictions on the outcome ranking on the populationwide level beyond transitivity and continuity if
the conditional mean outcome functions $\mu_0(q)$ and $\mu_1(q)$ are well-behaved. In
other words, for any population outcome function $\mu(q)$, it can be interpreted to
come from an environment with some external effects. For two treatments, the
proof of this simply involves choosing $\mu_0 = 0$ and $\mu_1(q) = \mu(q)/q$. A similar argument applies for more than two treatments. Therefore, the functional form of
external effects must be imposed in order for one to infer them from populationwide outcomes. However, one can always identify them from outcomes
conditional on treatments as the two-stage randomization scheme suggests.

The "internalization" principle of this two-step randomization concerns the
units of randomization for the allocations q in the first step. After those units
have been selected, the traditional randomization of the treatments d within
the larger units is applied. To make this more precise, consider a population of
N groups and $K + 1$ treatments as discussed before. Then the outcome means
are written most generally as a function of all groups treatment allocations
$\mu^g(q)$, as discussed before. The partition $\Psi = (\Psi_1, \dots, \Psi_J)$ of the groups
would again be defined as external effects operating within elements of the partition but not between them. The unit of randomization in the first stage of the
randomization should then be the elements of the partition Ψ. By randomly
assigning different treatment allocations across the elements of the partition,
we generate the independent variation in the external effects necessary to identify them.

We define a two-stage randomization plan (TSRP) $Q \equiv (q^1, \dots, q^C)$ to be
treatment allocations assigned to elements of the partition where $q^c = (q_{c1},
q_{c2}, \dots q_{cK+1})$ denotes the treatment allocations in community c across treat-
ments 1 through $K + 1$, $c = 1, 2, \dots, C$. Such a plan Q involves both random
assignment of treatment allocations across communities as well as the assignment of individual treatments within communities. Thus a standard experiment with random assignment is conducted within each community, with the
randomization allocating treatment according to the shares specified by the
vector q^c, as well as such vectors of treatment allocations being randomly as-

signed to communities. The question of interest here is how a TSRP should be designed to identify both private and external effects which generalizes the standard concern of identification of private effects only. An illustrative and simple example of the value of a TSRP to identify external treatment effects is when contrasting it with traditional randomization of two treatments. Consider choosing a standard randomized trial within each community. Assume that the entire community is in the experiment with half the community getting the treatment and half of it getting the control, as is commonly done when identifying private treatment effects. Such allocations have been derived to be optimal in terms of achieving the highest level of precision. They would entail a TSRP Q which had the allocations $q^c = (1/2, 1/2)$ for all communities. The problem is that this creates no variation to identify the external effects, as we need variation in allocations and not only treatments to identify their impact. Any allocation that is "optimal" to identify private treatment effects should not be replicated across the communities, because regardless of its features, no variation in allocations across communities is generated.

To consider identification by TSRPs, we limit ourselves to the following specification of outcome means

$$\mu_d^g(q) = \gamma_d^g + \sum_{d=0}^{K} \beta_d^g q_d^g + \alpha^g.$$

This says that the mean outcome for a given treatment and sub-population depends additively on the treatment assigned, the external effects, and the sub-population itself (community fixed effect). Since a TSRP has treatments randomly assigned within communities and treatment allocations randomly assigned across communities, differences in the private effects are identified from variation in treatment assignments within a community.

$$\mu_d^g(q) - \mu_{d'}^g(q) = \gamma_d^g - \gamma_{d'}^g.$$

On the other hand, due to the randomization of allocations across communities, the external treatment effects are identified from variation across these communities across the same treatment

$$\mu_d^g(q^g) - \mu_d^g(p^g) = \sum_{d=0}^{K} \beta_d^g q_d^g - \sum_{d=0}^{K} \beta_d^g p_d^g.$$

Sufficient variation in the observable treatment shares would enable one to identify the unobservable external effects. For example, when there are only two treatments, variation in the share of treated identifies the external effect operating on a given treatment according to

$$\beta_d^g = \frac{\mu_d^g(q) - \mu_d^g(p)}{q - p}.$$

To illustrate, consider an example in which the TSRP has the share of the population randomly vaccinated at 80%, $p = 0.80$, in some communities but 20%, $q = 0.20$, in others. Assume that in the more vaccinated communities the controls incurred less infections so that the difference in infection rates among the unvaccinated controls were, say, 20%; $\mu_0(p) - \mu_0(q) = 0.20$. On the other hand, consider when the difference was negligible for vaccinated individuals across vaccination rates, possibly due to an effective vaccine; $\mu_1(p) - \mu_1(q) = 0$. The random assignment of communities then enables one to infer the external effects

$$\beta_0^g = \frac{\mu_0^g(q) - \mu_0^g(p)}{q - p} = \frac{0.20}{0.60} = 1/3 \text{ and } \beta_1^g = \frac{\mu_1^g(q) - \mu_1^g(p)}{q - p} = 0.$$

ESTIMATION OF EXTERNAL TREATMENT EFFECTS

Consider when there are n observed units within each of C communities and one is to choose the shares of treated $(q_1, \ldots, q_C)$ in those communities. The $2 \times C$ layout has different treatment allocations corresponding to columns and different treatments corresponding to rows. The first row therefore maps out the mean values among treated $\mu_1(q)$ for different shares of treated and the second row maps out the mean values of the controls $\mu_0(q)$ for the same share.

The outcome means in Table 11.1 corresponds to those of Figures 11.1 and 11.2 concerning the two functions $\mu_1(q)$ and $\mu_0(q)$. Each cell contains the outcome mean for that particular allocation (column) and treatment (row). (More general external effects may always be separated in a similar manner using allocation-treatment cells.) The differences in outcome means across columns in a given row indicates the external effect within a treatment—the top row being the external effects for the treated and the bottom row those of the controls. The differences in outcome means across rows in a given column indicate the

Table 11.1. Outcome Means by Allocations and Treatments

Treatments (Rows)	Allocations (Columns)		
	$\mu_1(q_1)$	..	..	$\mu_1(q_C)$
	$\mu_0(q_1)$	..	..	$\mu_0(q_C)$

private effect holding the treatment allocation constant. Consider the additive (means-adjusted) specification

$$\mu_1(q) = \alpha_1 + \beta_1 q$$

$$\mu_0(q) = \alpha_0 + \beta_0 q$$

where observations on each allocation-treatment cell have variance σ^2. Running the regressions within treatment groups then gives rise to the variance of the estimator of the external effect (slope coefficient) as

$$V(\hat{\beta}_d) = \frac{\sigma^2}{v_q}, \qquad d = 0,1$$

where

$$v_q = \sum_{c=1}^{C}(q_c - q^{-2})$$

is the variance in the regressor made up of the treatment shares. If the private treatment effect estimator is the average private effect across allocations, its variance is

$$V(\hat{\alpha}_1 - \hat{\alpha}_0) = \frac{1}{C^2}\sum_{c=1}^{C}V(\hat{\alpha}_{c1} - \hat{\alpha}_{c0}) = \frac{1}{C^2}\sum_{c=1}^{C}\frac{\sigma}{n^2}\left[\frac{1}{q_c^2} + \frac{1}{(1-q_c)^2}\right].$$

This displays the trade-off in efficiently estimating the private versus external effect through the variation of treatment shares across communities. In other words, there is a tension here between getting efficient estimates of the private effect versus the external effect. The private effect is most efficiently estimated by having treatment shares in the middle. Indeed, splitting the sample equally between controls and treated, $q_c = 1/2$ for all $c = 1, \ldots, C$, minimizes $V(\hat{\alpha}_1 - \hat{\alpha}_0)$. This is in contrast to the external treatment effect, which is most efficiently estimated by having extreme values of the shares of treated for the standard reason that slope coefficients are more efficiently estimated the greater the variation in the regressor. The variance of the private effect rises with a

$$X = \begin{pmatrix} 1 & 1 \\ \vdots & \vdots \\ 1 & 1 \\ 1 & 0 \\ \vdots & \vdots \\ 1 & 0 \\ & \\ \vdots & \vdots \\ & \\ 1 & 1 \\ \vdots & \vdots \\ 1 & 1 \\ 1 & 0 \\ \vdots & \vdots \\ 1 & 0 \end{pmatrix} \begin{matrix} \left.\vphantom{\begin{matrix}1\\ \vdots \\ 1\end{matrix}}\right\} nq_1 \\ \left.\vphantom{\begin{matrix}0\\ \vdots \\ 0\end{matrix}}\right\} n(1-q_1) \\ \\ \\ \left.\vphantom{\begin{matrix}1\\ \vdots \\ 1\end{matrix}}\right\} nq_C \\ \left.\vphantom{\begin{matrix}0\\ \vdots \\ 0\end{matrix}}\right\} n(1-q_C) \end{matrix} \quad \begin{matrix} q_1 \\ \vdots \\ \\ \\ \vdots \\ q_1 \\ \vdots \\ \\ q_C \\ \vdots \\ \\ \\ \vdots \\ q_C \end{matrix}$$

Figure 11.3. Regressor matrix for experiment estimating private and external effects.

mean-preserving spread of the treatment shares as opposed to the variance of the external effect, which falls. This trade-off in efficiency in estimating the two effects arises because of the unique aspect that the value sampled of one covariate, the share treated, determines the size of the sample by which another covariate, the private effect, can be estimated.

More general specifications, including interactions between treatments and controls, operate the same way. In general we have observations on (y, d, q) by having n observations in each community on the outcome y, all of which has the share of treated q, but nq observations of which are treated and $n(1-q)$ observations which are controls. For a specification of the conditional mean as a function of treatments and allocations $E[Y|d,q]$, the matrix of regressor values $(1, x_1, x_2) = (1, d, q)$ would be as indicated in Figure 11.3.

The data resulting from a TSRP will thus be comprised of n observations from each covariate value as represented by the treatment share. The unique feature is that the sample size of the other covariate is induced by the level of the first: $d = 1$ is observed for nq observations and $d = 0$ for the remaining $n(1-q)$ observations. In other words, the treatment allocations within a community also determine the precision by which private effects can be estimated in that community. More specifically, the variance of the private and external effects estimators is given by the usual formula for a multiple regression $V\{\hat{\beta}\} =$

$\sigma^2(X'X)^{-1}$. This determines the objective function for the most efficient design and the corresponding quadratic form specifying the weights the investigator wants to assign to different types of errors.

CONCLUDING REMARKS

This chapter discussed the definition and identification of external treatment effects as well as the experimental designs to detect them. Such effects were defined as treatment allocations of other individuals affecting outcomes of a given individual. It was argued that group based macrorandomization, as opposed to randomizing treatments across individuals, was useful for identifying external treatment effects and that this was important for differentiating implementation effects from experimental effects. The types of effects were illustrated in the context of HIV vaccination evaluations.

The chapter suggests some future research questions. Since the chapter dealt with experimental design only where treatment allocations could be controlled, a corresponding analysis of external effects for observational studies, in which treatment allocations are chosen by those observed, seems warranted. In particular, standard discussions of instrumental variables that provide exogenous variation of only treatments, as opposed to treatment allocations, do not fully deal with the identification problems introduced by external effects discussed here. Future research might therefore fruitfully address the exact limitations of such standard instrumental variable solutions and propose remedies to overcome them as well as the limitations of the present analysis, given observational issues and issues of noncompliance. However, even under such circumstances, external effects might alter in significant ways how experimental evaluations should be interpreted as well as what they imply about the full-scale implementation of treatments, whether estimated through instrumental variable methods or not.

ACKNOWLEDGMENTS

I am thankful for comments from the two volume editors as well as Michael Boozer, Joseph Hotz, Tony Lancaster, and from seminar participants at the 1997 European Commission Conference "Community AIDS Trials in Africa" in Seville, Spain, as well as the 1998 SIMS conference "Quantitative Evaluation of HIV Prevention Programs" in Divonnes-les-Bains, France.

REFERENCES

1. Philipson T. External treatment effects and program implementation bias. Technical Working Paper 250, National Bureau of Economic Research, 2000.
2. World Bank. *Confronting AIDS: Public Priorities in a Global Epidemic.* Rev. ed. New York: Oxford University Press, 1999.
3. Harris J. Macro-effects in social experiments. In *Social Experimentation,* edited by J. Hausman and D. Wise, NBER, University of Chicago Press, 1986.
4. Garfinkel I, Manski C. Microexperiments and macro effects. In *Evaluating Training and Welfare Programs,* edited by Garfinkel, I., and C. Manski, Cambridge: Harvard University Press, 1992.
5. Manski C. *Identification in the Social Sciences,* Cambridge and London: Harvard University Press, 1995.
6. Manski C. The mixing problem in program evaluation. *Review of Economic Studies;* 64 (4) October 1997, 537–553.
7. Halloran E, Struchiner C, Longini I. Study designs for evaluating different efficacy and effectiveness aspects of vaccines. *American Journal of Epidemiology* 1997; 146 (10): 789–803.
8. Magder L, Brookmeyer R. Analysis of infectious disease data from partner studies with unknown source of infection. *Biometrics* 1993; 49:1110–1116.
9. Datta S, Halloran E, Longini I. Efficiency of estimating vaccine efficacy for susceptibility and infectiousness: Randomization by individual vs household. Forthcoming, *Biometrics* 1999; 55:792–798.
10. Brookmeyer R, Gail MH. *AIDS Epidemiology: A Quantitative Approach.* Oxford: Oxford University Press, 1994.
11. Donner A, Klar N. Methods for comparing event rates in intervention studies when the unit of allocation is a cluster. *American Journal of Epidemiology* 1994; 140:279–289.
12. Philipson T., Desimone J. Experiments and subject sampling. *Biometrika* 1997; 84: 221–234.

Chapter 12 Estimation
of Vaccine Efficacy
for Prophylactic HIV Vaccines

Ira M. Longini, Jr., Michael G. Hudgens, and M. Elizabeth Halloran

The current generation of prophylactic human immunodeficiency virus (HIV) vaccines are now in phase III vaccine trials. In this chapter, we use simulations to explore the feasibility of measuring different important protective effects of these vaccines in a particular population structure. The simulation population is motivated by a cohort of injecting drug users (IDUs) in Bangkok, Thailand,[1,2] in which a phase III trial of the recombinant envelope protein vaccine glycoprotein (gp) 120 is now in the field.[3]

HIV vaccines could have at least three important protective effects: (a) they could reduce the susceptibility to infection of vaccinated people, that is, vaccine efficacy for susceptibility (VE_S); (b) they could reduce the rate of disease progression in vaccinated people who get infected, that is, vaccine efficacy for disease progression (VE_P); (c) they could reduce the level of infectiousness to others of vaccinated people who get infected, that is, vaccine efficacy for infectiousness (VE_I). The current paradigm for measuring the VE_S is the doubly blinded randomized placebo-controlled trial. Such a trial is designed to ensure a balance in exposure to infection of the vaccinated and unvaccinated (placebo) groups. In addition, the VE_P is estimable with this trial design by comparing the disease progression rates for vaccinated compared to unvaccinated infected people. The classical design does not permit estimates of the VE_I. However, if we include sexual partnerships where at least one partner is exposed to infection from outside of the partnership, then we can estimate the transmission probability or secondary attack rate (SAR) by conditioning[4] on the reported contacts between infected and susceptible people. In this case, both the VE_S and the VE_I are estimable.[5-9] Since estimation of the VE_P is straightforward, we concentrate on methods for jointly estimating the VE_S and VE_I.

METHODS

Basic Study Design

Our design is motivated by the planned phase III HIV vaccine trial in a cohort of IDUs in Bangkok Metropolitan Authority (BMA).[1,2] We assume that the primary participants are exposed to HIV infection by sharing uncleaned needles with people of unknown infection status. At any time, a proportion of the primary participants have unprotected sex with a steady sexual partner. This steady sexual partner has negligible exposure to infection from partners other than the primary participant.

For a phase III doubly blinded randomized placebo-controlled HIV vaccine trial, we assume that a predetermined number of IDUs are recruited as primary participants and that vaccine and placebo are randomly assigned such that about one-half of them receive vaccine. Their self-reported steady sexual partners also are followed for infection status, but do not receive vaccine or placebo. We have previously referred to such a design as a nonrandomized partner design.[7,8]

The primary participants and their identified steady sexual partners are examined at enrollment and every six months thereafter until the end of the trial.[9] The exams will consist of HIV tests and self-reported monthly needle-sharing and unprotected sexual contact rates since the last exam. The vaccination status and the results of these exams constitute sufficient data to estimate the VE_S and VE_I.

Vaccine Efficacy and Transmission
Probabilities

We assume that the vaccine has a leaky[10,11] (multiplicative per-contact) effect on both susceptibility and infectiousness. We choose the leaky effect since HIV vaccines are likely to give only partial protection against the multiple strains of

HIV that circulate in the community.[12] Thus, we let θ denote the ratio of a vaccinated person's susceptibility to infection per needle-sharing contact with an unvaccinated infected person compared to an unvaccinated person. Then vaccine efficacy for susceptibility is $VE_S = 1 - \theta$. For infectiousness, we let ϕ denote the ratio of an infected vaccinated person's infectiousness per needle-sharing or sexual contact compared to the infectiousness of an unvaccinated infected person. Then vaccine efficacy for infectiousness is $VE_I = 1 - \phi$.

We define p_1 as the probability that an unvaccinated susceptible person is infected by an unvaccinated infected person due to a single needle-sharing act with that person. We assume that infection prevalence in the population where IDUs share needles is constant with value π. Thus, the probability that an unvaccinated susceptible person is infected by an unvaccinated person of unknown infection status due to a single needle-sharing act with that person is πp_1. The probability per needle-sharing act that a vaccinated susceptible person is infected by an unvaccinated person of unknown infection status is $\theta \pi p_1$. The primary participants provide information about $\theta = 1 - VE_S$ and p_1, since vaccine and placebo are randomized to the primary participants. We define p_2 as the probability that an unvaccinated susceptible person is infected by an unvaccinated infected person due to a single sex act with that person. The per-sex-act probability that an unvaccinated susceptible person is infected by a vaccinated infected steady partner is ϕp_2. Since steady partners will have known infection status, the partnerships provide information about p_2 and $\phi = 1 - VE_I$.

We assume that the rth primary participant and his or her steady partner are HIV tested at times $t_0 = 0, t_1, t_2, \ldots, t_{T_r}$, where $T_r + 1$ is the total number of exams. We let $\tau_r = 1, \ldots, T_r$ indicate time interval $(t_{\tau_r - 1}, t_{\tau_r}]$. Let $n_{r\tau_r}$ be the number of needle-sharing acts that the rth primary participant had in time interval τ_r. The primary participant has vaccination status v_r, where $v_r = 0$ for unvaccinated and $v_r = 1$ for vaccinated. We define the probability of infection for the primary participant in time interval τ_r as

$$\gamma_{v_r}(\tau_r) = 1 - (1 - \theta^{v_r} \pi p_1)^{n_{r\tau_r}}. \tag{1}$$

For unprotected sexual contact with a steady partner, we let $m_{r\tau_r}$ be the number of unprotected sex acts that the rth primary participant has with his or her steady partner over the time interval τ_r. If the primary participant does not have a steady sexual partner or does not have unprotected sexual contact with a steady partner during the time interval τ_r, then $m_{r\tau_r} = 0$. If the primary participant is infected during time interval τ_r, we also define $m'_{r\tau_r}$ as the number of such sex acts with the steady sexual partner in the interval when the primary participant is infected, where $m'_{r\tau_r} \leq m_{r\tau_r}$. We note that $m'_{r\tau_r}$ may not be observable if infection occurs within the interval τ_r. We define $\beta_{v_r}(\tau_r)$ as the probability that if the primary participant with vaccination status v_r is infected, then the partner will be infected by the primary participant in interval τ_r. Then,

$$\beta_{v_r}(\tau_r) = 1 - (1 - \phi^{v_r} p_2)^{m'_{r\tau_r}}. \tag{2}$$

The probability $\beta_{v_r}(\tau_r)$ is the partnership secondary attack rate due to $m'_{r\tau_r}$ sexual contacts.

Define the three infection status states (i,j), $i = 0, 1$ (primary participant) and $j = 0, 1$ (steady partner) as $0 = (0, 0)$, $1 = (1, 0)$, $2 = (1, 1)$, at each time interval $\tau_r = 1, 2, \ldots, T_r$ (see Figure 12.1). We assume that the steady sexual partner is at risk of infection only from the primary participant so that $(0, 1)$ is not a possible state. Then we define the one-step transition probability $P^{ab}_{vr}(\tau_r)$ as the probability that a partnership, where the primary participant has vaccination status v_r, makes a transition from state a to state b in time interval τ_r. The one-step transition probabilities are as follows

$$P^{00}_{v_r}(\tau_r) = 1 - \gamma_{v_r}(\tau_r), \tag{3}$$

$$P^{01}_{v}(\tau_r) = \gamma_{v_r}(\tau_r)[1 - \beta_{v_r}(\tau_r)], \tag{4}$$

$$P^{02}_{v_r}(\tau_r) = \gamma_{v_r}(\tau_r)\beta_{v_r}(\tau_r), \tag{5}$$

$$P^{11}_{v_r}(\tau_r) = [1 - \beta_{v_r}(\tau_r)], \tag{6}$$

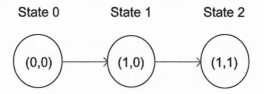

Figure 12.1. Transition diagram for primary participants and their steady partners. Transition from state 1 to state 2 is possible only if the primary participant is having unprotected sex with his or her steady sexual partner. Let "1" denote infection, and "0" not. Also let (i, j) denote the infection status of a primary participant $(i = 0, 1)$ and a steady partner $(j = 0, 1)$. The three infection states are denoted as $0 = (0, 0)$, $1 = (1, 0)$, and $2 = (1, 1)$. We assume that the steady sexual partner is only at risk of infection from the primary participant so that $(0, 1)$ is not a possible state.

$$P_{v_r}^{12}(\tau_r) = \beta_{v_r}(\tau_r), \tag{7}$$

$$P_{v_r}^{22}(\tau_r) = 1. \tag{8}$$

Correction for Exposure Bias

If a primary participant with a steady partner becomes infected in time interval τ_r, we do not observe $m'_{r\tau_r}$ in equation (2). Thus, there is a potential for miscalculation of the $0 \to 1$ and $0 \to 2$ transition probabilities. This involves the exposure of the sexual partner to the primary participant as modeled in equation (2). For the transition $0 \to 1$, we know that the primary participant became infected within the interval τ_r, and that the exposed partner escaped being infected by the primary participant. We observe $m_{r\tau_r}$ contacts between the partners, but only a fraction of those contacts are after the primary participant became infected in the time interval. If we use $m_{r\tau_r}$ instead of $m'_{r\tau_r}$ in equation (2), then the value for the number of contacts with the infected partner is too large. This will result in an underestimate of p_2 and, thus, an overestimate of $\phi = 1 - VE_p$, which is multiplied by p_2. The same problem occurs with the $0 \to 2$ transition. We need to use an estimate of $m'_{r\tau_r}$, that is, the true number of such sex acts that are with the steady partner when the primary participant is infected. We define $\bar{\beta}_{v_r}(\tau_r)$ as equation (2) evaluated at the estimates of $m'_{r\tau_r}$. Then the transition probabilities for the transitions $0 \to 1$ and $0 \to 2$ are

$$P_{v_r}^{01}(\tau_r) = \gamma_{v_r}(\tau_r)[1 - \bar{\beta}_{v_r}(\tau_r)], \tag{9}$$

$$P_{v_r}^{02}(\tau_r) = \gamma_{v_r}(\tau_r)\bar{\beta}_{v_r}(\tau_r). \tag{10}$$

This is an interval censoring problem, since the exact contact on which the index became infected is known to have occurred only during the $m_{r\tau_r}$ contacts in interval τ_r.

To derive the expression for $\bar{\beta}_{v_r}(\tau_r)$, let $N(x)$ be the random variable for the first contact from which the primary participant is infected, given that an infection has occurred by the xth contact. Then $N(x)$ has the truncated geometric probability mass function

$$P[N(x) = n] = \frac{\theta^{v_r}\pi p_1(1-\theta^{v_r}\pi p_1)^{n-1}}{\sum_{n=1}^{x}\theta^{v_r}\pi p_1(1-\theta^{v_r}\pi p_1)^{n-1}} = \frac{\theta^{v_r}\pi p_1(1-\theta^{v_r}\pi p_1)^{n-1}}{1-(1-\theta^{v_r}\pi p_1)^x}, \quad n = 1, 2, \ldots, x. \tag{11}$$

For example, if we observe a $0 \to 1$ transition during τ_r (6 months), we know that the primary participant is infected from one of the $n_{r\tau_r}$ outside contacts. Thus the distribution of the first contact causing infection of the primary participant in τ_r is given by $N(n_{r\tau_r})$. Since we are given monthly contact patterns, assume that during τ_r the contact patterns are the same for each month. For the development that follows below, we will assume that duration of τ_r is 6 months, although the model can be derived for general τ_r. Then, let $n_\mu = n_{r\tau_r}/6$ be the number of outside contacts of the primary participant during any month of τ_r. Similarly let $m = m_{r\tau_r}/6$ be the number of within-couple contacts for any given month within τ_r. If we let J be the random variable for the month in which the primary participant is infected, then

$$P[J = j] = \sum_n P[N(n_{r\tau_r}) = n], \quad j = 1,2,\dots,6, \tag{12}$$

where we sum over the n_μ contacts of month j.

Now suppose the primary participant is initially infected during month j. Partition the $n_\mu + m_\mu$ contacts within month j into three bins: contacts prior to n (the infectious contact), the nth contact itself, and all contacts thereafter. The probability the partner escapes infection from the infected primary participant within month j is given by

$$1 - \bar{B}_{v_r}(j) = \sum_{n=1}^{n_\mu} \left[P[N(n_\mu) = n] \sum_{m=0}^{m_\mu} \left(\frac{\binom{n-1+m_\mu-m}{m_\mu-m}\binom{n_\mu-n+m}{m}}{\binom{n_\mu+m_\mu}{m_\mu}} (1 - \phi^{v_r} p_2)^m \right) \right]. \tag{13}$$

For any remaining month in τ_r following month j, the escape probability is

$$1 - \bar{B}_{v_r} = (1 - \phi^{v_r} p_2)^{m\mu}, \tag{14}$$

so that the partner's escape probability from the infected primary participant over the 6-month period τ_r is given by

$$1 - \tilde{B}_{v_r}(\tau_r) = \sum_{j=1}^{\tau_r} P[J = j][1 - \bar{B}_{v_r}(j)](1 - \bar{B}_{v_r})^{\tau_r - j}. \tag{15}$$

Then, (15) is used in the transition probabilities (9, 10).

Inference

We are interested in estimating the parameters θ, ϕ, p_1, and p_2 from the observed transition sequences and numbers of observed needle-sharing and sexual contacts.

We let $s_{r\tau_r}$ be the state of the rth primary participant at the end of interval τ_r, with $s_{r0} = 0$ for the designs considered in this chapter. The numbers of needle-sharing and sexual contacts for the rth primary participant in time interval τ_r are $n_{r\tau_r}$ and $m_{r\tau_r}$, respectively. Then the observed history for the rth primary participant and his or her partner through time interval τ_r is given by the array

$$\mathcal{H}_{r\tau_r} = [v_r, s_{r1}, \ldots, s_{r\tau_r}, n_{r1}, \ldots, n_{r\tau_r}, m_{r1}, \ldots, m_{r\tau_r}]. \tag{16}$$

The likelihood function up to time τ_r for the rth primary participant is

$$L_r(\theta, \phi, p_1, p_2 | \mathcal{H}_{r\tau_r}^v) = \prod_{l=1}^{\tau_r} P_{v_r}^{s_{rl-1}, s_{rl}}(l), \tag{17}$$

where the transition probabilities (3–10) are evaluated with respect to $\mathcal{H}_{r\tau_r}$. We note that for the $0 \rightarrow 1$ and $0 \rightarrow 2$ transition probabilities, we use equations (11–15) to calculate that actual number of sexual contacts with an infected primary participant, $m'_{r\tau_r}$, from the observed number, $m_{r\tau_r}$ in (16).

When we have h primary participants, the complete observed histories up to time T are given by $\mathcal{H}_T = [\mathcal{H}_{1T}, \ldots, \mathcal{H}_{hT}]$. Then the likelihood function is

$$L(\theta, \phi, p_1, p_2 | \mathcal{H}_T) = \prod_{r=1}^{h} L_r(\theta, \phi, p_1, p_2 | \mathcal{H}_{rT_r}). \tag{18}$$

Standard Survival Analysis

The VE_S can be estimated using a standard Cox model. In this case the hazard rate for primary participant r in time interval τ_r is

$$\lambda_{v_r}(\tau_r) = \lambda(\tau_r) e^{\beta_1 v_r + \beta_2 n_{r\tau_r}}, \tag{19}$$

where $\lambda(\tau_r)$ is the baseline hazard rate and β_1 and β_2 are the regression coefficients associated with the vaccine and needle-sharing effects, respectively. For model (19), our measure of the VE_S is

$$VE_S = 1 - e^{\beta_1}. \tag{20}$$

Then β_1 and β_2 are estimated using a Cox hazards regression model with time-dependent variables.[13] The estimate of β_1 is substituted into (20) to obtain VE_S. The model (19) is misspecified for the relationship between risk of infection and the number of needle-sharing contacts given by (1). We do not know of any standard survival model for estimating VE_I.

Table 12.1. Needle-Sharing Frequencies: Steady-State
Probabilities

Category	Frequency	Probability
1	None	0.80
2	Monthly	0.15
3	Weekly	0.03
4	Daily	0.02

Simulations

We pattern the simulation population roughly on the BMA cohort. We use months as our time units, and we assume that exams are conducted every 6 months for 36 months. For primary participants, we partition the frequency of needle-sharing, n_{rt_r}, into four categories: (a) those who do not share needles, i.e., $n_{rt_r} = 0$; (b) those who share needles about once a month, i.e., $n_{rt_r} = 6$; (c) those who share needles about once a week, i.e., $n_{rt_r} = 24$; and (d) those who share needles about once a day, i.e., $n_{rt_r} = 180$. Table 12.1 shows a plausible steady-state proportion of primary participants in each of the four needle-sharing frequency categories. The mean needle sharing rate from the frequencies in Table 12.1 is 0.87 needles shared per month. Since there is likely to be some movement among categories, we propose the six-month one-step transition matrix shown in Table 12.2. Thus, if a primary participant is in category 1 now, the probability that he or she will still be in that category six months later is 0.95, and the probability that he or she will be in category 2 is 0.05. The matrix is constructed so that changes can be made only to adjacent categories. In addition, the matrix is constructed so that it will produce the proportions in Table 12.1 as a steady-state distribution.[14]

We also partition the frequency of unprotected sex acts with a steady part-

Table 12.2. Needle-Sharing Frequencies: Transition Matrix

Initial State	Subsequent State			
	1–none	2–monthly	3– weekly	4–daily
1–none	0.95	0.05	0	0
2–monthly	0.27	0.67	0.06	0
3–weekly	0	0.34	0.33	0.33
4–daily	0	0	0.50	0.50

Table 12.3. Unprotected Sex Acts with Steady Partners:
Steady-State Probabilities

Category	Frequency	Probability
1	None	0.50
2	Monthly	0.33
3	Weekly	0.12
4	Daily	0.05

ner, $m_{r\tau_r}$, into the same four categories as above. Table 12.3 gives a plausible steady-state proportion of primary participants in each of the four sex-act frequency categories. For example, at steady state, 50% of the primary participants have no unprotected sex with a steady sexual partner. The mean rate of unprotected sex acts from the frequencies in Table 12.3 is 2.31 sex acts per month. Table 12.4 gives a six-month one-step transition matrix that produces the steady-state distribution in Table 12.3. Transition matrices have been used by other investigators to describe changes in risk.[15]

For all the simulations, we assume that we recruit 2500 primary participants.[3] Vaccine and placebo are randomized on the person level so that equal numbers of trial primary participants get vaccine and placebo. Thus, we have 1250 primary participants per arm. We assume that the vaccine trial runs for three years, and that the annual loss to follow-up is 20% for the first year, 15% for the second year, and 10% during the third year.

We assume that it will take three injections to stimulate the immune system fully so that the maximum protective levels of VE_S and VE_I are achieved. We further assume that injections are given at months 0 (upon entry), 1, and 6, and that maximum protection is reached immediately after the third injection.

Table 12.4. Unprotected Sex Acts with Steady Partners: Transition Matrix

Initial State	Subsequent State			
	1–none	2–monthly	3– weekly	4–daily
1–none	0.80	0.20	0	0
2–monthly	0.30	0.55	0.15	0
3–weekly	0	0.40	0.50	0.10
4–daily	0	0	0.20	0.80

Table 12.5. Vaccine-Induced Protection over Time

Injection	Month	Effect
1	0	0
2	1	ψVE
3	6	VE

$0 \leq \psi \leq 1$

Table 12.5 summarizes the pattern of increasing protection that we assume for both VE_S and VE_I. Thus, immediately after the first injection there is no protection; immediately after the second injection both vaccine efficacies are multiplied by a factor ψ ($0 \leq \psi \leq 1$); and maximum protection is achieved immediately after the third injection. We assume that any subsequent injections after the third do not increase protection above the maximum, but can prevent waning of the protective effects. Since we conduct exams every six months, we need to approximate this increase in protection during the first six months. We substitute the parameters $\bar{\psi}VE_S$ and $\bar{\psi}VE_I$ for VE_S and VE_I in equations (1,2), where $\bar{\psi}$ is a weighted average of the reduced protection over the first six months. Thus, $\bar{\psi} = \frac{5}{6}\psi = 0.833\psi$. We add $\bar{\psi}$ to the parameters to be estimated with the likelihood function (18). In the case of the standard survival model (19), we add $\bar{\psi}$ as an additional time dependent covariate.

We simulate the system using previously described Monte Carlo methods.[9] We carry out 200 simulations for each set of parameters.

RESULTS

Calibration of the Model

The cumulative infection rate, or attack rate (AR), in the BMA cohort is estimated to be approximately 8 per 100 person-years of follow-up. Thus we calibrate our baseline simulation in the placebo group to have an AR close to 8% for the first year of follow-up. We use the actuarial estimator of the AR, that is, one minus the survival function.[16] Thus, our estimator for the AR takes loss to follow-up into account. The estimate of HIV prevalence in IDUs in the BMA cohort has been found to be consistently about 30%, thus, we set $\pi = 0.30$. We have no information on SAR from IDUs to their sexual partners, but male-to-female seroconcordant partner studies in Thailand indicate that the partner-

Table 12.6. Statistics for the Placebo Arm

Exam Month	Number at Risk[a]	Cumulative Number Infected		Primary AR		SAR
		Primary	Partner	6 mo.	Cum.	
0	1250					
6	1119	45	6	4.1	4.1	14.0
12	960	80	16	3.6	7.5	20.1
18	854	99	26	2.2	9.5	26.4
24	769	114	36	1.9	11.3	31.4
30	716	127	45	1.9	13.0	35.4
36	666	139	54	1.9	14.6	38.9

[a]Number of primary participants at risk of infection and not lost to follow-up during the six-month interval.

Note: Based on 200 simulated vaccine trials with 1250 primary participants in the arm. The transmission probability is preset at $p = 0.05$.

ship SAR could range from 27% to 46%.[17,18] We varied p_1 and p_2 until we were able to simulate a baseline epidemic in the placebo group with the above characteristics. This was achieved when $p_1 = p_2 = p = 0.05$. We let $p_1 = p_2 = p$ for the results given below. This reduces the number of parameters that we need to estimate to four: $\theta, \phi, \bar{\psi}, p$. We set the vaccine efficacies to $VE_S = 1 - \theta = 0.4$ and $VE_I = 1 - \phi = 0.6$. We set $\psi = 0.5$ so that $\bar{\psi} = 0.42$.

Table 12.6 gives the statistics for the placebo arm averaged over the 200 simulations relying on the baseline characteristics given above. The average AR is 7.5% for the first year and 14.6% for the whole trial. An average of 139 primary participants became infected over the course of the trial. We note that the six-month attack rate decreases from a high of 4.1% in the first six months of the trial to a low of 1.9% in the last six months of the trial. This is due to frailty effects in the fixed cohort. An average total of 54 partners are infected by primary participants by the end of the trial. Thus, the SAR averages 38.9% by the end of the trial. Table 12.7 gives statistics for the vaccine arm.

Estimated Parameters

Table 12.8 gives the estimated parameters, their standard errors, and power of the statistical tests. Continuing with the case when $p = 0.05$, the VE_S, VE_I, and $\bar{\psi}$ are all well estimated. The power to reject $H_0 : VE_S = 0$ and $H_0 : VE_I =$

Table 12.7. Statistics for the Vaccine Arm

Exam Month	Number at Risk[a]	Cumulative Number Infected		Primary AR		SAR
		Primary	Partner	6 mo.	Cum.	
0	1250					
6	1118	41	5	3.7	3.7	11.1
12	964	68	9	2.8	6.4	13.5
18	863	83	14	1.7	8.0	17.0
24	782	97	19	1.7	9.6	19.9
30	728	108	25	1.6	11.0	23.0
36	680	119	30	1.5	12.4	25.5

[a]Number of primary participants at risk of infection and not lost to follow-up during the six-month interval.
Note: Based on 200 simulated vaccine trials with 1250 primary participants in the arm. The parameters are preset at $p = 0.05$, $VE_S = 0.40$, $VE_I = 0.60$, and $\psi = 0.50$.

0 is 1.00 for both hypothesis tests. However, the power to reject $H_0 : \psi = 1$ is only 0.36. Table 12.9 gives the empirical 95% confidence intervals (CIs) on VE_S, VE_I and $\bar{\psi}$, that are [0.22, 0.56], [0.37, 0.74] and [0.00, 1.00], respectively. Tables 12.8 and 12.9 give the statistics on the estimated parameters for values of p ranging from 0.100 to 0.010. When $p = 0.010$, transmission is quite low. The average AR in the placebo arm is only 8.2% for the whole trial, and an average of 63 primary participants became infected over the course of the trial. In this case, the average partnership SAR in the placebo arm is only 16% with an average total of 12 partners infected by primary participants by the end of the trial. From Table 12.8, we see that the VE_S, VE_I, and $\bar{\psi}$ are still well estimated despite the small number of events. The power to reject $H_0 : VE_S = 0$ and $H_0 : VE_I = 0$ is still good for both hypothesis tests. However, there is considerable lack of precision. From Table 12.9, we see that the 95% confidence intervals on VE_S and VE_I are [0.16, 0.57] and [0.08, 0.90], respectively.

Time-Varying Vaccine Effects

Table 12.10 shows estimates of VE_S and VE_I under different models for the first six months of the trial. The first row shows the results when all the data over the full 36 months of the trial are used, and when $\bar{\psi}$ is estimated as above. The second row gives the results when the first six months of data are ignored. In this case, on average the first 46 infections in primary participants and the first six

Table 12.8. Estimated Parameters, Standard Errors, and Power of Statistical Tests

Transmission Probability p	Placebo			VE_S		VE_I		$\bar{\psi}$	
	AR	Number of cases	SAR	MLE (sd)	Power	MLE (sd)	Power	MLE (sd)	Power
0.100	19.0	183	50.1	0.41 (0.07)	1.00	0.60 (0.07)	1.00	0.41 (0.24)	0.41
0.050	14.6	139	38.9	0.40 (0.08)	1.00	0.60 (0.09)	1.00	0.43 (0.29)	0.36
0.025	11.5	109	28.1	0.39 (0.09)	1.00	0.59 (0.13)	0.99	0.45 (0.33)	0.30
0.010	8.2	75	16.0	0.39 (0.11)	0.94	0.58 (0.22)	0.80	0.42 (0.38)	0.27

Note: Based on 200 simulated vaccine trials with 1250 primary participants per arm. The parameters are preset at $VE_S = 0.40$, $VE_I = 0.60$, $\bar{\psi} = 0.42$.

Table 12.9. 95% Confidence Intervals

Transmission Probability	VE_S		VE_I		$\bar{\psi}$	
p	MLE	95% CI	MLE	95% CI	MLE	95% CI
0.100	0.41	0.26–0.52	0.60	0.43–0.69	0.41	0.00–0.84
0.050	0.40	0.22–0.56	0.60	0.37–0.74	0.43	0.00–1.00
0.025	0.39	0.23–0.54	0.59	0.31–0.78	0.45	0.00–1.00
0.010	0.39	0.16–0.57	0.58	0.08–0.90	0.42	0.00–1.00

Note: Based on 200 simulated vaccine trials with 1250 primary participants per arm. The parameters are preset at $VE_S = 0.40$, $VE_I = 0.60$, and $\bar{\psi} = 0.42$.

partners infected in the placebo arm are not used in the estimation. We note that ignoring data for the first six months does not result in any appreciable bias in the VE_S and VE_I estimators, but does result in a small loss of efficiency as reflected by an increase in standard deviation. The third row shows the results when we ignore the time-varying effects of vaccination and analyze the data as if the VE parameters were constant throughout the study. To accomplish this, we set $\psi = 1$ in the likelihood function. We see that the precision is good, but we get negatively biased estimates of the VE parameters, especially for VE_S.

Standard Survival Analysis

We first investigate the effects of estimating VE_S without specifying the covariate for the frequency of needle-sharing contact, in this case, $\beta_2 = 0$ in the Cox survival model (19). The statistics for different values of p are given in Table 12.11. We note that the VE_S is severely underestimated. For example, when $p = 0.05$, we have $\widehat{VE}_S = 0.21$, when the preset value is 0.40. Because of this negative bias, the power to reject $H_0 : VE_S = 0$ is low. Table 12.12 shows the

Table 12.10. Vaccine Efficacy Under Three Models

Model	VE_S			VE_I		
	MLE	sd	95% CI	MLE	sd	95% CI
$\bar{\psi}$ estimated	0.40	0.08	0.22–0.56	0.60	0.09	0.37–0.74
1st six months ignored	0.39	0.10	0.20–0.56	0.58	0.10	0.34–0.75
$\psi = 1$	0.34	0.07	0.17–0.47	0.57	0.08	0.40–0.72

Note: Statistics based on 200 simulated vaccine trials with 1250 primary participants per arm. The parameters are preset at $p = 0.05$, $VE_S = 0.40$, $VE_I = 0.60$, and $\bar{\psi} = 0.42$.

Table 12.11. Statistics for Standard Cox Model Without Numbers of Needle-Sharing Contacts as a Covariate

Transmission Probability p	VE_S			
	MLE	sd	95% CI	Power
0.100	0.27	0.10	0.10–0.41	0.82
0.050	0.21	0.10	0.04–0.38	0.52
0.025	0.22	0.13	0.12–0.41	0.41
0.010	0.26	0.14	0.04–0.44	0.57

Note: Based on 200 simulated vaccine trials with 1250 primary participants per arm. VE_S is preset at 0.40.

statistics for different values of p when we add the covariate for the frequency of needle-sharing contact. Adding the covariate decreases the negative bias, but the bias is still large for the higher values of p. In the case where $p = 0.05$, we have $\widehat{VE}_S = 0.29$.

DISCUSSION

We have shown that the VE_S can be estimated with reasonable precision from a vaccine trial similar in size to the one being planned in Thailand. For estimation of the VE_S, we looked at a range of 75 to 183 total infections among primary participants in the unvaccinated arm. We have shown that if the study population is augmented with steady sexual partners of the primary participants, then the VE_I also can be estimated with reasonable precision. For esti-

Table 12.12. Statistics for Standard Cox Model with Numbers of Needle-Sharing Contacts as a Covariate

Transmission Probability p	VE_S			
	MLE	sd	95% CI	Power
0.100	0.31	0.08	0.17–0.44	0.98
0.050	0.29	0.10	0.11–0.43	0.85
0.025	0.35	0.10	0.18–0.48	0.92
0.010	0.38	0.11	0.19–0.55	0.93

Note: Based on 200 simulated vaccine trials with 1250 primary participants per arm. VE_S is preset at 0.40.

mation of the VE_I, we looked at a range of 16.0% to 50.1% partnership SARS in the unvaccinated arm.

We have also shown that estimation of the VE parameters should take the buildup of immunity over the first three injections explicitly into account. We accomplish this by allowing the estimation of a reduction factor for the vaccine efficacies over the first six months of the trial. We show that ignoring the first six months of data results in some loss of precision, and that ignoring the initial time-dependent vaccine effects results in considerable negative bias in the VE parameters.

In our simulations, there are considerable heterogeneities in the needle-sharing frequencies (Tables 12.1 and 12.2) and frequencies of unprotected sex acts with steady partners (Tables 12.3 and 12.4). If such heterogeneities exist in the actual vaccine trial cohorts, then failure to take them into account by modeling or stratification will lead to attenuated VE estimates.[19,20] This effect is made apparent in Table 12.11, where a Cox survival model is used to estimate the VE_S without taking such heterogeneity into account. In our analysis, we take these heterogeneities explicitly into account by entering the observed numbers of needle-sharing and sexual contacts into the likelihood function through equations (1, 2). In addition, it is well known that unmeasured heterogeneities lead to decreasing incidence over time for fixed cohorts. We observe this phenomenon in our simulations (see Tables 12.6 and 12.7). In the actual BMA cohort, other events not reflected in the simulations, such as increased exposure during periodic incarceration,[21] could lead to increases in incidence for specific time periods. Nonetheless, if such unmeasured heterogeneities are present, then infection incidence could substantially decrease over a three-year trial. It may be necessary to recruit further participants during the trial to ensure that there are enough infections for adequate power and precision.

We have made the assumption of a leaky vaccine effect to derive a general model for estimating the VE parameters for multiple unknown strains of HIV. This should be adequate for the primary analysis of the HIV vaccine trial in Thailand. However, secondary analyses will involve estimating strain-specific effects. There are two HIV subtypes, B and E, circulating among IDUs in Bangkok. Thus, for the primary analysis, we would estimate an overall VE_S and VE_I, and then, for a secondary analysis, we would estimate subtype-specific vaccine efficacies.[22] Further estimates for variants within subtype also could be made. In addition, secondary analyses could involve time-varying effects, which would be appropriate if the mix of circulating strains changed over the course of the vaccine trial.

We have not dealt with estimation of vaccine efficacy for disease progression, VE_p, in this chapter. When assessing the VE_p, the outcome of interest is a clinical endpoint, such as AIDS diagnosis, or a marker for disease progression, such as the rate of $CD4^+$ T-lymphocyte decline. Standard methods for clinical trials can be employed to compare the progression rate of infected vaccinated people to the rate of infected unvaccinated people (see Rida).[6]

We present a method for estimating the VE parameters that takes the major risk factors for infection, such as numbers of needle-sharing and sexual contacts, into account. With respect to estimating the VE_S, we demonstrate that use of the Cox survival model results in an underestimate of VE_S even when the number of needle-sharing contacts is entered into the model (see Table 12.12). This occurs because the functional relationship between the number of needle-sharing contacts and the risk of infection is misspecified. Thus, when vaccine trial data are analyzed, we suggest that the method of analysis should be appropriate for the underlying infection process, as is the method that we outline here. Although we have considered a vaccine trial design where the VE_S is estimated for needle-sharing exposure and the VE_I is estimated for sexual exposure, other designs could involve sexual exposure for the VE_S or needle-sharing exposure for the VE_I. Although the methods proposed here are completely applicable to these other designs as well, the level of the VE_S and VE_I could vary with the type of exposure.

ACKNOWLEDGMENTS

We would like to thank the following investigators for providing information about the BMA cohort and for their participation and suggestions: Dr. Dwip Kitayaporn, Dr. Timothy D. Mastro, and Mr. Philip A. Mock of the HIV/ AIDS Collaboration, Bangkok; and Dr. Suphak Vanichseni and Dr. Kachit Choopanya of the BMA, Bangkok. We also would like to thank Dr. Donald Francis of VaxGen, Inc., for his input and suggestions concerning the HIV vaccine trial in the BMA cohort. This research was partially supported by NIH grants R01-AI32042, R01-AI40846, and T32-AI07442-06.

REFERENCES

1. D Kitayaporn, S Vanichseni, TD Mastro, K Choopanya, S Raktham, S Sujarita, DC Des Jarlais, C Wasi, S Subbarao, P Mock, WL Heyward, and J Esparza. HIV-1 incidence, subtypes, and follow up in a prospective cohort of injecting drug users (IDUs) in

Bangkok, Thailand. In *12th World AIDS Conference,* Geneva, June 28–July 3, 1998. Abstract no. 13127.

2. D Kitayaporn, S Vanichseni, TD Mastro, K Choopanya, DC Des Jarlais, C Wasi, S Raktham, N Young, P Mock, WL Heyward, and J Esparza. Characteristics of injecting drug users (IDUS) infected with HIV-1 subtypes B and E in a prospective cohort in Bangkok, Thailand. In *12th World AIDS Conference,* Geneva, June 28–July 3, 1998. Abstract no. 13144.

3. M Balter. Impending AIDS vaccine trial opens old wounds. *Science,* 279:650, 1998.

4. ME Halloran and CJ Struchiner. Causal inference for infectious diseases. *Epidemiology,* 6:142–151, 1995.

5. JS Koopman and RJ Little. Assessing HIV vaccine effects. *American Journal of Epidemiology,* 142:1113–1120, 1995.

6. WN Rida. Assessing the effect of HIV vaccination on infectiousness. *Statistics in Medicine,* 15:2393–2404, 1996.

7. IM Longini, S Datta, and ME Halloran. Measuring vaccine efficacy for both susceptibility to infection and reduction in infectiousness for prophylactic HIV-1 vaccines. *Journal of Acquired Immune Deficiency Syndromes and Human Retrovirology,* 13:440–447, 1996.

8. S Datta, ME Halloran, and IM Longini. Augmented HIV vaccine trial designs for estimating reduction in infectiousness and protective efficacy. *Statistics in Medicine,* 17: 185–200, 1998.

9. IM Longini. Chain binomial models. In P Armitage and T Colton, editors, *The Encyclopedia of Biostatistics,* 593–597. Wiley, New York, 1998.

10. ME Halloran, MJ Haber, and IM Longini. Interpretation and estimation of vaccine efficacy under heterogeneity. *American Journal of Epidemiology,* 136:328–343, 1992.

11. PG Smith, LC Rodrigues, and PEM Fine. Assessment of the protective efficacy of vaccines against common diseases using case-control and cohort studies. *International Journal of Epidemiology,* 13:87–93, 1984.

12. PW Berman, AM Gray, T Wrin, JC Vennarl, DJ Eastman, GR Nakamura, DP Francis, DH Schwartz, G Gorse, and MJ McElrath. Genetic and immunologic characterization of viruses infecting MN-rgp120-vaccinated volunteers. *Journal of Infectious Diseases,* 176:384–397, 1997.

13. P Andersen and R Gill. Cox's regression model for counting processes: A large sample study. *Annals of Statistics,* 10:1100–1120, 1982.

14. CL Chiang. *An Introduction to Stochastic Processes and Their Applications.* Krieger, Huntington, N.Y., 1980.

15. SM Blower, GJP van Griensven, and EH Kaplan. An analysis of the process of human immunodeficiency virus sexual risk behavior change. *Epidemiology,* 6:238–242, 1995.

16. CL Chiang. *The Life Table and Its Applications.* Krieger, Malabar, Fla., 1984.

17. C Kunanusont, HM Foy, JK Kreiss, S Rerks-Ngarm, P Phanuphak, S Raktham, CP Pau, and NL Young. HIV-1 subtypes and male-to-female transmission in Thailand. *Lancet,* 345:1078–1083, 1995.

18. T Nagachinta, A Duerr, V Suriyanon, et al. Risk factors for HIV-1 transmission from

HIV-seropositive male blood donors to their regular female partners in northern Thailand. *AIDS,* 11:1765–1772, 1997.

19. IM Longini and M E Halloran. A frailty mixture model for estimating vaccine efficacy. *Applied Statistics,* 45:165–173, 1996.

20. ME Halloran, IM Longini, and CJ Struchiner. Estimation and interpretation of vaccine efficacy using frailty mixing models. *American Journal of Epidemiol,* 144:83–97, 1996.

21. K Hiranras, S Vanichseni, D Kitayaporn, K Choopanya, DC Des Jarlais, S Raktham, W Subhachaturas, P Mock, and TD Mastro. Incarceration as a continuing HIV risk factor among injecting drug users in Bangkok. In *12th World AIDS Conference,* Geneva, June 28–July 3, 1998. Abstract no. 23209.

22. PB Gilbert, SG Self, and MA Ashby. Statistical methods for assessing differential vaccine protection against human immunodeficiency virus types. *Biometrics,* 54:799–814, 1998.

Chapter 13 Health Policy Modeling: Epidemic Control, HIV Vaccines, and Risky Behavior

Sally Blower, Katia Koelle, and John Mills

The HIV epidemic, which was first recognized in the early 1980s, became one of the great health crises of the late twentieth century. The United Nations Combined AIDS Program (UNAIDS) estimates that globally 16,000 HIV infections occur every day, and that there are more than 33 million persons infected.[1] As many as 40 million persons were infected by the year 2000; this is a global prevalence approaching 1%. The majority of HIV cases (perhaps 95%) are in citizens of the developing world.[1] Although antiretroviral chemotherapy can control HIV infection in an individual, at least temporarily, the cost and complexity of current antiretroviral regimens precludes their use by the majority of HIV-infected subjects. Behavioral modification (through education and other means) has so far had only a limited impact on the worldwide spread of HIV infection except in very defined groups. Thus, control of the HIV epidemic is likely to be achieved only through development of HIV vaccines. In this chapter we use mathematical models to predict the epidemiological consequences of a variety of HIV vaccines that are under development. We demonstrate how mathematical models can be used as health policy tools: to design control strategies that will result in the elimination of HIV, and to predict the epidemiological consequences of changes in risk behavior that may occur with the introduction of mass vaccination against HIV. We begin by discussing the current obstacles to HIV vaccine development and then review current HIV vaccine strategies.

OBSTACLES TO HIV VACCINE DEVELOPMENT

Vaccines have been used for nearly three centuries to control communicable diseases, beginning with the use of vaccinia (a "naturally attenuated" poxvirus) to prevent smallpox infection. More recently, recombinant DNA technology has been used to produce a vaccine against hepatitis B virus infection. The majority of the successful vaccines against viral infections have been live attenuated vaccines (e.g., measles, mumps, rubella, smallpox, and yellow fever). Some other immunization strategies have also been extraordinarily successful; for example, the use of the hepatitis B virus surface antigen subunit vaccine. Smallpox vaccine (vaccinia) was used selectively in the 1970s in a coordinated and successful global campaign to eradicate smallpox virus; eradication was formally confirmed by the World Health Organization in 1980. A worldwide effort to eradicate polio is well under way (the disease has already been eradicated in the Americas, Europe, and Australasia), and the eradication of measles, mumps, rubella, and hepatitis A and B virus infections is theoretically possible through intensive deployment of existing vaccines. Despite vigorous and well-funded research efforts, in some instances extending over decades, there are some viral infections for which vaccines have not been developed: respiratory syncytial virus, hepatitis C virus, and herpes simplex virus, to name a few. Considerable obstacles have been encountered in the search for an effective HIV vaccine. Here we discuss the obstacles that have arisen due to the genetic heterogeneity of HIV and to the protective immune response to HIV infection.

HIV Genetic Heterogeneity

HIV, a primate lentivirus (family *Retroviridae*), exhibits a very high degree of genetic heterogeneity that has hindered the development of an effective vaccine. There are two major types of HIV: HIV-1 and HIV-2. These two types are only about 50% related at the amino acid sequence level. HIV-1 is the predominant type among the two (accounting for more than 99% of all reported cases of AIDS and HIV infection). HIV-1 appears to be more easily transmissible than HIV-2, and also has a shorter incubation period (the interval between infection and development of AIDS).[2] Both types of HIV were derived from related primate lentiviruses that first infected humans hundreds of years ago.[2] HIV-2 evolved from simian immunodeficiency viruses (SIV) infecting macaques, while HIV-1 arose from SIV viruses infecting chimpanzees.[2,3] The two major HIV types are further divided into subtypes (also called clades), based on the nucleotide and amino acid sequence of the major retroviral genes, *env, pol,* and *gag.* There are three groups of HIV-1 subtypes: M, O, and N. The M (main) group, which comprises virtually all known HIV-1 strains, includes nine subtypes (A–I). The O (outlier) and N (non-M, non-O) groups presently consist of a heterogeneous collection of about 100 HIV strains that are highly unrelated to the M group (>40% sequence divergence at the genomic level in the *env* gene).[2] Closely related strains of HIV that are classified within the same subtype usually show sequence divergence of <20% in the *env* gene, whereas the variation among subtypes is between 30% and 20%. Variation is less in the *gag* and *pol* genes.[2]

HIV subtypes have been defined by sequence relatedness (i.e., on the basis of genetic differences), but not by immunological testing (i.e., not by functional differences). However, differences between subtypes have been detected both by antibody reactivity and by susceptibility to cytotoxic T-lymphocyte (CTL) lysis *in vitro.*[3–5] The differences among subtypes are most pronounced in the *env* gene; thus it is not surprising that antibody reactivity appears to be the most sensitive nonmolecular test for differentiating clades. However, the correlation between subtypes as determined by sequence analysis ("sequence subtypes") and "immunologic subtypes" as determined by antibody reactivity is poor.[5] CTLs, particularly those directed against *gag* and *pol* epitopes, are usually very broadly reactive;[2,4] subtyping as defined by CTL reactivity likewise may not correlate with either sequence subtyping or antibody subtyping.[2] Thus, it is currently unclear whether the genetic differences among subtypes will present a significant problem when designing HIV vaccines that are effective against multiple subtypes. Phase III clinical trials in Thailand and in the United States are testing the efficacy of a bivalent subunit HIV vaccine against subtypes B and E. Genetic heterogeneity that is the result of strain diversity is unlikely to pose as great an obstacle to HIV vaccine development, because HIV vaccines are being developed against a "cocktail" of strains and not a single strain.

The Protective Immune Response to HIV

Developing a vaccine against HIV has been hindered because the correlates of resistance to HIV have not yet been identified and because the immunological response to HIV infection is only partially understood. Immune responses are generally divided into two components, humoral immune responses (antibodies) and cellular responses (primarily CTLs). With respect to viral infections, as a general rule humoral immune responses *prevent new infections,* while cellular immune responses *control existing infections.*[6] In general, effective vaccines against other infections have been developed in two stages. The first stage involves understanding the immune response to infection and identifying the correlates of resistance to infection. The second stage involves designing the vaccine by stimulating the relevant immune components. For example, polio and hepatitis B virus vaccines were given with the view to eliciting neutralizing antibodies, as it was clear from both human and animal studies that neutralizing antibody would prevent infection. With HIV, it remains unknown as to whether resistance to infection is mediated by neutralizing antibody, CTLs, or other factors; hence, the appropriate target for a vaccine is unclear.

Dissection of the correlates of protective immunity to HIV has also been hampered by a lack of adequate experimental models, and by the technical difficulties in quantifying HIV-specific neutralizing antibody and CTLs. The available data, largely derived by extrapolation from the SIV-macaque and HIV-chimpanzee models, suggest a role for both neutralizing antibody and CTLs in preventing HIV infection of humans.[7,8] HIV-specific CTLs control HIV replication once infection is established and may also have a role in preventing infection.[7,9] The evidence that CTLs control HIV replication once infection is established (as is true for the majority of viral infections) is very sound. During primary infection of humans or macaques, resolution of the initial, high-grade viremia coincides with the CTL response, but not with the neutralizing antibody response.[9] Further, ablation of the CD8 lymphocyte subset (which contains the bulk of CTLs), markedly increases viral replication in SIV-infected macaques.[10] The most compelling evidence for the role of CTLs in resistance to infection comes from studies of individuals highly exposed to HIV who have remained uninfected. These subjects have developed an HIV-specific CTL response, but they lack serum antibody and have no other evidence of HIV infection.[7,9] It is hypothesized that these patients were infected with HIV but the infected cells were eradicated by a CTL response very shortly thereafter (aborting the infection), prior to the development of HIV antibodies. Similar observations have been made in macaques given very low doses of HIV-2.[11] The importance of the CTL response in resistance to HIV infection is also supported by experiments with a variety of vaccines in the SIV-macaque system.[7,9,12] As the immune response to HIV becomes more completely understood, it should aid

Table 13.1. Examples of HIV Vaccines and Vaccine Strategies Currently Under Development

Immunogens	Immunizing Strategies
Nonreplicating immunogens (viral proteins are not synthesized *in vivo*)	*Single immunogen* (e.g., envelope glycoprotein: DNA)
Whole HIV virions rendered non-infectious	*Nonreplicating immunogens with adjuvants* (e.g., envelope glycoprotein with alum)
Envelope glycoproteins (virion "subunits")	*"Prime-boost"* strategies (in which the immune system is primed with one
"Live" immunogens (those synthesizing viral proteins *in vivo*)	immunogen, then boosted with another)
Attenuated HIV	DNA protein
Recombinant live vector (viruses—vaccinia, fowlpox viruses, polio; bacteria—salmonella, BCG)	Virus vector-protein DNA-virus vector
Plasmid DNA	

vaccine design by identifying what type of immune response an effective HIV vaccine needs to induce.

Current HIV Vaccine Strategies

A variety of HIV vaccine strategies are currently in development (Table 13.1). As the initial hypothesis was that HIV infection could be prevented by neutralizing antibodies, and some data supported that hypothesis, the earliest vaccine efforts were focused on eliciting neutralizing antibodies by administration of purified, usually recombinant, HIV envelope proteins (gp160, gp120, gp41, or similar).[8,13] Although these strategies showed some success in animal models, including primate models, the phase I/II data in humans suggested that antibodies that could neutralize primary isolates (those initiating HIV-infection in patients) were inconsistently elicited by these preparations.[13] Despite this discouraging preliminary data, phase III studies of recombinant gp120 vaccines are now being conducted by VaxGen. In the United States, a study incorporating two subtype B envelope proteins is being conducted in high-risk subjects, while a bivalent (B/E subtype) product is under study in injecting drug users in Thailand.

The HIV vaccine strategies that are currently of most interest utilize recombinant viral vectors expressing one or more HIV proteins, or plasmid DNA constructed to express HIV proteins.[7] These recombinant viral vectors are usually poxviruses, specifically attenuated derivatives of vaccinia virus such as "modified vaccinia Ankara" (MVA) or one of several fowlpox viruses. These vectors are frequently being used in a "prime-boost" strategy, in which the immune system is primed with DNA or a viral vector, and then boosted with DNA or viral vector, or with recombinant envelope protein.[7] The poxvirus vectors have also been used to express peptide CTL epitopes for HIV as well as HIV proteins. One strategy which focuses on eliciting both neutralizing antibodies to the HIV envelope, as well as CTLs toward envelope and other HIV proteins, uses priming with a DNA vaccine or poxvirus recombinant followed by boosting with recombinant HIV envelope proteins (the boost is important because DNA and poxvirus vaccines are not very efficient at inducing antibodies).[7] Although this strategy has induced protective immune responses in primates, it is viewed with some skepticism. It is felt that the antibodies produced by this strategy may be of no better quality than those produced using immunization with the recombinant envelope proteins alone.[13] Nonetheless, because of the encouraging primate data,[14] clinical trials of this strategy are also under way.

Another strategy, for which there is also primate data suggesting efficacy, is priming the immune system with a DNA vaccine expressing HIV proteins, followed by boosting with a recombinant poxvirus, primarily avipox.[7] In pig-tailed macaques (*M. nemistrina*), this strategy induced very high levels of CTL (with weak antibody responses, as would be expected from this vaccine strategy) and it has protected against HIV and SIV challenge.[7,12] Clinical trials of DNA-avipox prime-boost strategies are planned to begin within a year. Also under consideration are poxvirus vectors containing HIV genes along with cytokine genes, with the goal of directing the resulting immune response toward the TH1 or TH2 compartments.[15]

To date, most effective viral vaccines that have been used successfully in mass vaccination programs have been live attenuated vaccines (e.g. polio, smallpox, and measles). However, proposals to develop a live attenuated HIV vaccine have been extremely controversial. The principal—and entirely realistic—concern is safety. Such vaccines would initiate a lifelong HIV infection and would thus have a lifelong potential for causing disease. These concerns have been heightened recently by reports of macaques experimentally infected with attenuated strains of SIV developing AIDS, and of immune deterioration in a cohort of Australian subjects naturally infected with an attenuated strain of HIV (with a *nef*-LTR deletion).[16,17] Proponents of the live attenuated vaccine approach for HIV argue: (i) that the best protection that has been achieved in primates against challenge with virulent strains of SIV has been with live attenuated SIV vaccines,[7] and (ii) that there is substantial evidence from humans as well as from a variety of higher primate models that attenuated variants of primate lentiviruses can be prepared. Furthermore, a robust live attenuated HIV vaccine strategy has several advantages: the vaccine could be manufactured cheaply and easily (as a DNA plasmid containing an infectious molecular clone), and protection could be achieved with a single dose. Which if any of the several vaccine strategies that are currently under development will be the most effective is currently unclear.

HIV VACCINE MODELS

HIV vaccines are being designed on the basis of the immunological protective response that they induce in individuals. However, if one wishes to understand and to predict the epidemiological consequences of HIV vaccination strategies one must use epidemic control models. An epidemic control model consists of a series of equations that are formulated based upon specific biological assumptions about the pathogenesis of HIV, the complex transmission processes that generate the epidemic, and the individual-level and population-level effects of the vaccine. Hence, an epidemic control model contains explicit mechanisms that translate the risk behavior of an individual into a population-level outcome such as incidence or prevalence. Thus, epidemic control models can be used as health policy tools to predict and to evaluate the epidemiological consequences of specific vaccines and particular vaccination strategies. Models are also useful tools for designing epidemic control strategies and for evaluating trade-offs among a variety of different medical and behavioral interventions.

Prophylactic Vaccines: Providing Only
Protection Against Infection

Blower and McLean published the first epidemic control model for HIV vaccines.[18-21] They used their model to predict the potential epidemiological impact of mass vaccination when used for both eradicating and noneradicating control of HIV epidemics in gay communities.[18-21] Their model reflects the biology of prophylactic vaccines and assumes that prophylactic vaccines could have three biological mechanisms of action ("take," "degree," and "duration") by which they could fail to protect against HIV-infection:

"Take." The term *take* specifies the fraction of vaccinated individuals in whom some level of protective immunological response is induced by the vaccine. Thus, the value of "take" can vary from zero (if a protective immune response is not induced in any of the vaccinated individuals) to 1.0 (if a protective immune response is induced in all of the vaccinated individuals).

Degree. The term *degree* specifies the degree of vaccine-induced protection against HIV-infection (i.e., the reduction in the probability of infection given exposure) that is induced in those individuals in whom the vaccine "takes;" degree can vary from zero (no protection) to 1.0 (complete protection).

Duration. The duration of vaccine-induced immunity (which is assumed to decay exponentially) is specified by the parameter ω; $1/\omega$ represents the average duration of vaccine-induced immunity. This term reflects the fact that the vaccine-induced immunity can wane in vaccinated individuals in whom the vaccine "took" and induced a certain degree of protection.

The epidemiological impact of a perfect prophylactic vaccine can be evaluated by using this model and assuming that the vaccine would "take" in everyone who is vaccinated (i.e., "take" = 1.0), induce complete protection against infection to every exposure (i.e., "degree" = 1.0), and that the vaccine-induced immunity would never wane ($\omega = 0$). However, it is virtually certain that any prophylactic HIV vaccine will be imperfect (i.e., "take" < 1.0 and/or "degree" < 1.0 and/or duration of vaccine-induced immunity will wane with time). The model can also be used to predict the epidemiological impact of these imperfect prophylactic vaccines if the vaccine fails to protect against infection by any one, or any combination, of the three biological mechanisms (take, degree, and duration).

If a mass vaccination campaign utilizes an imperfect vaccine, then HIV infections can occur in four groups:

1. individuals who were not vaccinated (i.e., the vaccination coverage level was less than 100%).
2. individuals who were vaccinated but in whom the vaccine did not "take,"
3. individuals who were vaccinated and in whom the vaccine "took," but in whom the vaccine-induced immunity waned, and
4. individuals who were vaccinated, in whom the vaccine "took" and did not wane, but who received only partial protection (degree < 1.0) upon exposure.

In this model it is assumed that if individuals in groups 2, 3, and 4 become HIV-infected then the natural history of infection and disease will be the same as in unvaccinated individuals (group 1) who become HIV-infected. The model consists of four ordinary differential equations, which specify the rate of change over time of the number of individuals in each of four states: susceptible (X), successfully vaccinated (V), HIV-infected (Y), and AIDS (A). The equations that specify this model are given elsewhere.[18,19]

Prophylactic Vaccines: Providing Protection
Against Infection and Altered Pathogenesis

Here we extend the Blower and McLean vaccine model to develop a new model to evaluate potential prophylactic HIV vaccines that both protect against infection and influence the natural history of HIV infection in "successfully" vaccinated individuals who subsequently become HIV-infected. We define an individual to be "successfully" vaccinated if they are vaccinated, the vaccine "takes," and the vaccine-induced immunity does not wane (Figure 13.1). However, "successfully" vaccinated individuals can subsequently become HIV-infected, if their degree of protection is less than 1.0 (Figure 13.1). We assume that the vaccine could influence the infectiousness and/or the rate of disease progression in these "successfully" vaccinated HIV-infected individuals. We define an individual to be a vaccine failure if they were vaccinated and either the vaccine did not "take" or the vaccine-induced immunity waned (Figure 13.1). We assume that the vaccine failures who subsequently become HIV-infected would have the same level of infectiousness and rate of disease progression as unvaccinated HIV-infected individuals (Figure 13.1).

Our model consists of five ordinary differential equations, which specify the rate of change over time of five categories of individuals: susceptible individuals (who are unvaccinated or vaccine failures) (X), "successfully" vaccinated individuals (V), HIV-infected individuals who were previously "successfully" vaccinated (Y_V), HIV-infected individuals who were never vaccinated or who were vaccine failures (Y_U), and AIDS cases (A). The size of the sexually active community is specified by N (where $N = X + V + Y_V + Y_U$). New susceptible individuals enter the sexually active community at rate π, and they leave at an average rate μ. A fraction p of newly susceptible individuals are vaccinated, and the vaccine "takes" (i.e., produces a protective immunological response) in a fraction ε of those vaccinated; therefore, the fraction of new susceptibles that enter the susceptible pool is $(1 - \varepsilon p)$, and the fraction that is "successfully" vaccinated is εp. Susceptible individuals become HIV-infected at rate $\lambda c X$, where λ is the average per capita risk of infection and c is the average number of new sex partners acquired per unit time. The average per capita risk of infection (λ) is calculated as the product of two factors: the per partnership transmission probability and the fraction of the community that is infected and infectious. Thus, $\lambda = [\beta_U (Y_U/N) + \beta_V (Y_V/N)]$, where β_U represents the per partnership transmission probability of Y_U individuals and β_V represents the per partnership transmission probability of Y_V individuals. Vaccine-induced immu-

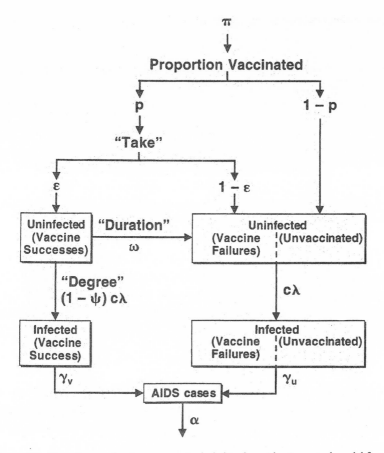

Figure 13.1. Flow diagram for the processes included in the epidemic control model for HIV vaccination described in equations (1)–(5). The model can be used to evaluate potential prophylactic HIV vaccines that both protect against infection and influence the natural history of HIV infection in "successfully" vaccinated individuals who subsequently become HIV-infected. Individuals are defined to be "successfully" vaccinated if they are vaccinated (p), the vaccine "takes" (ε), and the vaccine-induced immunity (ω) does not wane. "Successfully" vaccinated individuals can subsequently become HIV-infected, if their degree of protection (ψ) is less than 1.0. The vaccine can influence both the infectiousness (β_v) and/or the rate of disease progression (γ_v) in these "successfully" vaccinated HIV-infected individuals. Individuals are defined as vaccine failures if they are vaccinated (p), and either the vaccine does not "take" (ε) or the vaccine-induced immunity wanes (ω). Vaccine failures who subsequently become HIV-infected have the same level of infectiousness (β_U) and rate of disease progression (γ_U) as unvaccinated HIV-infected individuals. The model consists of five ordinary differential equations, which specify the rate of change over time of five categories of individuals: susceptible individuals (unvaccinated and vaccine failures), uninfected "successfully" vaccinated individuals, infected "successfully" vaccinated individuals, infected individuals who were never vaccinated or who were vaccine failures, and AIDS cases. This model is described by equations (1)–(5).

nity in the "successfully" vaccinated wanes at a rate ω; thus the average duration of vaccine-induced immunity is $1/\omega$ years, and the number of "successfully" vaccinated individuals entering the susceptible pool (per unit time) is ωV. Hence, the rate of change in the number of susceptible individuals (X) per unit time is specified by:

$$dX/dt = (1 - \varepsilon p)\,\pi - \mu\,X - \lambda\,c\,X + \omega\,V. \tag{1}$$

The fraction of new susceptibles in whom the vaccine "takes" enter the "successfully" vaccinated state at rate $\varepsilon p\pi$. They may leave this state for one of three reasons: they may leave the community (at average rate μ), their vaccine-induced immunity may wane (at an average rate ω), or they acquire HIV-infection. The degree of vaccine-induced protection against HIV infection is ψ; thus, their probability of becoming HIV-infected is $\lambda\,c\,(1 - \psi)$. Hence, the rate of change in the number of "successfully" vaccinated individuals (V) per unit time is specified by:

$$dV/dt = \varepsilon p\pi - \mu\,V - \omega\,V - (1 - \psi)\,c\lambda\,V. \tag{2}$$

"Successfully" vaccinated individuals (i.e., individuals in whom the vaccine "took" and did not wane) who become HIV-infected enter the infectious class Y_V. Individuals leave this class if they leave the sexually active community (at average rate μ) or as they progress to AIDS (at average rate γ_V). Thus the rate of change in the number of infectious individuals (Y_V) per unit time is specified by:

$$dY_V/dt = \lambda\,c\,(1 - \psi)\,V - (\mu + \gamma_V)\,Y_V. \tag{3}$$

Unvaccinated individuals and vaccine failures (i.e., individuals in whom the vaccine either did not "take," or in whom the vaccine "took" but waned) who become HIV-infected enter the infectious class Y_U. Individuals leave this infectious class if they leave the sexually active community (at average rate μ) or if they progress to AIDS (at average rate γ_U). Thus the rate of change in the number of infectious individuals (Y_U) per unit time is specified by:

$$dY_U/dt = \lambda\,c\,X - (\mu + \gamma_U)\,Y_U. \tag{4}$$

The number of AIDS cases (A) per unit time increases at rate $\gamma_V Y_V + \gamma_U Y_U$ (due to the incidence of disease) and decreases as AIDS patients leave the community (at average rate μ) or die of AIDS (at rate α):

$$dA/dt = \gamma_V Y_V + \gamma_U Y_U - (\mu + \alpha)\,A. \tag{5}$$

Prophylactic Vaccines:
The Two-Subtype Problem

The two previously discussed HIV vaccine models can be used to assess the epidemiological impact of HIV vaccines if only a single subtype is circulating. However, in many developing countries two subtypes of HIV are present. In most developed countries there is an overwhelming predominance of one subtype, but a second subtype could become established. Previously, Porco and Blower have developed and analyzed three mathematical models that can be used to assess the epidemiological consequences of imperfect prophylactic HIV vaccines for geographical locations where more than one subtype is present.[22,23] Their models allow the vaccine to provide a degree of protection against infection by one subtype and differential vaccine-induced cross-immunity against a second subtype.[22,23] Each of the three two-subtype models includes a different biological mechanism of action for the differential protective effect of cross-immunity: differential degree,[22] differential take,[23] and differential infectivity.[23] Porco and Blower have used their models to calculate (by deriving analytical expressions) the vaccination coverage levels, the vaccine efficacy levels, and the degree of vaccine-induced cross-immunity that would be necessary to control an HIV epidemic that is generated by two subtypes.[22,23] The equations that describe these models, the analytical equilibrium results, and the transient dynamics of these models are presented elsewhere.[22,23] This theoretical framework can also be extended to include more than two subtypes of HIV.

USING TRANSMISSION MODELS
AS HEALTH POLICY TOOLS

Transmission models can be used as health policy tools in a variety of ways.[24–30] Here we discuss two ways HIV epidemic control models can be used: to design vaccination strategies that will result in the eradication of HIV and to predict the epidemiological consequences of risk behavior change that occur concurrently with a mass vaccination campaign.

Designing Vaccination Strategies
to Eliminate HIV

PROPHYLACTIC VACCINES: PROVIDING ONLY PROTECTION AGAINST INFECTION

Previously, Blower and McLean[18–21] used their model to derive a new measure of HIV vaccine efficacy (ϕ) that was based upon the three assumed possible biological mechanisms of action of the vaccine—"take" (ε), "degree" (ψ), and "duration" (ω):

$$\phi = \frac{\varepsilon \psi \mu}{\mu + \omega} \tag{6}$$

where: $1/\mu$ = the average length of the sexual lifespan of an individual.

Any specified level of vaccine efficacy (ϕ) can be achieved by a wide variety of different vaccines that could work in many different ways, since the efficacy (ϕ) of the vaccine is determined by a combination of the "take," "degree," and "waning" effect[18-21] (equation 6). Vaccine efficacy (ϕ) is extremely sensitive to the duration of protection; consequently, HIV vaccines that wane quickly will have a low efficacy.[18-21] If the efficacy of a vaccine is low mainly due to the rapid waning of protection then the effectiveness of a mass vaccination program can be easily increased simply by revaccination. However, if the efficacy of the vaccine is low mainly due to "take" or "degree" effects, then the effectiveness of a mass vaccination program could be improved only by increasing coverage levels and/or developing more effective vaccines.

Blower and McLean used their new efficacy measure to quantify the relationships among vaccination coverage levels, vaccine efficacy levels, and the severity of the epidemic,[18-21] where severity of the epidemic was specified by the basic reproductive number, R_0. The basic reproductive number, R_0, is the average number of secondary cases of HIV infection produced by one infectious case during the individual's lifetime, in a community where everyone is susceptible (equation 7).[18-21]

$$R_0 = \frac{c\beta_U}{\mu + \gamma_U} \tag{7}$$

where: c = the average number of sex partners per unit time,

$\quad \beta_U$ = the transmission probability of HIV per sexual partnership from an unvaccinated individual, and

$\quad \gamma_U$ = the average progression rate to AIDS in an unvaccinated individual.

Blower and McLean[18-21] also calculated an analytical expression for the vaccinated reproductive number (R_p) for their model (equation 8); R_p is the average number of secondary cases of HIV infection produced by one infectious case during the case's lifetime, in a community where a mass vaccination program against HIV is in place.

$$R_p = R_0 (1 - p\phi) \tag{8}$$

where: p = proportion of the population that is vaccinated.

Blower and McLean used their expression for R_p to derive an expression for the critical vaccination coverage (p_c); where p_c was defined to be the minimum proportion of the community that has to be vaccinated in order to eradicate an HIV epidemic (i.e., p_c was derived by setting $R_p = 1.0$):

$$p_c = \left(\frac{1}{\phi}\right)\left(1 - \frac{1}{R_0}\right). \tag{9}$$

Thus, equation 9 can be used to calculate the critical vaccination coverage for any vaccine efficacy level (ϕ) and epidemic severity level (R_0). It may be seen from equation 9 that HIV vaccines of low to moderate efficacy will only be able to eradicate HIV epidemics if very high vaccination coverage levels are obtained. However, low to moderate efficacy vaccines would significantly reduce the prevalence and incidence of HIV, even if the achieved coverage levels were below that of the critical vaccination coverage level.

PROPHYLACTIC VACCINES: PROVIDING PROTECTION AGAINST INFECTION
AND VACCINE-ALTERED PATHOGENESIS

The vaccinated reproductive number (R_p) for the model described by equations 1–5 is given in equation 10:

$$R_p = S(1 - \psi) R_V + (1 - S) R_0 \tag{10}$$

S is the probability that an individual is (and remains) "successfully" vaccinated—the individual is vaccinated, the vaccine "takes," and the vaccine-induced immunity does not wane during the individual's sexual lifespan (Figure 13.1); hence, $S = (p\varepsilon)(\mu/(\mu + \omega))$.

R_V is the average number of secondary cases of HIV-infection that are produced by one "successfully" vaccinated individual who becomes infected during his lifetime. Hence, $R_V = (c\beta_V)/(\mu + \gamma_V)$; where c = the average number of sex partners per unit time, β_V = the transmission probability of HIV infection per sexual partnership from a "successfully" vaccinated infected individual, and γ_V = the average progression rate to AIDS in a "successfully" vaccinated infected individual.

In this model, an infected individual can be in one of two infectious states (Y_V and Y_U), each of which generates a different number of secondary cases (Y_V generates R_V cases and Y_U generates R_0 cases). The probability that the infected individual will be in the Y_V state is the probability that the individual will be "successfully" vaccinated and become infected due to the degree effect; thus, this probability equals $S(1 - \psi)$ (Figure 13.1). The probability that the individual will be in the Y_U state is the probability that the individual either will be unvaccinated or will be a vaccine failure (a vaccinated individual in whom the vaccine either did not "take" or waned); this probability equals $(1 - S)$ (Figure 13.1). Thus, the vaccinated reproductive number (R_p) equals the average number of secondary cases produced by each infectious state weighted by the probability that the initial infected individual would be in that particular infectious state (equation 10).

By setting R_p (given in equation 10) equal to 1.0, the critical vaccination coverage (p_c) that would be required to eradicate an HIV epidemic can be derived:

$$p_c = \left(\frac{\mu + \omega}{\varepsilon \mu}\right)\left(\frac{1 - R_0}{(1 - \psi)R_v - R_0}\right). \tag{11}$$

The analytical expression for the critical vaccination coverage level given in equation 11 appears more complex than the analytical expression for the critical vaccination coverage level given in equation 9; however, if the vaccine does not alter either the transmissibility or the progression rate of HIV-infection (i.e., $\beta_V = \beta_U$ and $\gamma_V = \gamma_U$) then equation 11 collapses to equation 9.

Equation 11 can be used to calculate the critical vaccination coverage that is necessary to achieve eradication for any vaccine that can both protect against infection (with a "take," degree, and/or duration effect) and that can also alter transmissibility and/or the progression rate of HIV infection in those individuals who are "successfully" vaccinated and subsequently become HIV-infected (Figure 13.1). The biological characteristics of such vaccines could produce three possible outcomes: $R_0 > R_V$, $R_0 \sim R_V$, and $R_V > R_0$. The first outcome $(R_0 > R_V)$ will occur if the vaccine reduces transmissibility of HIV (i.e., $\beta_U > \beta_V$) and/or increases the progression rate to AIDS (i.e., $\gamma_V > \gamma_U$) in "successfully" vaccinated individuals who become infected. The second outcome $(R_0 \sim R_V)$ will occur if either the vaccine has little to no effect on transmissibility and disease progression rates or the vaccine alters both transmissibility and disease progression rates but the effects (in terms of R_V) cancel each other out. The third outcome $(R_V > R_0)$ will occur if the vaccine increases the transmissibility of HIV (i.e., $\beta_V > \beta_U$) (which seems unlikely) and/or decreases the progression rate to AIDS (i.e., $\gamma_U > \gamma_V$) (which seems plausible).

For all three outcomes, the critical coverage level necessary to achieve eradication will decrease with an increase in the "take" effect and/or the duration effect of the vaccine (see equation 11), as occurred with the previous vaccine model. Thus, vaccines that have a high "take" and a low waning rate must be developed if HIV epidemics are to be eradicated. However, the importance of the degree effect in determining the critical vaccination coverage level will depend upon which of the three outcomes occurs. The importance of the degree effect for two of the outcomes ($R_0 \sim R_V$ and $R_V > R_0$) is relatively straightforward; increasing the magnitude of the "degree" effect decreases the vaccination coverage that is necessary to eradicate HIV (Figure 13.2A). However, if R_V is considerably less than 1.0 (which can occur only when $R_0 > R_V$, because $R_0 > 1$),[19] then the effect of degree on the critical vaccination coverage is substantially less pronounced (Figure 13.2A). Under these conditions the magnitude of the "degree" effect has little influence on the critical vaccination coverage, because the only effect of "degree" is to partition "successfully" vaccinated individuals between the uninfected state (when they cannot transmit HIV) and the infected state (when they can transmit HIV) (Figure 13.1). If the "successfully" vaccinated HIV-infected individuals can generate only an extremely low number of secondary cases ($R_V \ll 1.0$), then the magnitude of the degree effect cannot significantly alter p_c (see equation 11 for R_p). These results imply that if $R_V \ll 1.0$ then it would be unnecessary to develop a vaccine that had a high degree effect to eradicate HIV (Figure 13.2A). It seems highly unlikely that vaccines that accelerate the progression rate to HIV (i.e., $\gamma_V > \gamma_U$) in "successfully" vaccinated individuals would be used as epidemic control agents; consequently, $R_V \ll 1.0$ would occur only as the result of vaccines that reduced the transmissibility of HIV (i.e., $\beta_U > \beta_V$).

When designing epidemic control strategies it is always best to have multiple goals and not aim only for disease eradication.[25] The magnitude of the degree effect is not important in determining the number of individuals who need to be vaccinated in order to achieve the goal of eradication when $R_V \ll 1.0$. This is because the eradication criterion (p_c) is based upon herd immunity effects, and uninfected and infected "successfully" vaccinated individuals are approximately equivalent in generating herd immunity. However, if the vaccine does not completely prevent progression to AIDS in the "successfully" vaccinated HIV-infected individuals, then it will be necessary to develop vaccines that induce as high a degree of protection as possible in the "successfully" vaccinated individuals in order to achieve the additional goals of minimizing the incidence of AIDS and the AIDS death rate.

PROPHYLACTIC VACCINES: THE TWO-SUBTYPE PROBLEM

For the case of two subtypes, it is necessary to derive vaccinated reproductive numbers for each subtype; where $R_p^{(1)}$ is the vaccinated reproductive number for subtype 1 and $R_p^{(2)}$ is the vaccinated reproductive number for subtype 2.

A

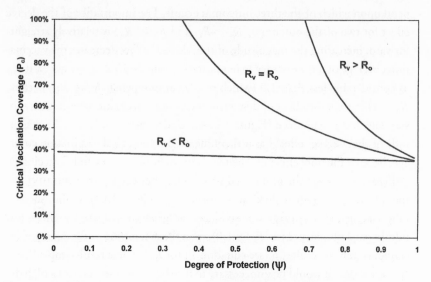

Figure 13.2A. The minimum critical vaccination coverage (p_c) needed in order to eradicate an HIV epidemic as a function of the degree of protection (ψ) for three different hypothetical HIV vaccines. The three vaccines differ with respect to the average number of secondary cases of HIV infection that are produced by one "successfully" vaccinated HIV infected individual: $R_V < R_0 (R_V = 0.15)$, $R_V \sim R_0 (R_V = 1.5)$, and $R_V > R_0 (R_V = 3.0)$. The average number of secondary cases of HIV infection produced by an unvaccinated HIV-infected individual (R_0) for each vaccine is 1.5. Other parameters are: vaccine "take" (ψ) = 0.95, the average length of the asymptomatic period for infected individuals (vaccinated as well as unvaccinated) ($1/\gamma$) = 10 years, the per partnership transmission probability of HIV from an unvaccinated individual (β_U) = 0.1, the per partner transmission probability of HIV from a "successfully" vaccinated HIV-infected individual differs for each of the three vaccines ($\beta_V = 0.1\beta_U$, $\beta_V = \beta_U$, and $\beta_V = 2\beta_U$), vaccine-induced immunity is lifelong, the average sexual life span ($1/\mu$) = 30 years and the number of new sex partners per year (c) = 2.

Analytical expressions for $R_p^{(1)}$ and $R_p^{(2)}$ have been derived previously [22,23] and are given in equations 12 and 13.

$$R_p^{(1)} = R_0^{(1)} (1 - p\varepsilon) + R_0^{(1)} p\varepsilon (1 - \zeta_1) \qquad (12)$$

$$R_p^{(2)} = R_0^{(2)} (1 - p\varepsilon) + R_0^{(2)} p\varepsilon (1 - \zeta_2) \qquad (13)$$

where: $R_0^{(1)}$ = the basic reproductive number of subtype 1
$R_0^{(2)}$ = the basic reproductive number of subtype 2
p = the vaccination coverage level

B

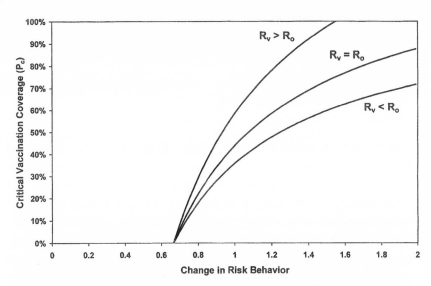

Figure 13.2B. The minimum critical vaccination coverage (p_c) needed in order to eradicate an HIV epidemic as a function of the change in risk behavior for the three HIV vaccines shown in Figure 13.2A. The same parameter values are used as in Figure 13.2A. Risk behavior is defined as the number of new sex partners per year (c) multiplied by the per partner transmission probability of HIV (β). The change in risk behavior = (new level of risk behavior) / (old level of risk behavior).

ε = the fraction of the vaccinated individuals in whom there is a protective immunological response (i.e., the "take")

ζ_1 = the degree of protection that the vaccine confers against infection by subtype 1 in the individuals who are effectively vaccinated, where the proportion effectively vaccinated = $p\varepsilon$

ζ_2 = the degree of cross-immunity (i.e., the "degree" of protection that the vaccine confers against infection by subtype 2 in the individuals who are effectively vaccinated, where the proportion effectively vaccinated = $p\varepsilon$).

To derive the eradication criteria for HIV epidemics that are generated by two subtypes, one must calculate the critical vaccination coverage for each subtype $(p_c^{(1)}$ and $p_c^{(2)})$ independently, and then vaccinate at the higher of the two critical vaccination coverage levels.[22,23] Consequently, vaccination coverage levels have to be high enough to eradicate each subtype independently.[22,23] Eradication will be possible only if a vaccine is applied at a high coverage level, has a high "take" and also induces a high degree of cross-immunity between subtypes.[22,23]

Predicting the Epidemiological Consequences of Risk Behavior Changes and Mass Vaccination Campaigns Against HIV

One of the main problems to consider when designing HIV epidemic control strategies is predicting the epidemiological consequences of changes in HIV risk behaviors that may occur in concurrence with a mass vaccination campaign. In the previous section we showed how to calculate the critical vaccination coverage level required to eradicate HIV epidemics, assuming that the level of risk behavior would remain unchanged. Here we consider the problem of HIV eradication when risk behavior changes. Previously, we have demonstrated how the vaccinated reproductive rate (R_p) can be used to derive an analytical expression for the minimum vaccination coverage level (p_c) necessary to eradicate an HIV epidemic. R_p can also be used to identify which epidemic control strategies are functionally equivalent (i.e., which will produce the same epidemiological effect); hence, R_p can be used to quantify the trade-offs between any medical intervention (for example, vaccination) and behavioral interventions that change risk behavior.[19-21] In this section, we use R_p to evaluate the simultaneous effect of changes in risk behavior and mass vaccination on the severity of the epidemic; we examine the trade-offs between risk behavior change and mass vaccination via the critical vaccination coverage level.

PROPHYLACTIC VACCINES: PROVIDING PROTECTION ONLY AGAINST INFECTION

Blower and McLean linked their model with epidemiological data to determine the vaccine efficacy levels and the vaccination coverage levels required to eradicate the HIV epidemic in San Francisco.[19-21] They also assessed the tradeoff between vaccination and potential changes in risk behavior.[19-21] Their quantitative results showed that it would be unlikely that an HIV vaccine would be able to eradicate the San Francisco HIV epidemic unless they were combined with considerable reductions in risk behaviors. Furthermore, they demonstrated that under certain conditions mass vaccination could have the perverse outcome of increasing the severity of the HIV epidemic. The probability of such a perverse outcome occurring depends upon three factors: the degree to which the risk behavior is increased (D) (that is, D equals the new level of risk behavior divided by the initial level of risk behavior, and the level of the risk behavior is defined as the number of new sex partners per unit time multiplied by the transmission probability per partnership), the efficacy (ϕ) of the vaccine used, and the achieved coverage levels (C). If the inequality $D > 1 / [1 - \phi C]$ is satisfied, then a mass vaccination campaign against HIV could do more harm than good.[19] For example, a mass vaccination campaign could increase the severity of an HIV epidemic among gay men if risk behavior increased by a factor of 1.4 and 50% of the susceptibles were vaccinated with a 60% effective vaccine.

PROPHYLACTIC VACCINES: PROVIDING PROTECTION AGAINST INFECTION
AND VACCINE-ALTERED PATHOGENESIS

Similar results for the effect of risk behavior changes on the critical vaccination coverage can be obtained from an analysis of our new model in which the vaccine can both prevent infection and alter the pathogenesis of HIV infection in "successfully" vaccinated individuals. In Figure 13.2B, we plot, for the three hypothetical vaccines shown in Figure 13.2A, the effect of changes in risk behavior on the critical vaccination coverage. Decreasing risk behavior would make it easier to eradicate an HIV epidemic (i.e., the critical vaccination coverage levels are lower); obviously, if risk behavior decreases sufficiently an epidemic would end even without a vaccine (Figure 13.2B). Conversely, increasing risk behavior would make it harder to eradicate HIV, and if risk behavior increased markedly then it would become impossible to eradicate HIV even if high efficacy vaccines were available (Figure 13.2B).

We have also evaluated the short-term epidemiological consequences of vaccines and changes in risk behavior. The efficacy of the vaccine is a measure of its protective capacity when administered under ideal conditions (i.e., during phase III clinical trials), and we have previously shown that ϕ can be used as a new measure of vaccine efficacy.[18–21] The effectiveness of a vaccine is a measure of the actual field performance of the vaccine in the "real world"; consequently, the effectiveness is a function of the achieved coverage level, any changes in risk behavior that may occur, and the efficacy of the vaccine. We have applied our new model to predict the short-term effectiveness of mass vaccination campaigns on the HIV epidemic in the gay community in San Francisco. For our modeling, we used the appropriate epidemiological parameters to reflect the current HIV epidemic in the gay community in San Francisco, with an HIV seroprevalence of 30% and an annual incidence rate of 1% to 3%. For our analyses we ran the model with and without mass vaccination and then calculated effectiveness ($E(t)$):

$$E(t) = 1 - \frac{C_V(t)}{C_U(t)} \tag{14}$$

where: $C_V(t)$ = the cumulative number of HIV infections at time t with mass vaccination

$C_U(t)$ = the cumulative number of HIV infections at time t without vaccination.

We predicted the effectiveness of HIV vaccines of moderate (50%) to high (80%) efficacy with either low (50%) or high (90%) coverage levels, assuming that risk behavior did not change after the mass vaccination program was introduced (Figure 13.3A). If $E(t) > 0$ then the vaccine program was beneficial, if $E(t) = 0$ then the vaccine program had no effect, and if $E(t) < 0$ then the vaccine program was detrimental. Obviously, a vaccine that has a high efficacy applied at a high coverage level has a very high effectiveness (Figure 13.3A). However, even vaccines with a moderate level of efficacy (50%) if applied at a high coverage level (90%) can have substantial effectiveness (Figure 13.3A). We also predicted the effectiveness of these two vaccines if risk behavior decreased by 50% at the same time that the mass vaccination program was initiated (Figure 13.3B). Not surprisingly, under these circumstances all vaccines worked better. Notably, if vaccination was accompanied by a reduction in risk behavior then even a moderately effective (50%) vaccine at low coverage (50%) substantially reduced the number of new HIV infections (Figure 13.3B).

We then evaluated the effectiveness of a moderately effective (50%) vaccine at low (50%) or high (90%) coverage levels, assuming that risk behavior increased by 50% (Figure 13.4A). For these predictions we evaluated the effectiveness of two hypothetical vaccines that failed in two different ways. Both vaccines had an efficacy of 50%, but one vaccine had a partial "take" effect (i.e., the "take" was 50% and the degree effect was 100%—therefore, 50% of the vaccinated were completely protected at every exposure and 50% of them were completely unprotected at every exposure) and the second vaccine had a partial "degree" effect (i.e., the "take" was 100% and the degree was 50%—therefore, 100% of the vaccinated were protected in 50% of their exposures). As before, increasing levels of risk behavior reduced the effectiveness of both vaccines (Figure 13.4A). However, if risk behavior increased by 50% when a moderately effective vaccine (50%) was applied at a low coverage level (50%) then the net effect of the vaccine program was perverse, as the number of new HIV infections increased (Figure 13.4A). When risk behavior increased, the partial "take" vaccine had a greater effectiveness than the partial "degree" vaccine (Figure

A

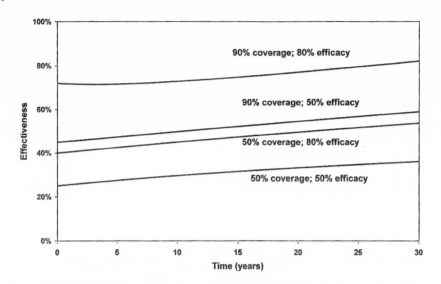

B

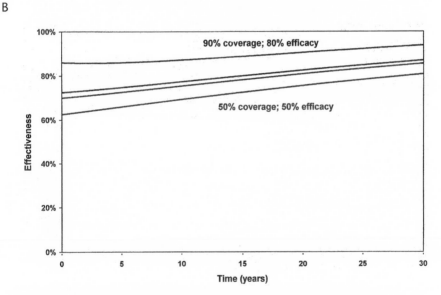

Figure 13.3. Effectiveness of two HIV vaccines (that are 50% and 80% effective) in lowering the incidence of HIV in the gay community in San Francisco when applied at coverage levels of 50% and 90%. (A) Risk behavior remains stable after the introduction of the vaccine, with the average number of new sex partners per year = 1.8. (B) Risk behavior decreases 50% when mass vaccination begins at $t = 0$. In both (A) and (B) the degree of protection of the vaccine $(\psi) = 1.0$, the average sexual life span $(1/\mu) = 30$ years, the average survival time from an AIDS diagnosis to death $(1/\alpha) = 20$ months, the per partnership transmission probability $(\beta_U = \beta_V) = 0.1$, the average length of the asymptomatic period for infected individuals (vaccinated as well as unvaccinated) $(1/\gamma) = 10$ years, and the average duration of vaccine-induced immunity = 20 years.

A

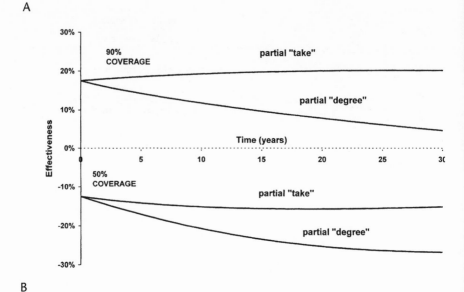

B

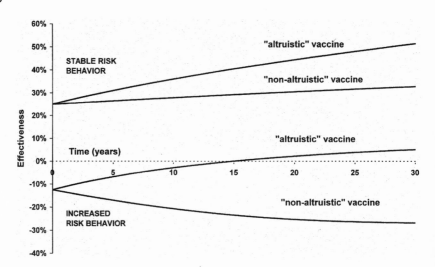

Figure 13.4.

13.4A). Since the partial "degree" vaccine provided only a degree of protection upon exposure, the effectiveness of the partial "degree" vaccine decreased sharply over time (Figure 13.4A).

We also predicted the effectiveness of two other hypothetical vaccines, both inducing a 50% "degree" of protection against infection, but in addition one vaccine had an "altruistic" effect (the vaccine reduced the infectiousness of "successfully" vaccinated HIV-infected individuals by 100-fold). The vaccines were applied at low coverage levels (50%), and risk behavior was either maintained at a stable level or increased by 50% (Figure 13.4B). As before, increasing risk behavior decreased effectiveness of both vaccines (Figure 13.4B). However, under conditions of increased levels of risk behavior, the effectiveness of the "non-altruistic" vaccine decreased with time (due to the degree effect, as in Figure 13.4A); but the effectiveness of the "altruistic" vaccine increased with time. Effectiveness increased because transmission decreased with time. Transmission decreased because the number of "successfully" vaccinated HIV-infected individuals increased over time and these individuals had a very low level of infectiousness.

PROPHYLACTIC VACCINES: THE TWO-SUBTYPE PROBLEM

To eradicate HIV epidemics that are generated by two subtypes, it is necessary to vaccinate at the higher of the two critical vaccination coverage levels[22,23] (see Figures 13.5A and 13.5B). Thus, the effect of risk behavior change on eradication, when more than one subtype is present, can be complex. If an HIV vaccine induces a high degree of cross-immunity then changes in risk behavior will have similar effects on the two subtypes (Figure 13.5A) and the results are the same as previously discussed for a single subtype. Increasing risk behavior will increase the critical vaccination coverage levels required to eradicate an HIV epidemic and may make it impossible to achieve that goal (i.e., the value of p_c becomes greater than 1.0) (Figure 13.5A). Conversely, decreasing levels of risk behavior lower the critical vaccination coverage levels required to achieve erad-

---

Figure 13.4. Effectiveness of HIV vaccines in lowering the incidence of HIV in the gay community in San Francisco. (A) Two vaccines are considered. Both vaccines had an efficacy (ϕ) of 50%, but one vaccine had a partial "take" effect (i.e., the "take" (ε) was 50% and the degree (ψ) was 100%—therefore, 50% of the vaccinated were completely protected at every exposure and 50% of them were completely unprotected at every exposure) and the second vaccine had a partial "degree" effect (i.e., the "take" (ε) was 100% and the degree (ψ) was 50%—therefore, 100% of the vaccinated were protected in 50% of their exposures). For both vaccines the average duration of vaccine-induced immunity is 20 years. Mass vaccination at $t = 0$ is accompanied by a 50% increase in risk behavior. Vaccine effectiveness is considered for two coverage levels: 50% and 90%. (B) The effectiveness of an "altruistic" vaccine is considered, where an "altruistic" vaccine is defined to be a vaccine which lowers the per partnership transmission probability of HIV from an infected "successfully" vaccinated individual (β_V). An "altruistic" vaccine (where $\beta_V = 0.01$ β_U) is compared with a "non-altruistic" vaccine (where $\beta_V = \beta_U$). Two cases are considered: stable levels of risk behavior and a 50% increase in levels of risk behavior.

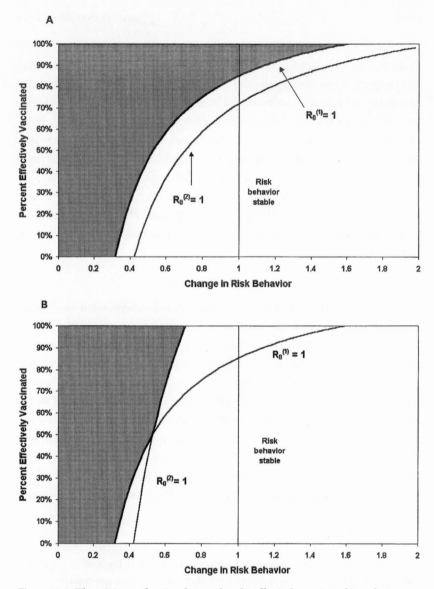

Figure 13.5. The minimum fraction that needs to be effectively vaccinated in order to eradicate HIV for the two-subtype differential "degree" model is plotted against changes in risk behavior that occur when the mass vaccination campaign is introduced. The fraction that needs to be effectively vaccinated is defined as the proportion vaccinated (p) multiplied by the "take" (ε) of the vaccine. The reproductive numbers of both subtypes must be less than 1.0 for HIV eradication to occur. Hence, the fraction that needs to be effectively vaccinated is shown by the gray area that lies above the greatest of the two reproductive numbers. Without a change in behavior (i.e., at change in risk behavior = 1.0), the reproductive number for subtype 1 ($R_0^{(1)}$) is 3.2, and the reproductive number of subtype 2 ($R_0^{(2)}$) is 2.4. In both (a) and (b), the vaccine confers an 80% degree of protection against subtype 1 (i.e., $\zeta_1 = 0.8$). In (A), the vaccine induces a high degree of cross-immunity ($\zeta_2 = 0.8$) against subtype 2, whereas in (B), the vaccine induces a low to moderate degree of cross-immunity ($\zeta_2 = 0.4$) against subtype 2.

ication (Figure 13.5A). However, if the vaccine induces a moderate to low degree of cross-immunity, then the effects of changes in risk behavior can be more complex (Figure 13.5B). Under these conditions, the critical vaccination coverage levels are higher, the epidemic is more sensitive to changes in risk behavior, and the possibility of achieving eradication is substantially reduced (compare Figure 13.5A with Figure 13.5B).

DISCUSSION

An effective HIV vaccine has yet to be developed, and in contrast to the successful immunization efforts against many other viral infections, there are inadequate immunological clues from human and animal studies as to how such a vaccine might be constructed. HIV represents a formidable challenge to vaccine development, as it employs almost every strategy used by other viruses to evade the immune system, as well as a few which appear to be unique to HIV.[7,12] It is gratifying that there is now an active, global, and relatively well-funded effort to find an HIV vaccine, as well as promising preclinical data from primate models of HIV infection that some vaccine strategies may prevent HIV infection. However, there is only one candidate HIV vaccine being investigated for efficacy in clinical trials, a subunit envelope vaccine, and there is considerable skepticism within the scientific community that this particular strategy will be effective.[12] It is imperative that the immunogens and vaccine strategies which have been shown to be promising in preclinical studies be moved rapidly into phase I and II studies in humans, and into phase III efficacy studies if shown to be safe and promising, and that further innovative vaccine strategies be developed through basic research.

We have demonstrated how epidemic control models can be used to design vaccination strategies that will result in the elimination of HIV and to predict the outcomes of mass vaccination campaigns with HIV vaccines of varying efficacy. We have also used our models to predict the epidemiological consequences of changes in risk behavior during mass vaccination campaigns in terms of both the long-term effects on elimination and the short-term effects on effectiveness. Our results have implications for clinical trial design, for vaccine design, and for design of epidemic control strategies. If phase III clinical trials of candidate HIV vaccines are conducted in the traditional manner, the results will provide a measure of only the number of infections that were prevented due to the vaccine. Our results illustrate that if HIV vaccines are imperfect (i.e., with an efficacy of less than 100%), as is likely to be the case, and if increases in risk behavior are also likely, then it is essential that the phase III clinical trials not only estimate the reduction of the incidence rate due to the vaccine but also determine the biological mechanisms of failure of the vaccine. Phase III clinical trials must also try to measure the degree of cross-immunity that the vaccines induce among HIV subtypes. Currently, new statistical methods are being designed to estimate the different biological mechanisms of failure within a phase III trial and to determine the optimal trial design.[31-33] If these new statistical methods are applied it will be possible to use the results from the phase III trials to predict the interaction of the vaccination program with changes in risk behavior, and hence to predict (as we have done here) the effectiveness of HIV vaccines in the "real world."

Our results also have implications for the design of vaccines. We have shown that any specified level of vaccine efficacy (ϕ) can be achieved by a wide variety of vaccines that could work in many ways; however, a highly effective vaccine should have a high "take," a high "degree," and a low rate of waning. Vaccine efficacy is extremely sensitive to the duration of protection; vaccines that wane quickly will have a low efficacy. If the vaccines are to be used against multiple subtypes, they should also induce a high degree of cross-immunity if used against very different immunological subtypes. Furthermore, some vaccines will be more effective than other vaccines if risk behavior increases. For example, we have shown that if risk behavior increases, then "take" and "altruistic" vaccines will have a greater effectiveness than "degree" vaccines. Increases in risk behavior are more likely to occur, as the result of mass vaccination, in some risk groups than others. Therefore, it is possible that we should consider designing different vaccines for different risk groups.

We have used our results to design HIV epidemic control strategies. We have shown that eradication will be possible only if a vaccine is applied at a high coverage level, has a high efficacy, and induces a high degree of cross-immunity between subtypes. However, even moderately efficacious vaccines, applied at low coverage levels, could significantly reduce the incidence of HIV if risk behavior remains stable or decreases. Conversely, if risk behavior increases then vaccine effectiveness will be substantially reduced. Furthermore, if risk behavior increases by too much, then a perverse effect will occur and the incidence and the prevalence of HIV infection could increase following a mass immunization program. To date, no vaccines have been developed against any sexually transmitted disease; thus, until now it has not been necessary to deal with the problem of imperfect vaccines and increases in risk behavior. Our results highlight the importance of developing HIV prevention programs that utilize both mass vaccination and risk reduction interventions. We suggest that epidemic control models are the appropriate health policy tools to design such integrated prevention programs.

ACKNOWLEDGMENTS

We are grateful to Travis Porco for earlier discussions of this work and for the derivation of equations 10 and 11. We thank Hayley Gershengorn and Elad Ziv for their thoughtful comments on this chapter. We also thank Jake and Dan Freimer for their insights. SMB gratefully acknowledges the financial support of NIAID/NIH. JM gratefully acknowledges financial support from the Australian National Council on AIDS and Related Diseases to the National Center on HIV Virology Research and the Research Fund of the Macfarlane Burnet Center for Medical Research.

REFERENCES

1. *UN AIDS/WHO: AIDS Epidemic Update, December 1998.* Geneva, Joint United Nations Program on HIV/AIDS, 1998.
2. Subbarao S, Schochetman G. Genetic variability of HIV-1. *AIDS* 1996; 10A:S1–23.
3. Gao F, Bailes L, Chen Y-L, et al. Origin of HIV-1 in *Pan troglodytes troglodytes.* Presented at the Keystone Symposium on HIV Vaccine Development, January 7–13, 1999, Keystone, Colorado, Abstract No. 005.
4. Dorrell L, Dong T, Ogg G, et al. Distinct recognition of non-clade B HIV-1 epitopes by cytotoxic T cells from donors infected in Africa. Presented at the Keystone Symposium on HIV Vaccine Development, January 7–13, 1999, Keystone, Colorado. Abstract No. 109.
5. Nyambi P, Nadas A, Gorny MK, et al. Immunotyping of HIV-1: An approach to immunologic classification of HIV. Presented at the Keystone Symposium on HIV Vaccine Development, January 7–13, 1999, Keystone, Colorado, Abstract No. 120.
6. Whitton JL, Oldstone MBA. Immune response to viruses. Chapter 12 in *Fields Virology,* third edition, edited by Fields BN, Knipe DM, Howley PM. Philadelphia: Lippincott-Raven, 1996; 345–374.
7. Letvin NL. Progress in the development of an HIV-1 vaccine. *Science* 1998; 280:1875–80.
8. Haigwood NL, Zolla-Pazner S. Humoral immunity to HIV, SIV and SHIV. *AIDS* 1998; 12A:S121–132.
9. Johnson RP, Siliciano RF, McElrath MJ. Cellular immune responses to HIV-1. *AIDS* 1998; 12A:S113–120.
10. Schmitz JE, Kuroda MJ, Lifton MA, et al. The role of CD8+ lymphocytes in the control of primary and chronic SIV infection. Presented at the Keystone Symposium on AIDS Pathogenesis, January 7–13, 1999, Keystone, Colorado, Abstract No. 336.

11. Putkonen P, Makitalo B, Bottiger D, Biberfeld G, and Thorstensson R. Protection of human immunodeficiency virus type 2-exposed seronegative macaques from mucosal simian immunodeficiency virus transmission. *J Virol* 1997; 71:4981–4984.
12. Kent SJ, Anne Z, Best SJ, Chandler JD, Boyle DB, and Ramshaw IA. Enhanced t-cell immunogenicity and protective efficacy of a human immunodeficiency virus type 1 vaccine regimen consisting of consecutive priming with DNA and boosting with recombinant fowlpox virus. *J Virol* 1998; 72:10180–10188.
13. Burton DR, Moore JP. Why do we not have an HIV vaccine and how can we make one. *Nature Medicine,* 1998; 4:495–531.
14. Zolla-Pazner S, Burda S, Belshe R, et al. Prime/boost immunization of humans induces antibodies that react with many HIV-1 clades and neutralize several X4- and R5- and dual-tropic primary isolates. Presented at the Keystone Symposium on HIV Vaccine Development, January 7–13, 1999, Keystone, Colorado, Abstract No. 420.
15. Ramsay AJ, Ruby J, Ramshaw IA. The modulation of immune responses by cytokines encoded in recombinant vaccine vectors. In *Strategies in Vaccine Design,* edited by Ada GL. CRC Press, Boca Raton, Florida, 1995, 174–91.
16. Learmont JC, Geczy A, Mills J, et al. Limmunologic and virologic status after 14–18 years of infection with an attenuated strain of HIV-1—A report from the Sydney Blood Bank Cohort (SBBC HIV-1). *NEJM,* 1999; 340:1715–1722.
17. Baba TW, Liska V, Khimani AH, et al. Live attenuated, multiply deleted simian immunodeficiency virus causes AIDS in infant and adult macaques. *Nature Medicine,* 1999; 5:194–203.
18. McLean A and Blower SM. Imperfect vaccines, herd immunity and HIV. *Proc Roy Soc London Series B* 1993; 253:9–13.
19. Blower SM and McLean AR. Prophylactic vaccines, risk behavior change and the probability of eradicating HIV in San Francisco. *Science* 1994; 265:1451–1454.
20. Blower SM and McLean AR. AIDS: Modelling epidemic control. *Science* 1995; 267: 252–253.
21. McLean AR and Blower SM. Modelling HIV vaccination. *Trends Microbiol* 1995; 3: 458–463.
22. Porco TC and Blower SM. Designing HIV vaccination policies: Subtypes and cross-immunity. *Interfaces* 1998; 28(3):167–190.
23. Porco TC and Blower SM. HIV vaccines: The effect of the mode of action on the coexistence of HIV subtypes. *Mathematical Population Studies* 2000; 8(2):205–229.
24. Blower SM, Small PM and Hopewell P. Control strategies for tuberculosis epidemics: New models for old problems. *Science* 1996; 273:497–500.
25. Blower SM and Gerberding JL. Understanding, predicting and controlling the emergence of drug-resistant tuberculosis: A theoretical framework. *Journal of Molecular Medicine* 1998; 76:624–636.
26. Blower SM, Porco TC and Darby G. Predicting and preventing the emergence of antiviral drug resistance in HSV-2. *Nature Medicine* 1998; 4(6):673–678.
27. Blower SM, Koelle K and Lietman T. Antibiotic resistance—to treat . . . [Letter to the editor]. *Nature Medicine* 1999; 5(4):358.
28. Blower SM and Dowlatabadi H. Sensitivity and uncertainty analysis of complex mod-

els of disease transmission: An HIV model, as an example. *Internat Statist Rev* 1994; 62:229–243.

29. Blower SM, Hartel D, Dowlatabadi H, May RM, and Anderson RM. Drugs, sex and HIV: A mathematical model for New York City. *Phil Trans Roy Soc Series B* 1991; 321:171–187.

30. Blower SM, Gershengorn HB and Grant RM. A tale of two futures: HIV and antiretroviral therapy in San Francisco. *Science* 2000; 287:650–654.

31. Longini IM, Datta S and Halloran ME. Measuring vaccine efficacy for both susceptibility to infection and reduction in infectiousness for prophylactic vaccines. *JAIDS* 1996; 13:440–447.

32. Longini IM, Sagatelian K, Rida WN and Halloran ME. Optimal vaccine trial design when estimating vaccine efficacy for susceptibility and infectiousness from multiple populations. *Statistics in Medicine* 1998; 17:1121–1136.

33. Longini IM and Halloran ME. A frailty mixture model for estimating vaccine efficacy. *Appl Statist* 1996; 45(2):165–173.

Chapter 14 Development and Validation of a Serologic Testing Algorithm for Recent HIV Seroconversion

Glen A. Satten, Robert S. Janssen, Susan Stramer, and Michael P. Busch

Owing to the long incubation period from infection to AIDS, researchers often ignore the fact that infection with HIV, the onset of infectivity, and a detectable antibody response on standard screening assays are not simultaneous. The time at which HIV antibody is first detectable in peripheral blood using an enzyme-linked immunoassay (EIA) can vary by manufacturer and generation of test (first-generation tests were replaced by second-generation tests in 1987, and third-generation tests or combination HIV-1/HIV-2 tests became available in 1992). Typically the differences in onset of detectability are fairly small. For example, DNA PCR can detect HIV infection on average about 5 days before p24 antigen can be detected, which in turn occurs on average about 5 days before a third-generation HIV 1/2 combination test can detect HIV antibodies.[1] However, for some events in early HIV infection the appropriate timescale may be weeks rather than days. For example, Satten and Sternberg estimate that on average about 44 days pass between seroconversion on an HIV 1/2 combi test and development of a 3-band positive Western blot assay result,[1] and Busch, Lee, and Satten et al. estimate that approximately 20 days separate seroconversion on a third-generation recombinant-based HIV 1/2 combi test and seroconversion on a second-generation whole-virus lysate assay.[2] Time periods between two time-ordered events in the very early stages of HIV infection are often called window periods, and persons are said to be in their window period if they have experienced the first but not the second of the two events. Because this language is somewhat imprecise, it is often necessary to specify exactly which window period is being referred to (e.g., individuals who have detectable virus by DNA PCR but do not yet test reactive on the p24 antigen assay are in their PCR-to-p24 window period).

Window periods are of interest for several reasons. Most cases of HIV transmission from transfusion of blood screened for HIV is due to donation by seroconverting donors who are in the window period between the onset of infectivity (currently believed to correspond to the onset of detectability of HIV DNA by PCR) and onset of detectability of p24 antigen (a core protein of HIV).[3-5] In addition, primary HIV syndrome (symptomatic expression of infection with HIV) and viremia (high virus titers associated with acute HIV infection) typically occur during the window period between PCR detectability and development of sufficient antibody response to be detected using a screening EIA. Early treatment during this same window period is currently thought to be an effective strategy for subsequent control of HIV disease.

From an epidemiologic viewpoint, window periods associated with early HIV infection also offer the opportunity to measure HIV incidence in a population by conducting a single cross-sectional survey. Because longitudinal measurement of HIV incidence is time-consuming, costly, and subject to follow-up bias, a method of estimating HIV incidence in a cross-sectional setting is highly desirable. Incidence of HIV infection can be estimated cross-sectionally using a window period of known mean duration ω; once such a window period is identified, incidence $\hat{I}$ is obtained by estimating the prevalence $\hat{P}$ of persons in the window and solving the equation $\hat{P} = \hat{I}\omega$. The first implementation of this strategy for estimating HIV incidence was carried out by Brookmeyer and Quinn, who used the window period between detectability of p24 antigen and detectability of antibodies to HIV and a mean window period duration of approximately $\omega = 22.5$ days.[6-7]

A window period must have a number of characteristics for optimal use in cross-sectional estimation of HIV incidence. First, the window period must not be too short. Short window periods, while highly specific for early HIV infection, require enormous sample sizes (or very high HIV incidence) before a reasonable number of people are observed in their window period. For this reason,

Brookmeyer and Quinn have used the p24 window primarily in India,[6] where recent introduction and subsequent rapid spread of HIV has resulted in high incidence in sentinel populations such as commercial sex workers. Conversely, the window period must not be too long. In order for the cross-sectional approach described above to work, it must be assumed that HIV incidence is constant over the length of the window period. Very long window periods result in violation of this condition, resulting in marker values which may reflect past rather than current patterns of HIV incidence.

If possible, the window period should start after detectable antibodies have developed (as detected using an EIA and confirmed by a Western blot). This is desirable for two reasons. First, most studies will already screen for HIV serostatus using the standard EIA/Western blot algorithm; if this is the case only HIV-positive specimens (typically a small subset of the survey) need be tested for window period status. Second, many interesting applications involve retrospective estimation of HIV incidence using stored specimens. In many such cases only HIV-positive sera were stored for further study. A final condition on the window chosen for estimating HIV incidence is that individuals should be unaware that they are in their window periods. For example, the p24-to-antibody detectability window corresponds to the period during which persons may experience flu-like symptoms of primary HIV infection. This may result in oversampling of persons in their p24 window period in surveys conducted in health-care settings and undersampling of such persons in other sampling settings (this argument has been used to explain why the yield of p24 antigen screening in the blood system has been lower than expected).

The approach we describe here uses the window period between seroconversion on a sensitive EIA and seroconversion on a specially developed less sensitive (or "detuned") assay which detects HIV antibodies on average 129 days after the sensitive EIA. Our approach was based on the following two insights. First, the time period between antibody detection using a third-generation EIA and a first-generation EIA could be used as a window period for estimating HIV incidence. Second, the first-generation EIA was developed to detect HIV antibodies as early as possible, and perhaps an assay could be developed which detected HIV antibodies as late as possible. To accomplish this we set about to "detune" an existing assay (the Abbott 3A11 assay), that is, to find conditions for which this assay would reliably detect antibodies to HIV months after the same assay could detect HIV antibodies when run under standard conditions. We refer to the assay when run under our new conditions as the 3A11-LS (for less sensitive), and refer to the use of the 3A11 (with confirmatory Western blot) and

3A11-LS assay as the serologic testing algorithm for recent HIV seroconversion (STARHS). Because persons are considered 3A11-reactive only if they also have a positive Western blot (corresponding to the usual screening algorithm), strictly speaking the window period we are using starts at the onset of Western blot reactivity (which occurs shortly after 3A11 seroconversion). However, since the Western blot is used only as a confirmatory assay, we will continue to refer to the start of the window period as the onset of 3A11 reactivity.

For the STARHS approach to be useful, we must obtain an estimate of the mean duration ω between 3A11 and 3A11-LS seroconversion. To have confidence in the STARHS approach to estimating incidence, we must validate our approach by comparing cross-sectionally calculated HIV incidence with longitudinally calculated incidence among the same persons. Finally, to ensure eventual and persistent seroconversion on the 3A11-LS assay, we must study persons with late-stage HIV disease. These issues were discussed in Janssen, Satten, Stramer, et al.,[8] the paper which introduced the STARHS approach. The purpose of this chapter is to elaborate on some of the statistical models and techniques used in that paper which were not described in detail there.

MODEL FOR ESTIMATING THE DISTRIBUTION
OF THE DURATION OF THE WINDOW PERIOD

Estimation of the mean and distribution of the times between 3A11 and 3A11-LS seroconversions requires data on 3A11, Western blot, and 3A11-LS assay results for serial specimens from a group of individuals. For practical reasons, such specimens are not collected daily; worse, the tendency is for frequency of specimen collection to be roughly inversely proportional to total duration of observation. Thus, specimens from three separate data sources were combined to estimate the distribution of times between seroconversion on the two assays: participants in the San Francisco Men's Health Study, attendees of an STD clinic in Trinidad, and repeat plasma donors in the United States.

Because the exact days of 3A11/WB and 3A11-LS seroconversion are not measured precisely, a mathematical model must be used to estimate the mean and interseroconversion times distribution. We assumed that for each individual and each assay there was a distinct time of seroconversion, before (after) which the individual's assay test results would be consistently nonreactive (reactive), and that the time of 3A11-LS seroconversion was no earlier than the time of 3A11/WB seroconversion. We also assumed that the times of specimen collection were independent of the (unknown) times of seroconversion on both assays. We further assumed that the time interval containing each individual's time of 3A11/WB seroconversion was short enough that incidence could be assumed constant throughout the interval. Finally, we assumed that the distribution of times between seroconversion was independent of the calendar time of 3A11/WB seroconversion.

The longitudinal data gathered from each individual can be summarized by three quantities: a_i, the time of the last 3A11/WB nonreactive test; b_i, the time of the first 3A11/WB reactive test; c_i, the time of the last 3A11-LS nonreactive test; and d_i, the time of the first 3A11-LS reactive test. By study enrollment criteria $b_i < \infty$ for all persons, and by study design for all persons $b_i \le d_i$, with equality only if $a_i = c_i$. Because a_i, b_i, c_i, and d_i are measured in days, we take the t_{i1} and t_{i2} to be integer-valued (discrete) random variables. If we let t_{i1} denote the unknown time of 3A11/WB seroconversion and t_{i2} denote the unknown time of 3A11-LS seroconversion, then the assumptions above imply that t_{i1} is uniformly distributed between a_i and b_i. Hence, the contribution to the likelihood for the ith person for the case $d_i < \infty$ is

$$L_i = \frac{1}{(b_i - a_i + 1)} \sum_{t_1 = a_i}^{b_i} \sum_{t_2 = c_i}^{d_i} f(t_2 - t_1) = \frac{1}{(b_i - a_i + 1)} \sum_{s = l_i}^{u_i} f(s) k_i(s)$$

where $\ell_i = \max(0, c_i - b_i)$, $u_i = d_i - a_i$ and $k_i(s) = \frac{1}{2}\{\min(2b_1 + s, 2d_i - s) - \max(2a_i + s, 2c_i - s)\}$, or

$$L_i = \frac{1}{(b_i - a_i + 1)} \sum_{t_1 = a_i}^{b_i} S(c_i - t_1 - 1)$$

for the case $d_i = \infty$, where $S(t) = 1 - \sum_{t'=0}^{t} f(t')$ for $t \ge 0$ and $S(-1) = 1$. The overall likelihood L is the product over contributions from the individual in the study.

We chose f to be an arbitrary function with mass at integers $0, 1, \ldots, K_{max}$ and maximized L with respect to parameters $f(j)$ using an E-M algorithm. Additional details and shortcuts which allow expedited treatment of the case $d_i = \infty$ are available elsewhere.[9] The E-M algorithm can be augmented by adding a smoothing step which replaces f at the rth E-M iteration by a smoothed version of f. This speeds convergence enormously and has negligible effect on the final estimate of

$$\hat{\omega} = \sum_{s=0}^{K_{max}} sf(s).$$

The estimate of $S(t)$ obtained by this procedure is shown in Figure 14.1, along with 95% pointwise bootstrap confidence intervals. The bootstrap pro-

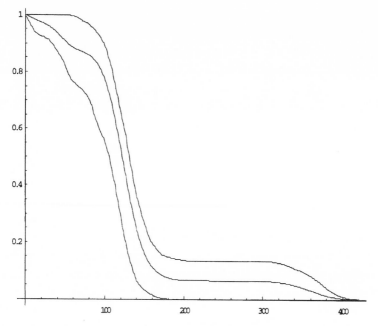

Figure 14.1. Estimated survival function for the duration of the window period between 3A11 and 3A11-LS seroconversion (cutoff = 0.75), with (pointwise) upper and lower 95% confidence bands.

cedure was conducted by generating 1000 independent and identically distributed resamplings of the data conditional on maintaining the same number of observations from each data source. Confidence intervals were obtained using the percentile method. The estimate of ω corresponding to our best estimate of $S(t)$ was 129 days; using the same bootstrap procedure, a 95% confidence interval for ω of (109, 149) was obtained.

CALCULATING CONFIDENCE INTERVALS
FOR INCIDENCE AND TRENDS IN INCIDENCE

As a result of testing with the 3A11-LA assay, individuals are placed into one of three categories: 3A11-nonreactive, 3A11-reactive/3A11-LS-nonreactive, and 3A11-LS-reactive. Denote the probabilities of these three categories by ϕ_1, ϕ_2, and ϕ_3. The prevalence of persons with early HIV infection is calculated using only data from persons who are 3A11-nonreactive and 3A11-reactive/3A11-LS-nonreactive, so that the appropriate prevalence is $\phi_2/(\phi_1 + \phi_2)$. The number of persons detected who are 3A11-LS-reactive is ancillary to this prevalence, and hence we condition our calculations on the number of persons detected who are 3A11-nonreactive and 3A11-reactive/3A11-LS-nonreactive. As the number of persons who are 3A11-reactive/3A11-LS-nonreactive is small compared to the number 3A11-nonreactive, we further assume a Poisson distribution for the number of persons who are 3A11-reactive/3A11-LS-nonreactive.

Incidence is estimated as the ratio of an estimated prevalence and the estimated duration of the window period. Hence, a confidence interval for incidence should account for uncertainty in both of these quantities. This is most easily accomplished using the Bonferroni method, in which the $100(1 - \alpha)\%$ confidence interval for HIV incidence is calculated by using $100(1 - \alpha/2)\%$ confidence intervals for the prevalence of persons in the window period and for the mean duration of the window period. Specifically, if n 3A11-reactive/3A11-LS-nonreactive specimens are detected out of N 3A11-nonreactive or 3A11-reactive/3A11-LS-nonreactive specimens tested, then an approximate $100(1 - \alpha/2)\%$ Poisson confidence interval for $(N I \omega)$ has limits

$$n^-_{\alpha/2} = \tfrac{1}{2}\chi^{-1}_{2n,\alpha/4} \text{ and } n^+_{\alpha/2} = \tfrac{1}{2}\chi^{-1}_{2(n+1),1-\alpha/4},$$

where $\chi^{-1}_{df,p}$ is the pth quantile of the chi-square distribution with df degrees of freedom. To obtain incidence I given $(N I \omega)$ we must divide by $N\omega$; hence, a $100(1 - \alpha)\%$ confidence interval for I is given by

$$\left(\frac{n^-_{\alpha/2}}{N\omega^+_{\alpha/2}}, \frac{n^+_{\alpha/2}}{N\omega^-_{\alpha/2}} \right)$$

where $(\omega^-_{\alpha/2}, \omega^+_{\alpha/2})$ is a $100(1 - \alpha/2)\%$ confidence interval for ω. From the bootstrap study described earlier, the 97.5% confidence interval for ω is (108, 154) days. An alternate procedure to account for the variability in ω would be to assume a prior distribution on ω.[10]

A major advantage of using the Poisson approximation is that values of $n^-_{\alpha/2}/\omega^+_{\alpha/2}$ and $n^+_{\alpha/2}/\omega^-_{\alpha/2}$ can be tabulated for various values of n. A table of such values for $n \leq 50$ would allow calculation of confidence intervals for HIV incidence in most studies.

VALIDATION OF THE STARHS ASSAY STRATEGY
INCIDENCE CALCULATIONS

Before the STARHS strategy can be used to estimate HIV incidence with any confidence, it must be validated in populations where longitudinally calculated incidence can also be obtained. A study in which longitudinally calculated inci-dence is compared with cross-sectionally calculated incidence among the same persons, and for which the study duration is short enough that incidence may be considered constant over the study period will be called a validation study. Janssen et al. report results from two validation studies.[8] We consider first the comparison of cross-sectional and longitudinal incidence in the San Francisco Men's Health Study (SFMHS). The SFMHS is a population-based cohort study with scheduled follow-up (waves) every six months. Janssen et al. compare ob-served incidence between the jth and $(j + 1)$th waves with cross-sectionally calculated incidence at the $(j + 1)$th wave. Note that only persons seen at both the jth and $(j + 1)$th waves contribute to the longitudinal calculation. Hence, for a proper comparison only persons seen at both the jth and $(j + 1)$th waves should be considered in the cross-sectional sample at the $(j + 1)$th wave. By comparing incidence only between successive waves, Janssen et al. also ensure that incidence is constant over the time periods under study.[8] They present 12 such comparisons in Table 14.2; the average of the 12 observed incidences was 1.4%/year, while the average of the 12 cross-sectionally calculated incidences was 1.5%/year.

The second validation study in Janssen et al. was conducted using data from repeat blood donors.[8] This study raises a new statistical issue: What type of cross-sectional estimation is valid when individuals are seen very frequently in the longitudinal study? In the SFMHS example above, persons were seen at two successive waves and contributed to the validation study if they were 3A11-nonreactive at the first wave. Suppose that instead of waves separated by 6 months, individuals (labeled i) were seen at times t_{i0} and t_{i1} that were very close together. Then the prevalence of persons at time t_{i1} in their window pe-riod would be distorted because it was known these persons were 3A11-nonre-active (i.e., not in their window period) at time t_{i0}. Hence, in longitudinal studies with frequent follow-up, it is necessary to develop techniques which take this effect into account. Satten et al. consider this case;[11] their approach is outlined here for the simple case where each person is seen only twice.

We assume that seroconversions are rare so that the person-time of follow-up does not need to be adjusted, the longitudinal estimator of incidence is $n/\Sigma_i \tau_i$, where $\tau_i = t_{i1} - t_{i0}$ is the amount of follow-up time contributed by the ith person and n is the number of seroconverters (persons who are 3A11-nonre-active at t_{i0} and 3A11-reactive at t_{i1}). Let β be the expected proportion of sero-converters who are in their window period at time t_{i1}. Then an estimator of in-cidence based on samples at time t_{i1} is $(n_d/\beta)/\Sigma_i \tau_i$, where n_d is the number of

3A11-reactive/3A11-LS-nonreactive specimens at time t_{i1}. Define $\bar{\tau} = \frac{1}{N}\Sigma_i\tau_i$; then this new estimator can be rewritten as $n_d/N\beta\bar{\tau}$. Assuming constant incidence (particularly reasonable if t_{i0} and t_{i1} are always close), the time of 3A11 seroconversion for a person who seroconverts between t_{i0} and t_{i1} is uniformly distributed between t_{i0} and t_{i1}. Hence, the value of β is easily computed to be

$$\beta = \int_0^\infty \left\{ \frac{1}{\tau}\int_0^\tau S(u)du \right\} dF_s(\tau)$$

where $S(u)$ is proportion of persons with window period longer than u, and $F_s(\tau)$ is the cumulative distribution of follow-up time τ_i among seroconverters. While β can be estimated from this last expression using the empirical distribution of follow-up times among seroconverters, it is preferable to derive an expression which uses the distribution of follow-up times among all donors, as this will allow much greater precision in estimation of β. To accomplish this, note that the probability that a given person seroconverts in an interval proportional to the length of that interval. Hence $F_s(\tau)$ is a length-biased version of $F(\tau)$, the distribution of follow-up times among all donors, that is, $dF_s(\tau) = \tau dF(\tau)/\mathcal{E}(\tau)$, where $\mathcal{E}(\tau) = \int \tau dF(\tau)$. Thus, β can be rewritten as

$$\beta = \int_0^\infty \int_0^\tau S(u)du\, dF(\tau)/\varepsilon(\tau) := \gamma/\varepsilon(\tau).$$

Finally, noting that $\tau/\mathcal{E}(\tau) \to 1$, we may estimate incidence using $n_d/N\hat{\gamma}$, where

$$\hat{\gamma} = \int_0^\infty \int_0^\tau S(u)du\, d\hat{F}(\tau),$$

and where $\hat{F}(\tau)$ is the empirical distribution of follow-up times among all donors. Note that if all observed values of τ_i are long enough that $\int_0^{\tau_i} S(u) = \bar{\omega}$, then this estimator of incidence reduces to the usual cross-sectional incidence estimator (as in the case of the SFMHS validation study, in which τs were typically 6 months apart). Using this approach, Janssen et al. estimated HIV incidence in repeat blood donors (where τ_i may be as short as 56 days) to be 2.95×10^{-5}/year [95% confidence interval (1.14-6.53)] compared with the longitudinally observed incidence 2.60×10^{-5}/year [95% confidence interval (1.49-4.21)].

SAMPLE SIZE CALCULATIONS

Sample size calculations can be carried out with two possible goals in mind: hypothesis testing or point estimation. Sample size calculations for testing hypotheses about changes in HIV incidence over time or differences in HIV inci-

Table 14.1. Data Layout in a 2 × 2 Table for Comparing HIV Incidence Between Two Populations (One Which Has Experienced an Intervention and a Control Population)

	Intervention	Control	
3A11-reactive/3A11-LS-nonreactive	n_1	n_2	n
3A11-nonreactive	$N_1 - n_1$	$N_2 - n_2$	$N - n$
	N_1	N_2	N

dence between subgroups can be calculated using standard techniques. Suppose we wanted to be able to detect the difference between an incidence of 0.1%/year and 0.2%/year with probability 0.80 in two populations. Because the prevalence of 3A11-reactive 3A11-LS-nonreactive persons is nearly equal to the disease odds (as long as recent infection is rare), the sample size required could be calculated by noting that the analysis can be carried out by testing whether the odds ratio in the 2 × 2 table shown in Table 14.1 is equal to 1.0. Note that by testing the ratios of incidence as in Table 14.1 (rather than differences) the value of ω drops out, so that uncertainty in the estimated value of ω does not contribute to the confidence interval width and sample size calculations for this type of calculation. Assuming column-based sampling, the cell occupation probabilities are $I_j \cdot \omega$ and $1 - I_j \cdot \omega$ for the first and second rows of the jth column, respectively. Sample size calculations to detect a change in HIV incidence in the same population, measured in two cross-sectional surveys at different times, can also be calculated using similar reasoning.

Sample size calculations for point estimation of HIV incidence are somewhat more difficult, because the uncertainty in the estimated value of ω should be accounted for. Following Kupper and Hafner,[12] we calculate sample sizes so that $100^*(1 - \alpha)\%$ confidence interval width goals are met with probability $(1 - \beta)$. Assume that n, the number of 3A11-reactive but 3A11-LS-nonreactive specimens follows a Poisson distribution with parameter pN where N is the number of persons with 3A11-LS nonreactive test results. Let $100^*(1 - \alpha)\%$ confidence limits for n be denoted by $n_\alpha^\pm$. Then, our sample size determination is to find the smallest N such that

$$Pr\left[\frac{n_{\alpha/2}^+}{N\omega_{\alpha/2}^-} - \frac{n_{\alpha/2}^-}{N\omega_{\alpha/2}^+} \le d\right] \ge 1 - \beta \tag{1}$$

where the Bonferroni correction has been applied. In calculating confidence intervals, we use the approximate limits

$$n^-_{\alpha/2} = \tfrac{1}{2}\chi^{-1}_{2n,\alpha/4} \text{ and } n^+_{\alpha/2} = \tfrac{1}{2}\chi^{-1}_{2(n+1),1-\alpha/4}$$

as discussed earlier.

Let $y(x)$ be the solution to

$$\frac{\chi^{-1}_{2(y+1),1-\alpha/4}}{\omega^-_{\alpha/2}} - \frac{\chi^{-1}_{2y,\alpha/4}}{\omega^+_{\alpha/2}} = x. \tag{2}$$

Because the left-hand side of (2) is monotone increasing in y, values of $n \leq y(2Nd)$ will correspond to confidence interval widths which are shorter than d. Hence, (1) is satisfied whenever

$$\sum_{j=0}^{[y(2Nd)]_-} \frac{(pN)^j}{j!} e^{-pN} \geq 1 - \beta \tag{3}$$

where $[w]_-$ is the smallest integer $\leq w$. Equation (3) may be rewritten as

$$\frac{\Gamma([(y(2Nd)]_- + 1, pN)}{\Gamma([y(2Nd)]_- + 1, 0)} \geq 1 - \beta \tag{4}$$

where

$$\Gamma(\alpha, x) = \int_x^\infty t^{a-1} e^{-t} dt.$$

Some sample sizes calculated using this criterion are shown in Table 14.2. It may seem initially odd that for fixed d, larger sample sizes are required as incidence increases. However, the proper comparison is apparently on the percent scale. For example, if I/d is held fixed at 1, then the resulting sample sizes are 47,780 for $I = 0.5\%$, 23,890 for $I = 1\%$ and 4,780 for $I = 5\%$.

Because of these results, it may be more appropriate to calculate sample sizes for fixed confidence interval width on the log scale. This turns out to be easier as well. In this case, we require that

$$Pr\left[\log\left\{ \frac{n^+_{\alpha/2}}{N\omega^-_{\alpha/2}} \right\} - \log\left\{ \frac{n^-_{\alpha/2}}{N\omega^+_{\alpha/2}} \right\} \leq 2\log d \right] \geq 1 - \beta \tag{5}$$

The choice of constant $2 \log d$ allows the interpretation for d that the upper limit is two factors of d greater than the lower limit; to the extent that the intervals are symmetric on the log scale, we may infer that the lower limit is $1/d$ and the upper limit d times the point estimate. To determine the minimum sample size satisfying (5), let $z(x)$ be the solution to

$$\frac{\chi^{-1}_{2(z+1),1-\alpha/4}}{\chi^{-1}_{2z,\alpha/4}} = x. \tag{6}$$

Table 14.2. Sample Size Calculations Based on Equation 1

	d	Sample Size
Incidence = 0.5%	0.5	47,780
	1.0	8,350
	2.0	2,120
Incidence = 1.0%	0.5	744,430
	1.0	23,890
	2.0	4,180
	3.0	1,900
Incidence = 5.0%	2.5	149,090
	3.0	38,750
	4.0	10,230
	5.0	4,780

d = Confidence interval width (%).

As the left-hand side of (6) is a monotonic decreasing function of z, (5) is satisfied whenever

$$\sum_{j=\left[z\left(d^2\omega_{\alpha/2}^-/\omega_{\alpha/2}^+\right)\right]_-+1}^{\infty} \frac{(pN)^j}{j!} e^{-pN} \geq 1-\beta. \tag{7}$$

Equation (7) may be rewritten as

$$\frac{\gamma\left(\left[z(d^2\omega_{\alpha/2}^-/\omega_{\alpha/2}^+)\right]_-+1, pN\right)}{\Gamma\left(\left[z(d^2\omega_{\alpha/2}^-/\omega_{\alpha/2}^+)\right]_-+1, 0\right)} \geq 1-\beta \tag{8}$$

where

$$\gamma(a,x) = \int_0^x t^{a-1} e^{-t} dt,$$

from which the sample size can be easily determined. Note (8) is easier to use than (4) because only one evaluation of z using (6) is required, while (4) requires repeated evaluation of (3). Sample sizes calculated using (5) were reported in Janssen et al.[8]

Analogous calculations for one-sided confidence intervals may also be carried out. Finally, if for some reason an investigator has fixed limits A and B which should contain the confidence interval with probability no less than $1 - \beta$, then a sample size based on ensuring that

$$Pr\left[\frac{n_{\alpha/2}^+}{N\omega_{\alpha/2}^-} \leq B \text{ and } \frac{n_{\alpha/2}^-}{N\omega_{\alpha/2}^+} \geq A\right] \geq 1 - \beta$$

can be carried out in a similar way.

DETERMINING THE EFFECT OF A PREVENTION
PROGRAM ON HIV INCIDENCE

The STARHS assay approach can be used to implement studies that make direct measurements of the effect of a prevention program or other intervention on HIV incidence. For example, suppose we wish to determine if an intensive counseling intervention results in fewer HIV infections. Prior to the intervention, we conduct a serosurvey and find n_1 persons with discordant 3A11/3A11-LS results and $N_1 - n_1$ persons who are 3A11-nonreactive. After the conclusion of the campaign, another survey is conducted and we find n_2 persons with discordant 3A11/3A11-LS results and $N_2 - n_2$ persons who are 3A11-nonreactive. Then we can test whether the campaign had an effect on the number of recently infected persons by estimating the odds ratio of Table 14.1.

For more complicated problems involving many covariates and interactions between covariates, logistic regression can be used to model the odds of being recently infected versus being uninfected. Logistic regression has been frequently used to find factors associated with HIV prevalence. By using the STARHS approach, risk factors can be identified that are directly associated with incident HIV cases, rather than prevalent infection.

DISCUSSION

The STARHS approach allows calculation of HIV incidence in a population in a single cross-sectional survey, by determining the prevalence of persons who have a 3A11-reactive result but who have not yet developed a high enough antibody response to have a reactive 3A11-LS assay. The 3A11-LS assay, specially created for this purpose, is a "detuned" version of the 3A11 assay. Some advantages of this approach are that only specimens with a 3A11-reactive result (confirmed by Western blot) need be tested with the 3A11-LS assay and that there is a relatively long duration between 3A11 and 3A11-LS seroconversion.

In addition to estimating HIV incidence, the STARHS approach has other potential applications. Current belief is that the time period between infection and seroconversion corresponds to a peak period of HIV infectiousness.[13] Hence, partner notification strategies could be tailored to identifying social networks in which HIV transmission is actively occurring. Additionally, viral replication in lymphoid tissue remains as high immediately after seroconversion as before,[14] which gives a pathophysiologic basis for assigning persons identified by the 3A11-LS assay the same treatment regimen as persons initially identified as HIV-positive before seroconversion. Finally, the STARHS approach can be useful in recruiting persons into studies of treatment for recently infected persons; an example of this application is given in Janssen et al.[8]

We hope that the STARHS approach using the 3A11-LS assay is only the first step in developing robust tools to estimate HIV incidence. Further laboratory work on developing "less sensitive" or "detuned" assays which reliably detect HIV infection as late as possible would be welcome. In addition, the approach may be useful in other diseases, particularly hepatitis C. Some aspects of the STARHS approach still need further study. All specimens we have examined to date are from persons infected with HIV-1 subtype B. The validity of the STARHS approach should be independently evaluated for other subtypes: we plan to do this. Additionally, the effect of injection drug use or the high level of immune system activation characterizing persons in the developing world on time to 3A11-LS-seroconversion, and even establishment of the proportion who do eventually seroconvert, needs to be studied. In addition, the Centers for Disease Control and Prevention (CDC) are developing a comprehensive quality control program for laboratories which will be performing testing using the 3A11-LS assay under an investigational new device license recently granted to CDC by the FDA.

Prevention programs and other interventions designed to reduce the burden of HIV disease should be judged in part by the number of infections that they prevent. The simplest way to measure this is to determine the effect the program has had on HIV incidence. As a result, the STARHS approach is an important tool for evaluation of prevention programs.

REFERENCES

1. Satten G. A. Sternberg M. Fitting semi-Markov models to interval-censored data with unknown initiation times. *Biometrics* 1999; 55:507–513.
2. Busch M. P., Lee L. L. L., Satten G. A., Henrard D. R., Farzadegan H., Nelson K. E., Read S., Dodd R. Y., Petersen L. R. Time course of detection of viral and serological markers preceding HIV-1 seroconversion: Implications for blood and tissue donor screening. *Transfusion* 1995; 35:91–97.
3. Petersen L. R., Satten G. A., Dodd R., Bush M., Kleinman S., Grindon A., Lenes B., Karon J., and the HIV Lookback Study Group. Duration of time from HIV-1 infectiousness to detectable antibody. *Transfusion* 1994; 34:283–289.

4. Lackritz E. M., Satten G. A., Aberle-Grasse J., Dodd R. Y., Raimondi V. P., Janssen R. S., Lewis W. F., Notari E. P., Petersen L. R. Estimated risk of HIV transmission by screened blood in the United States. *New England Journal of Medicine* 1995; 333: 1721–1725.

5. Busch M. P., Satten G. A. Time course of viremia and antibody seroconversion following HIV exposure. *American Journal of Medicine* 1997; 102 (5B):117–124.

6. Brookmeyer R., Quinn T. C. Estimation of current human immunodeficiency virus incidence rates from a cross-sectional survey using early diagnostic tests. *American Journal of Epidemiology* 1995; 141:166–172.

7. Brookmeyer R., Quinn T. C., Shepherd M., Mehendale S., Rodrigues J., Bollinger R. The AIDS epidemic in India: A new method for estimating current human immunodeficiency virus (HIV) incidence rates. *American Journal of Epidemiology* 1995; 142:709–713.

8. Janssen R. S., Satten G. A., Stramer S., Rawal B. D., O'Brien T. R., Weiblen B. J., Hecht F. M., Jack N., Cleghorn F. R., Kahn J. O., Chesney M. A., Busch M. P. New testing strategy to detect early HIV-1 infection for use in incidence estimates and for clinical and prevention purposes. *Journal of the American Medical Association* 1998; 280:42–48.

9. Sternberg M., Satten G. A. Discrete-time nonparametric estimation for semi-Markov models of chain-of-events data with interval censoring and truncation. *Biometrics* 1999; 55:514–522.

10. Brookmeyer, R. Accounting for follow-up bias in estimation of HIV incidence. *Journal of the Royal Statistical Society* A, 1997; 160:127–140.

11. Satten G. A., Janssen R. S., Busch M. P., Datta S. Validating marker-based incidence estimates in repeatedly screened populations. *Biometrics* 1999; 55 (4):1224–1227.

12. Kupper L. L., Hafner K. B. How appropriate are popular sample size formulas? *American Statistician* 1989; 43:101–105.

13. Jacquez J. A., Koopman J. S., Simon C. P., Longini I. M., Jr. Role of the primary infection in epidemics of HIV infection in gay cohorts. *Journal of Acquired Immune Deficiency Syndrome* 1994; 7:1169–1184.

14. Pantaleo, G., Cohen O. J., Schacker T., et al. Evolutionary pattern of human immunodeficiency virus (HIV) replication and distribution in lymph nodes following primary infection: Implications for antiviral therapy. *Nature Medicine* 1998; 4 (3):341–345.

Chapter 15 Issues in Quantitative Evaluation of Epidemiologic Evidence for Temporal Variability of HIV Infectivity

Stephen C. Shiboski and Nancy S. Padian

Much recent attention has focused on the implications of possibly increased HIV transmission from individuals in the primary phase of infection for epidemic development and the design of prevention programs. The following quotations from articles illustrate this:

> The pattern of high contagiousness during the primary infection followed by a large drop in infectiousness may explain the pattern of epidemic spread seen in male homosexual cohorts in the early years of the epidemic.[1]

> The relatively short interval of high viral load during early infection followed by a long period of low viral load, suggests a special window of time during which focused HIV prevention efforts could be particularly effective.[2]

> Because direct epidemiologic evidence for this phenomenon is limited, biological observations of levels of virus in peripheral blood, mathematical epidemic models and indirect epidemiologic evidence have been the primary driving force behind discussions and recommendations in current literature on the subject.[2,3]

This chapter presents a framework for evaluating epidemiologic evidence for the variation of HIV infectivity, with a particular emphasis on assessing the importance of the primary infection period. In addition to reviewing recent results, we outline key concepts from simple probability models for transmission and basic principles of epidemiologic study design and data analysis. Monogamous couples form a natural unit for studying transmission risk because the source of infection can often be identified and exposure is limited to contact within the partnership. When multiple partners of unknown infection status are a possibility, more complex exposure scenarios generally preclude the possibility of direct investigation of factors affecting variation in infectivity. For these reasons, most of our discussion focuses primarily on results from partner studies of transmission in susceptible monogamous partners of known infected individuals. It is our hope that these results will be useful in informing decisions about implementation of prevention programs targeting individuals in the primary phase of infection.

We begin by defining infectivity and transmission probability and show how both depend on exposure and on properties related to infectiousness and susceptibility. Next, we briefly review the design of epidemiologic studies of transmission and introduce a framework for evaluating the information they provide about the nature of infectivity. Finally, we review results from several existing studies of heterosexual transmission and discuss the results and implications.

MODELS FOR SEXUAL TRANSMISSION OF HIV

Before we cover particular issues about assessing evidence for the importance of primary infection, we review some key quantities and concepts from the epidemiology of sexual transmission.

Definition of Infectivity

The fundamental epidemiologic quantity linking transmission to infectious properties of infected individuals is the infectivity, or per-exposure infection probability. Because it depends on a well-defined quantification of exposure (i.e., a single exposed contact), this measure is a useful summary of average risk and is a pivotal building block in mathematical models of epidemic spread. For HIV, the definition of a unit of exposure varies with different routes of transmission. To simplify the presentation of ideas, we will concentrate on a single mode of sexual transmission in a partnership consisting of a known susceptible individual and a potentially infectious partner called the index case. We define a unit of exposure to mean a single sexual contact that carries a non-zero risk of transmission. Such a contact is termed *exposed*. Clearly the magnitude of the associated risk depends on both the degree of susceptibility of the uninfected partner and the degree of infectiousness of the infected partner. Since these properties in turn may depend on when contacts occur (e.g., relative to the time of infection of the infected partner), the infectivity can more generally be expressed as a function of time as well as of additional factors influencing susceptibility and/or infectiousness. These may include intrinsic factors related to properties of the infected and/or susceptible partner (e.g., past history of STD infection, viral load) and extrinsic factors related to characteristics of the partnership (e.g., use of contraception).

We will denote the infectivity for a contact occurring at time t as $\lambda(t)$. The choice of time scale depends on the application. Examples include chronological time, time-on-study, and time since infection of the infected partner (appropriate in the case of monogamous contact between an uninfected person and a known infected person). The last example is particularly relevant for relating infectivity to the stage of infection of the infected partner and will be the focus of much of the chapter. The special case where infectivity is constant (i.e., $\lambda(t) = \lambda$), with no between- or within-partnership variation due to the factors discussed above, is the most common representation used in practice. However unrealistic, a constant infectivity often is the only quantity that can be reliably estimated from available data, and still provides a useful measure of average risk to compare between different transmission settings. In addition, it serves as a null model to which more realistic models can be compared.

Models for Transmission Probabilities

Calculations of risk for realistic exposure scenarios need to account for the possibility of multiple contacts, some of which may be noninfectious (i.e., contacts that occur before the index case becomes infected). The transmission probability for a given exposure history is a model for the risk of infection conditional on the reported exposure. The simplest scenario is a monogamous partnership consisting of a susceptible person in contact with a partner of known infection status. We define the risk associated with a single sexual contact between a susceptible individual and such a partner to be:

$$p(t) = I(t) \times \lambda(t)$$

Here, $I(t)$ is a binary indicator of the partner's infection status (i.e., $I(t) = 1$ when the partner is infected), $\lambda(t)$ is the infectivity defined above, and t represents chronological time. For a noninfectious contact (i.e., for $I(t) = 0$), $p(t) = 0$, while for an exposed contact $p(t) = \lambda(t)$, as required by our definition of infectivity. Now consider a series of k contacts in the same partnership: If complete information on the infectivity and infection status is available for all contacts, and if we assume that infection outcomes of successive contacts are mutually independent, the probability P of becoming infected given exposure consisting of k contacts occurring at times $t_1, t_2, \ldots, t_k$ can be written:

$$P = 1 - \prod_{j=1}^{k}[1 - p(t_j)] = 1 - \{[1 - p(t_1)] \times [1 - p(t_2)] \times \cdots \times [1 - p(t_k)]\}. \quad (1)$$

The product of terms in brackets on the right-hand side of this equation is the *escape probability* of avoiding infection in k contacts, each with a different, independent infection probability given by the time and contact-specific transmission probability $p(t)$. The transmission probability P is thus the complement of the escape probability. From the definition of $p(t)$, contacts where the partner of the susceptible is noninfectious carry zero risk. Thus, P includes terms only for exposed contacts. Note that transmission probability retains specific information about time variation in infectivity through the component terms. In practice, detailed information about timing and the nature of specific contacts is not available and a simpler transmission model must be used. Notice in particular that if the infection status indicator $I(t)$ is not observed, the appropriate model must depend on the probability that a given contact is exposed. Next, we consider simplifications that reflect the information available in data from typical partner studies of transmission in monogamous couples consisting of a defined infectious partner, or index case (known to be infected first), and susceptible partner.

CONSTANT INFECTIVITY MODEL

If the infectivity is assumed to be a constant λ for all contacts, the above transmission model simplifies considerably to:

$$P = 1 - (1 - \lambda)^l, \quad (2)$$

where l is the number of exposed contacts out of the total number reported (k). If the infectiousness of particular contacts is not observed (i.e., the time of infection of the index case is unknown) then l can not be determined and this model is inappropriate. In this case, additional information about the distribution of possible periods of infectiousness is required. The constant model is the most commonly applied model for HIV transmission, not because it provides a realistic description of the process but because it represents the limit of what can be estimated using most available data. However, the assumptions of this model clearly preclude any inferences about more complex properties of infectivity.

TIME-VARYING INFECTIVITY MODELS

Many partner studies carry more information about exposure than is required for the constant model, including information about possible times of infection and disease stage of the index case. Although this is never complete enough to fit the transmission model (1), simplifying assumptions about the infectivity may lead to more feasible models. As an example, assume that the time of the index case infection is known, that distinct periods of varying infectiousness can be identified, that infectivity is constant within these periods, and that numbers of exposed contacts in these periods can be counted or estimated. For three such periods, with i_1, i_2, and i_3 exposed contacts, respectively, the transmission probability is:

$$P = 1 - [(1-\lambda_1)^{i_1}(1-\lambda_2)^{i_2}(1-\lambda_3)^{i_3}]$$ (3)

Because the actual numbers of contacts in particular time periods are rarely reported in retrospective data, these numbers must be estimated using the total numbers of reported contacts and assuming that the rate of contacts is constant over time.

An alternative approach is to make no assumptions about the actual form of the infectivity other than that it varies with time. Assuming a constant contact rate μ (as described above), the following transmission probability applies for a fixed interval of exposure with known duration t beginning with the (known) time of infection of the index case:

$$P = 1 - \exp\left[-\int_0^t \mu\lambda(s)\,ds\right]$$ (4)

As described above, when the time of infection of the index case is unknown, the number of exposed contacts must be estimated, and computation of the associated transmission probability is more complex (as discussed further in the next section). With the assumption that infectivity is constant over defined time intervals, the model below provides a very close approximation to the contact-based model (3):

$$P = 1 - \left[e^{-\mu t_1 \lambda_1} \times e^{-\mu(t_2-t_1)\lambda_3} \times e^{-\mu(t_3-t_2)\lambda_3}\right]$$

A critical feature to note about the time-based models is that the infectivity is assumed to vary deterministically with time, but not according to other (individual or partnership-level) factors. However, in contrast to the contact-based models, the time-based infectivity estimates allow direct inferences to be made regarding variations following the time of index case infection.

UNKNOWN INFECTION STATUS

The models developed above all depend on knowledge of the infection status indicator $I(t)$ in distinguishing which contacts are exposed. In most studies, this information is not available. In this case, assumptions and/or additional knowledge about the potential infection status of partners must be used in order to define an appropriate transmission probability. The standard statistical approach to account for this uncertainty is to compute the expected value of the transmission probability with respect to the distribution of the infection status indicator. To do this it is generally assumed that contacts occur uniformly throughout the period of contact between the partners. The infection status indicator takes on the value 1 when the partner becomes infected, and remains that way as long as the partner is infectious. For HIV, this is assumed to be indefinitely. Thus the key unknown quantity is the time of infection of the partner. If external information about the potential times of infection is known or can be estimated, this information can be used in defining the transmission probability. For each candidate infection time we can compute the appropriate number of exposed contacts and/or the exposure duration and contact rate and plug these into one of the models defined above. By averaging over all possible infection times and weighting the transmission probabilities by the likelihood of each, we obtain an overall transmission probability that reflects our state of knowledge. The uniformity assumption made above is vital to this definition when contact information is limited to a total number or rate for the entire contact duration. (This is usually the case.)

ADDITIONAL TRANSMISSION MODELS

A number of other transmission models can be defined using the basic expressions defined above. For example, models for contact with multiple partners usually assume independence of infection outcomes between partners and are based on products across partners of probabilities like those defined above. In these settings, information about partner-specific infection status is virtually never known, and assumptions about the prevalence of infection among partners must be invoked. A simple model of this kind, which assumes that prevalence among n partners contacted is a constant ρ, and that average contact rates (μ) and per-contact infectivity (λ) are also constant, is:

$$P = 1 - \left[1 - \rho(1 - e^{-\mu\lambda t})\right]^{n} \tag{5}$$

The expression in parentheses is the per-partner infectivity. No estimates of its components are possible without separate contact data for each partnership. Clearly, models with these simplifying assumptions can reveal very little about temporal variations in the per-exposure infectivity (λ). However, stratified versions that attempt to estimate separate per-partner infectivities for groups of partners distinguished by different infection prevalence and infectivity level may yield indirect information.

Another common generalization is to allow the infectivity in the above models to depend on additional observed and/or unobserved variables. This is usually accomplished via a proportional hazards or proportional odds assumption linking covariates to the transmission probability. Models with unobserved components (e.g., omitted covariates that are important factors explaining infectiousness and/or susceptibility) are said to reflect between partnership heterogeneity in infectivity not accounted for by observed factors. For more detail on the construction of transmission models for more complex exposure scenarios, consult Rhodes et al.[4]

APPLYING TRANSMISSION MODELS
TO EPIDEMIOLOGIC STUDIES

The Structure of Transmission Data Observed
in Epidemiologic Studies

A key feature that distinguishes epidemiologic studies of infectious disease from analogous studies of chronic diseases is the definition of exposure. Infection requires contact with infected individuals; therefore, any meaningful definition of exposure requires information about frequency and duration of contact, as well as some indication of whether or not contacts were potentially infectious. The structure of the models outlined above reinforces this point.

RETROSPECTIVE STUDIES

The basic exposure information collected in retrospective partner studies of monogamous couples includes a measure of duration and frequency of contact over a defined time period. Table 15.1 displays the data structure that might be

Table 15.1. Data Format for Transmission Prevalence by Exposure Duration from a Retrospective Study

Exposure Duration (Months)	1–10	11–20	...	91–100	...
Infection prevalence	p_{10}	p_{20}	...	p_{100}	...
Number exposed	n_{10}	n_{20}	...	n_{100}	...

obtained in a study in the case where index case infection times are known and the beginning and end of exposure can be unambiguously defined. (In cases where infection times are unknown, the information in the table must be estimated using additional information, as discussed above.) Each individual is categorized by infection status and reported duration of exposure at the time of recruitment. The resulting estimates of infection prevalence can be examined for trends with increasing exposure. Clearly, the amount of information provided about this relationship depends on the range of exposure durations reported. If no partnerships report exposure duration in a given range, the data provide no information about infection risk in this range. This point is critical in assessing the level of information provided about infectivity. One way of circumventing this difficulty is to adopt models for infection risk based on assumptions about how infectivity varies with time (e.g., the constant or piecewise constant models). However, the danger of these assumptions is that the model extrapolates over ranges of exposure duration not actually observed. The accuracy and validity of the resulting estimate is impossible to assess.

Another common characteristic of exposure data from retrospective studies is that contact information is self-reported and often reflects a very long time period. When the time of the infection of the index case can be determined, this information can be used to modify estimates of contact history. However, in most cases, neither partner has detailed knowledge of when the primary infected partner became infected. Consequently, it is impossible to accurately estimate the number of exposed contacts. The most commonly used approach to contact estimation is to assume that contacts occurred at a constant rate throughout the observed or estimated exposure period. In some studies more detailed information (e.g., a diary) is available including estimates of the number of contacts which occurred in particular periods. The reliability of both of these approaches must be seriously questioned considering the retrospective nature of the data.

PROSPECTIVE STUDIES

In contrast to retrospective studies, prospective follow-up of susceptible individuals in contact with potentially infectious partners can potentially provide the best direct estimates of changes in infectivity. This is because exposure and relevant covariate information can be assessed at frequent intervals with less potential for bias due to recall problems. However, improved estimates are rarely practical for two primary reasons: ethical considerations require counseling of serodiscordant couples in use of contraceptives, which typically results in few seroconversions among partners; and infection times of index cases are usually unknown, and observed exposure generally occurs well after these times. As a result, such data provide useful information only about variations in transmission rates in periods of exposure occurring well after the primary infection phase. The data structure from prospective studies is similar to standard survival outcomes and can be summarized in life-table form with transmission events expressed as a proportion of person-months of exposure duration. When index case infection times are unknown, additional information about when these may have occurred and about contact rates over the unobserved periods of exposure is necessary for estimation of infectivities and transmission probabilities.

Approaches to Statistical Analysis

For data from retrospective or prospective studies, the association between exposure and infection can be summarized using standard statistical techniques for epidemiologic data, including chi-square and log-rank tests, or logistic and proportional hazards regression if control for additional explanatory factors is desired. However, these techniques do not account for the following key features of the transmission models outlined above:

1. Prevalence of infection cannot decrease with increasing degree of exposure.
2. Zero exposure corresponds to zero infection risk.

In many instances, observed data may show apparent decreases in transmission risk with increasing exposure, or may indicate infection risk associated with no reported exposure. This may result from chance variation, selection effects, and/or measurement error in exposure information and should be corrected for in analyses. In these instances a conventional logistic or proportional hazards regression model for infection outcome, including degree of exposure as a covariate, may estimate a non-zero risk associated with no reported exposure, or decreasing risk with increasing exposure unless special modifications are made. In addition, the regression coefficients (e.g., log-odds ratios, log-relative hazards) for additional factors may not provide good estimates of risk unless exposure is adequately modeled.[5,6]

A more appropriate framework for analysis of transmission data is to base analyses on plausible transmission models such as those described earlier. These models are well suited to the structure of data collected from most studies, incorporate exposure information in a sensible way, and provide estimates of key parameters such as the infectivity. Consult Shiboski[7] for further details for references on statistical methods for monogamous couple studies. A number of alternative measures of transmission risk are reviewed in Brookmeyer and Gail.[8]

ASSESSING EVIDENCE FOR VARIATION IN INFECTIVITY

Direct and Indirect Evidence for Variation in Infectivity

Based on the background provided above, we can now outline several guiding principles that assist in evaluating infectivity information from epidemiologic studies of transmission. The major study ingredients required for direct inferences about infectivity are as follows:

1. infection status (cross-sectional or prospective),
2. estimates of the number of partners contacted and contacts with each,
3. duration of contact,
4. infection status of partners contacted, and
5. time of infection for infected partners.

Direct evidence for variation in infectivity generally requires an estimate of per-exposure infectivity and/or transmission probabilities with explicit control for duration and intensity of exposure, and detailed information on the placement of exposure of a susceptible person relative to the time of infection of the infected partner(s). Indirect evidence is provided by studies that do not include such assessments of exposure or actual estimates of infectivity but allow inferences to be made about the relationship between cumulative transmission risk and factors. For example, a number of cross-sectional studies of monogamous couples have observed that transmission was more common in partners of index cases with reduced CD4 lymphocyte counts at enrollment, leading to the inference that infectivity may be elevated in later stages of HIV disease.

REVIEW OF CURRENT EPIDEMIOLOGIC EVIDENCE

Although there is convincing evidence for temporal variations in viral levels from serial biological measurements of viral titers in plasma, current results reflect relatively small numbers of patients, and variability between individuals is not well understood. Further, the relationship between levels of the blood and genital fluids is not well established.[3] Thus, although these observations suggest that changes in viral load may mirror changes in infectiousness, additional data from epidemiologic studies is needed for confirmation.

A number of studies have been conducted which provide information about HIV infectivity and the possible relationship with the primary infection period. These can be roughly classified as providing either indirect or direct evidence about time variations in infectivity as defined above.[1,9] We now briefly review these results. As mentioned above, evidence can be crudely grouped into direct and indirect categories.

INDIRECT EVIDENCE FROM MATHEMATICAL MODELS

A number of authors have investigated the influence of temporal variations in infectivity on development of epidemics using deterministic epidemic models.[1,9-11] The earlier work noted that if infectivity was characterized by two periods of elevated infectivity before and after an intervening longer period of noninfectivity, then early epidemic growth is driven primarily by the initial period of high infectivity. The later work uses slightly different models to come to similar conclusions, but the authors go further to hypothesize that their model results are a likely explanation for the shape of the epidemic curve seen in San Francisco between 1987 and 1995. To produce these results, infectivity is assumed to be 200 times higher in the primary phase than in the middle phase of infection. In evaluating these claims, it is important to note that both modeling approaches assume that all infected individuals follow exactly the same pattern of infectiousness and that susceptibility is invariant as well. This is clearly an oversimplification given observed between-individual variability in biological observations of viral levels. Since variation of infectivity is implicitly assumed, these results do not provide any direct evidence for the phenomenon in question. However, these results combined with biological observations of individual-level variations of virus in plasma are widely considered the most compelling evidence for the importance of primary HIV infection in influencing epidemic spread.[2,3]

INDIRECT EVIDENCE FROM EPIDEMIOLOGIC STUDIES

Many epidemiologic studies of HIV transmission have addressed the issue of variability of infectivity. Initial examinations of variability focused on changes with different levels of exposure measured by contacts. Results from studies of monogamous couples generally show little or no relationship between increasing number of contacts and transmission risk.[12,13] Although these have frequently been interpreted to support the notion that transmission risk is unrelated to degree of exposure, complementary analyses of between-partnership variation have noted evidence for substantial heterogeneity not controlled for by measured risk factors.[14] In addition, subsequent analyses based on considerations from transmission models, such as those presented above, have observed some association. In addition, most results indicate that transmission risk does not increase according to the relationship prescribed in the constant infectivity model of equation (2),[2] and that early contacts seem to carry disproportionately more risk than contacts occurring later.[15,16] However, since these analyses do not control explicitly for duration of exposure or for the times of occurrence of contacts relative to the infection time of the index case, implications of the results for temporal variation are not conclusive.

Further indirect information about variations in infectivity comes from epidemiologic studies of transmission involving susceptible individuals contacting multiple partners. Very high estimates of per-partner infectivity (see model in Koopman et al.)[5] and transmission probabilities from studies conducted early in the U.S. epidemic among homosexual men[17,18] and among military recruits in Thailand[19] have been interpreted to reflect increased transmission from index cases in the primary stage of infection.[1,9] Conversely, relatively low estimates of per-contact infectivity (usually in the range 0.001–0.01) from studies of transmission among monogamous couples are hypothesized to be heavily influenced by low infectiousness of index cases in the asymptomatic period characterized by relatively low viral load (for a summary of infectivity estimates from a range of studies see Mastro et al.).[20]

In addition to the results cited above, a number of other observations indicate that transmission can occur readily from index cases in later stages of infection. A number of studies of heterosexual transmission in monogamous partnerships have observed increased transmission risk from index cases in later stages of disease.[20,21] A related result is the observation that much of the recent transmission among young men in San Francisco can be attributed to contacts with older partners who are likely to be in later stages of infection.[22] Another example is provided by the widely publicized case of a single index case infecting 13 of 41 female partners in New York State (at least half of which were known to have become infected several months after the index case could have last been in the primary phase of infection). Finally, a 1999 study[23] examines the relationship between heterosexual transmission in a study of 38 monogamous couples and HIV viral load in plasma among index cases. Although the results indicate increased transmission risk with higher viral load levels, the measurements of the latter were made at indeterminate times in the disease course of the index cases.

Taken together, these results provide reasonable evidence for variation of infectivity between partnerships and indirectly imply that variation with duration of infection of index cases is likely. However, the results do not necessarily imply that the bulk of transmission occurs from contacts during the primary (or any other single) infection phase. Indeed, observations from many of these studies and other well-publicized cases of heterosexual transmission indicate clearly that transmission can occur readily well after this stage.

DIRECT EVIDENCE FROM EPIDEMIOLOGIC STUDIES

Relatively few studies have attempted to estimate time variation in infectivity or transmission probabilities with explicit control for exposure frequency and duration, mainly owing to the lack of appropriate data. Here we review a number of results that we feel best represent the current state of direct evidence.

The best sources of direct information on changes in infectivity are studies of monogamous couples with identified index cases whose infection times are known. Two well-known CDC-sponsored studies of transmission among partners of index cases infected via contaminated blood products provide perhaps the best examples. We will denote these the Peterman[24] and HATS (Heterosexual AIDS Transmission Study) studies[21] and refer readers to the original papers for detailed descriptions. Although small (51 and 31 couples, respectively), these studies provide perhaps the best information on HIV infectivity in the monogamous heterosexual setting. Since couples in these studies were typically formed prior to infection of the index case, and sexual contact was generally unprotected prior to the couple's knowledge of this event, many of the couples yield exposure intervals that overlap the primary infection period of the index case and extend as much as five years beyond. As discussed earlier, a key re-

Table 15.2. Infection Prevalence (Number of Couples) by Duration of Exposure for Two CDC-Sponsored Studies

| Study | Duration of Exposure (Months After Infection of Index Case) | | | | | | |
	1–20	21–40	41–60	61–80	81–100	101–180	Overall
HATS	0.00 (3)	0.333 (6)	0.143 (7)	0.500 (6)	0.167 (6)	0.000 (3)	0.226 (31)
Peterman	0.091 (11)	0.200 (20)	0.059 (17)	0.000 (3)	—	—	0.118 (51)

Table 15.3. Constant Infectivity Estimates and Tests of Linear Variation and
Uncontrolled Heterogeneity for Two CDC-Sponsored Partner Studies

Study	Infectivity (95% CI)	P (Time Variation)	P (Heterogeneity)
HATS	0.0009 (0.0004, 0.002)	0.13	0.017
Peterman	0.0008 (0.0004, 0.002)	0.28	0.001

quirement for estimation of infectivity is that the data contain a range of exposure durations and corresponding infection prevalences. For estimates to be informative about the primary infection stage, exposure durations of six months
or less must be represented (i.e., the first column of Table 15.1). Table 15.2 presents prevalence information for both studies in a format similar to Table 15.1.
The minimum reported duration by a couple with an infected partner was 23
and 20 months for the HATS and Peterman studies, respectively.

Previously[25] we presented infectivity estimates for both these studies and
summarized evidence for variability of infectivity. Table 15.3 presents constant
infectivity estimates for vaginal contacts along with tests of the hypotheses for
linear time variation (in the log infectivity), and random residual partnership
variation in addition to linear time variability. Evidence for (linear) time variability is not significant (based on a likelihood ratios test), but both studies display apparent heterogeneity across partnerships even after time variation is accounted for.

Figures 15.1 and 15.2 show infectivity estimates and corresponding escape
probability estimates as a function of time since infection of the index case for
the two CDC studies. Each plot includes a log-linear estimate and a smooth
semiparametric estimate whose form is determined by the data. Even more
elaborate models for time variation failed to significantly improve fit over the
constant infectivity model. Confidence intervals clearly show the uncertainty
in estimates, especially in the period immediately following infection of the index case. Evidence for substantial partnership-level heterogeneity remained for
all fitted models. In summary, these studies yield remarkably similar infectivity
estimates and both display evidence for significant partnership-level variation
in infectiousness and susceptibility. (These conclusions persist even after controlling for available covariates.) However, the small sample size and associated
great uncertainty preclude any strong conclusions about the nature of variation. In particular, the results do not support the hypothesis that infectivity
varies in a consistent pattern over time for all partnerships.

Larger monogamous couple studies with unknown times of index case in-

A

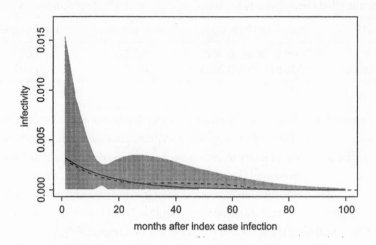

B

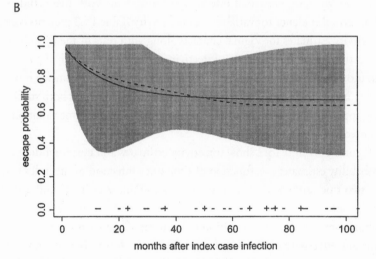

Figure 15.1. (A) Log-linear (solid line) and semiparametric (dashed line) infectivity estimates for the HATS study, including pointwise 95% confidence intervals (shaded) for the log-linear estimates. (B) Log-linear (solid line) and semiparametric (dashed line) escape probability estimates for the HATS study, including pointwise 95% confidence intervals (shaded) for the log-linear estimates. HIV serostatus and reported exposure duration for individual partners is indicated by the symbols along the horizontal axis.

A

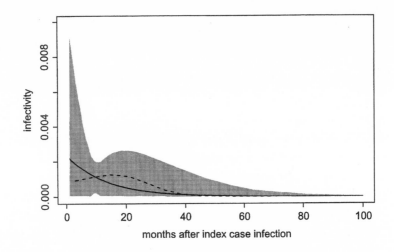

B

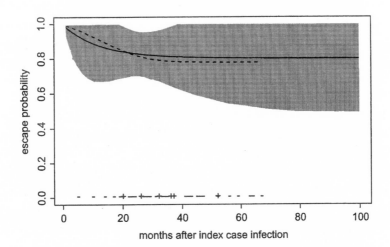

Figure 15.2. (A) Log-linear (solid line) and semiparametric (dashed line) infectivity estimates for the Peterman study, including pointwise 95% confidence intervals (shaded) for the log-linear estimates. (B) Log-linear (solid line) and semiparametric (dashed line) escape probability estimates for the Peterman study, including pointwise 95% confidence intervals (shaded) for the log-linear estimates. HIV serostatus and reported exposure duration for individual partners is indicated by the symbols along the horizontal axis.

fection can also provide useful information if data are supplemented with external information on possible distributions for these times. Focusing on the time variability of infectivity, analyses of such studies are presented in Shiboski and Padian, and Leynaert et al.[25,26]

Leynaert et al.,[26] in analysis of data from the European Study Group partner study, estimate infectivity separately for male-to-female anal and vaginal contacts using a model which assumes that infectivity progresses deterministically through three stages driven by the level of immunosuppression in the index case. The form of this model is quite similar to equation (3). Index case infection times are unknown, so in order to compute numbers of exposed contacts for each of these stages a distribution of infection times was adopted, estimated by combining information from population prevalence of infection with an external model for CD4 decline in index cases. Given the observed enrollment CD4 count for the index case, the model was used to produce an imputed distribution of possible infections times which was then applied to retrospectively estimate numbers of contacts occurring in each of the stages (assuming constant contact rates throughout). Under this scheme, an index case recruited with low CD4 counts is assumed to be more likely to have been infected before an index case recruited with higher CD4 counts. The basic analysis strategy was to compare the three-stage model for both types of contacts with a model assuming constant infectivity using likelihood ratio statistics. Although no evidence was seen for variation for vaginal contacts, a three-stage model fit significantly better than the constant counterpart for anal contacts. The infectivity estimates and 95% confidence intervals for the three stages and both types of contact are presented in Table 15.4.

The estimates in Table 15.4 are characterized by a great deal of uncertainty, especially in the early stage. This probably results from a lack of observations with very short durations of exposure (computed after accounting for possible index case infection times), as observed in the CDC studies discussed above. Thus, although there is evidence for a departure from constant per-contact risk (for anal contacts), the results shed very little light on the actual form of the infectivity in this period. In fact, an alternative model with constant infectivity for vaginal contacts and two separate constants for the middle stage and the combined late and early stages described the data equally well. At least three additional factors must be considered in interpreting these results: (1) it is likely that these data are characterized by substantial residual partnership-level heterogeneity which was not evaluated; (2) the fact that exposure assessments and estimates of infectivity implicitly assumed that index cases' disease progression

Table 15.4. Infectivity Estimates (and 95% Confidence Intervals) for Anal and Vaginal Contacts Occurring in Three Periods Following Infection of the Index Case from the European Study Group Partner Study

Type of Contact	Stage 1 (0–3 months)	Stage 2 (CD4 > 200)	Stage 3 (CD4 < 200)
Vaginal	0.0008 (0.0000, 0.0033)	0.0007 (0.0005, 0.0009)	0.0006 (0.0000, 0.0016)
Anal	0.1261 (0.0000, 0.3058)	0.0160 (0.0004, 0.0381)	0.3213 (0.0000, 0.7629)

A

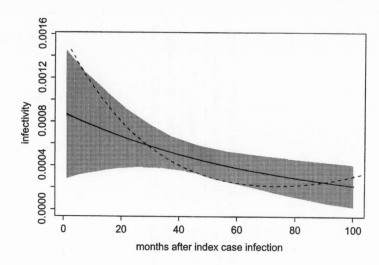

B

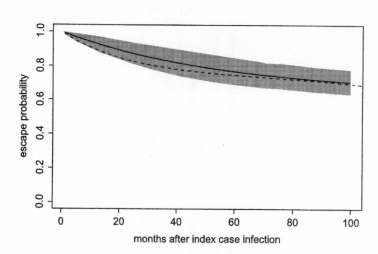

Figure 15.3. (A) Log-linear (solid line) and semiparametric (dashed line) infectivity estimates for the cps study, including pointwise 95% confidence intervals (shaded) for the log-linear estimates. (B) Log-linear (solid line) and semiparametric (dashed line) escape probability estimates for the cps study, including pointwise 95% confidence intervals (shaded) for the log-linear estimates.

and infectiousness follow the hypothesized three stage pattern makes it impossible to evaluate whether alternative models with fewer such assumptions would fit the observations equally well; (3) stage-specific estimates of anal and vaginal contact frequency are based on assumed constant contact rates and may be measured with considerable error. The authors of this study acknowledge these points in their conclusions.

The California Partners' Study (CPS) is another widely cited and analyzed source of transmission information for monogamous couples.[26,27] It shares many design features with the European Study Group study just described. In previous work[25] we estimated infectivity for vaginal contacts using methods similar to those described above for the CDC studies. Since index case infection times were unknown we accounted for this uncertainty using external information about chronological changes in HIV prevalence in Northern California. The constant infectivity estimate for these data is 0.0006 (95% C.I.: 0.0004, 0.0008). The p-values corresponding to the tests for linear time variation and heterogeneity (described above) are 0.017 and <0.001, respectively. Figure 15.3 displays infectivity and escape probability estimates for this study. There is apparent weak evidence for temporal variation, especially in the semiparametric estimate (dashed line). However, semiparametric alternatives failed to improve fit significantly compared to the log-linear model. Re-analysis of these data using an alternative (uniform) distribution for index case infection times did not change these conclusions because there were insufficient data on stage of disease of index cases at enrollment.

To summarize, although the results presented above give some support to the hypothesis that infectivity varies in time following index case infection, the tremendous uncertainty about estimates coupled with the evidence for partnership heterogeneity makes a number of alternate explanations for observed transmission rates equally plausible. In particular, relatively constant but heterogeneous infectivity can also lead to estimates with an apparent decline in risk over time.[25] Given the large uncertainty and the potential for measurement error in exposure data and model misspecification, the strongest conclusion that seems warranted from these results is that both temporal and partnership variability are likely to occur.

Use of Transmission Models in Computing
Infection Risks for Defined Exposures

All studies examined above display evidence for transmission occurring well after the primary infection period. An advantage of the transmission modeling

Table 15.5. Conditional Transmission Probability (and 95% Confidence Interval) for Three Durations of Exposure

Study	Exposure Duration		
	0–2 yrs	2–5 yrs	>5 yrs
CDC	0.27 (0.02, 0.52)	0.08 (0.00, 0.66)	0.010 (0.00, 0.21)
Peterman	0.17 (0.06, 0.28)	0.03 (0.00, 0.35)	0.002 (0.0, 0.06)
CPS	0.12 (0.07, 0.18)	0.12 (0.10, 0.15)	0.110 (0.04, 0.18)

Note: It is assumed exposure begins at the start of the interval and that average contact rate is approximately 7 per month.

approach is that the fitted model can be used to predict transmission risk under a variety of exposure scenarios. Table 15.5 presents estimates of transmission probabilities for a monogamous partner undergoing exposure of varying duration and starting at three different times following infection of the index case. The estimates and confidence intervals are derived from the parametric models for the studies presented in Figures 15.1, 15.2, and 15.3.

The estimates show that the transmission risk for an exposure length of two years beginning at the time of infection of the index case is between 0.12 and 0.27, which is two to five times higher than a three-year exposure beginning two years after the index case was infected. Although imprecise and applicable only to the setting of monogamous couples, these estimates provide useful information about risk for exposure to infected individuals in varying stages of infection. They indicate that a prolonged exposure to an index case in the period two to five years following infection may carry significant risk. They also indicate that risk for a similar exposure occurring in a two-year period immediately after index case infection is likely to be one to three times higher. Computation of analogous probabilities for a shorter period falling close to the time of index case infection (e.g., within three months) represents extrapolation of the model outside the range of observed data (as shown in Figures 15.1, 15.2, and 15.3), and is likely to yield highly unstable and unreliable estimates. For this reason, we believe that current results from epidemiologic studies do not justify quantitative statements about how high transmission risk is likely to be in the primary infection period.

DISCUSSION

Given the recent interest in the implications of variable infectivity on design and implementation of prevention programs, it is interesting to speculate on what the above results imply about the impact of a program targeted specifically at individuals in the primary phase of infection. Cates and colleagues[2] propose a series of goals and strategies to facilitate development of prevention programs targeted at individuals in the primary phase of infection, including:

1. development of methods for identifying individuals in the primary infection stage,
2. initiation of early antiretroviral therapy,
3. network notification of recent partners of individuals in the primary infection stage,
4. implementation of mass STD treatment programs, and
5. vaccine trials focused on impacting infectiousness.

As noted by the authors, success of these programs depends critically on the ability to effectively target individuals in the primary phase. Given that the length of this period is likely to be at most three months, this is likely to be difficult, especially in resource-limited settings. A further concern is that such programs can only be expected to succeed if the supposed pattern of infectiousness is distributed fairly uniformly in the population in question. Considering the evidence reviewed here, we believe that implementation of such programs is premature. The finding from mathematical models that epidemics of HIV are largely driven by individuals in the primary phase of infection depends on the assumption that all individuals possess the same pattern of variation in infectivity and that the level of infectiousness in this period is dramatically (e.g., as much as 200 times) higher than in other phases. These assumptions are not well supported by existing epidemiologic evidence.

The results reviewed in the previous section make it clear that there is still a great deal of uncertainty about the nature of infectivity given the available epidemiologic data. Although there is good evidence that infectivity is likely to be highly variable, support for a fixed pattern of infectiousness mirroring observations of levels of virus in plasma is relatively weak. A major flaw in arguments that infectivity follows this pattern deterministically is that they neglect to account for susceptibility and for additional factors which may influence transmission rates. This seems inappropriate, especially for situations where cofactors such as infection with other sexually transmitted diseases are prevalent. Two avenues of further investigation are needed to understand these issues better. The first is more extensive observations of individual-level changes in levels of virus in blood and genital secretions. Critical in this regard are estimates of between-individual variation in levels as a function of time following infection.

Second, additional epidemiologic investigations in settings where exposure, infectiousness and susceptibility can be better quantified are necessary for obtaining better estimates of infectivity.

REFERENCES

1. Jacquez JA, Koopman JS, Simon CP, Longini IM. Role of the primary infection in epidemics of HIV infection in gay cohorts. *J Acquir Immune Defic Syndr Hum Retrovirol* 1994; 7:1169–1184.
2. Cates W, Chesney MA, Cohen MS. Primary HIV infection—A public health opportunity. *J Amer Pub Health Assoc* 1997; 87:1928–1930.
3. Royce RA, Sena A, Cates W Jr, Cohen MS. Sexual transmission of HIV. *N Engl J Med* 1997; 336:1072–1078.
4. Rhodes PH, Halloran ME, Longini, IM. Counting process models for infectious disease data: Distinguishing exposure to infection from susceptibility. *J Royal Stat Soc B* 1996; 58:751–762.
5. Koopman JS, Longini IM, Jacquez JA. The role of early HIV infection in the spread of HIV through populations. *Am J Epidemiology* 1991; 133:1199–1209.
6. Shiboski S, Padian N. Population and individual based approaches to the design and analysis of epidemiological studies of STD transmission. *J Infect Dis* 1996; 174(suppl 2): S188–S200.
7. Shiboski S. Partner studies. In Armitage P, Colton T (eds.). *Encyclopedia of Biostatistics,* New York: John Wiley & Sons, 1998.
8. Brookmeyer R, Gail MH. *AIDS Epidemiology: A Quantitative Approach,* Oxford: Oxford University Press, 1994.
9. Koopman JS, Jacquez JA, Welch GW, Simon CP, Foxman B, Pollock SM, Barth-Jones D, Adams AL, Lange K. The role of early HIV infection in the spread of HIV through populations. *J Acquir Immune Defic Syndr Hum Retrovirol* 1997; 14:249–258.
10. Blythe SP, Anderson RM. Distributed incubation and infectious periods in models of the transmission dynamics of the human immunodeficiency virus (HIV). *IMA J Math Appl Med Biol* 1988; 5:1–19.
11. Blythe SP, Anderson RM. Variable infectiousness in HIV transmission models. *IMA J Math Appl Med Biol* 1988; 5:181–200.
12. Kaplan EH. Modeling HIV infectivity: Must sex acts be counted? *J Acquir Immune Defic Syndr Hum Retrovirol* 1990; 3:55–61.
13. Padian N, Shiboski S, Jewell NP. The association between number of exposures and rates of heterosexual transmission of human immunodeficiency virus (HIV). *J Infect Dis* 1990; 161:883–887.
14. Wiley JA, Herschkorn SJ, Padian NS. Heterogeneity in the probability of HIV transmission per sexual contact: The case of male-to-female transmission in penile-vaginal intercourse, *Stat Med* 1989; 8:93–102.
15. Downs AM, De Vincenzi I. Probability of heterosexual transmission of HIV: Relation-

ship to the number of unprotected sexual contacts. *J Acquir Immune Defic Syndr Hum Retrovirol* 1996; 11:388–395.

16. Padian NS, Shiboski SC, Glass SO, Vittinghoff E. Heterosexual transmission of HIV in northern California: Results from a ten year study. *Amer J Epidem* 1997; 146:350–357.

17. Grant RM, Wiley JA, Winkelstein W. Infectivity of the human immunodeficiency virus: Estimates from a prospective study of homosexual men. *J Infect Dis* 1987; 156: 189–193.

18. DeGruttola V, Seage GR, Mayer KH, Horsburgh CR. Infectiousness of HIV between male homosexual partners. *J Clin Epidemiol* 1989; 42:849–856.

19. Mastro TD, Satten GA, Nopkesorn T, Sangkharomya S, Longini IM. Probability of female-to-male transmission of HIV-1 in Thailand. *Lancet* 1994; 343:204–207.

20. Mastro TD, de Vincenzi I, et al. Probabilities of sexual HIV-1 transmission. *AIDS* 1996; 10 Suppl A:S75–S82.

21. O'Brien TR, Busch MP, Donegan E, Ward JW, Wong L, Samson SM, Perkins HA, Altman R, Stoneburner RL, Holmberg SD. Heterosexual transmission of human immunodeficiency virus type I from transfusion recipients to their sexual partners. *J Acquir Immune Defic Syndr Hum Retrovirol* 1994; 7:705–710.

22. Service SK, Blower SM. Linked HIV epidemics in San Francisco. *J Acquir Immune Defic Syndr Hum Retrovirol* 1997; 15:318–319.

23. Pedraza M-A, del Romero J, Roldan F, Garcia S, Ayerbe A-Y, Noriega AR, Alcami J. Heterosexual transmission of HIV-1 is associated with high viral load levels and a positive viral isolations in the infected partner. *J Acquir Immune Defic Syndr Hum Retrovirol* 1999; 21:120–125.

24. Peterman TA, Stoneburner RL, Allen JR, Jaffe HW, Curran JW. Risk of HIV transmission from heterosexual adults with transfusion-associated infections. *JAMA* 1988; 259: 55–63.

25. Shiboski SC, Padian NP. Epidemiologic evidence for time variation in HIV infectivity. *J Acquir Immune Defic Syndr Hum Retrovirol* 1988; 19:527–535.

26. Leynaert B, Downs AM, de Vincenzi I. Heterosexual transmission of human immunodeficiency virus: Variability of infectivity throughout the course of infection. *Amer J Epidem* 1998; 148:88–96.

27. Padian N, Marquis L, Francis DP, Anderson RE, Rutherford GW, O'Malley PM, Winkelstein W. Male-to-female transmission of human immunodeficiency virus. *JAMA* 1987; 258:788–790.

Index